Diagnostic Tests

made

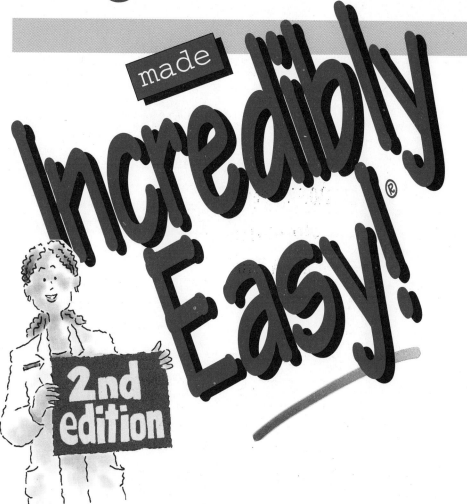

Incredibly Easy!®

2nd edition

Wolters Kluwer | Lippincott Williams & Wilkins
Health

Philadelphia · Baltimore · New York · London
Buenos Aires · Hong Kong · Sydney · Tokyo

Staff

Executive Publisher
Judith A. Schilling McCann, RN, MSN

Editorial Director
David Moreau

Clinical Director
Joan M. Robinson, RN, MSN

Art Director
Mary Ludwicki

Editorial Project Manager
Gabrielle Mosquera

Clinical Editor
Joanne M. Bartelmo, RN, MSN

Editors
Josephine M. Donofrio, Diane Labus

Copy Editors
Kimberly Bilotta (supervisor), Carol Brown,
Scotti Cohn, Shana Harrington, Dona Perkins,
Pamela Wingrod

Designer
Georg W. Purvis IV

Illustrator
Bot Roda

Digital Composition Services
Diane Paluba (manager), Joyce Rossi Biletz,
Donald Knauss, Donna S. Morris

Associate Manufacturing Manager
Beth J. Welsh

Editorial Assistants
Karen J. Kirk, Jeri O'Shea, Linda K. Ruhf

Indexer
Barbara Hodgson

DXTIE2E010508

Library of Congress Cataloging-in-Publication Data
Diagnostic tests made incredibly easy!. — 2nd ed.
    p. ; cm.
    Includes bibliographical references and index.

    1. Diagnosis. 2. Nursing assessment. 3. Nursing. I. Lippincott Williams & Wilkins.
    [DNLM: 1. Diagnostic Techniques and Procedures—Nurses' Instruction. 2. Diagnostic Techniques and Procedures—Problems and Exercises. WB 18.2 D536 2008]
RT48.5.D533 2008
616.07'5—dc22
ISBN-13: 978-0-7817-8690-4 (alk. paper)
ISBN-10: 0-7817-8690-8 (alk. paper)   2008002664

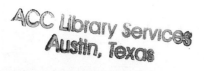

Contents

Contributors and consultants

Carla McCaghren Allen, MEd, BHS, RT(R)(CT)
Clinical Assistant Professor
University of Missouri
Columbia

Kim D. Cooper, RN, MSN
Nursing Department Chair
Ivy Tech Community College
Terre Haute, Ind.

Lillian Craig, RN, MSN, FNP-C
Adjunct Faculty
Oklahoma Panhandle State University
Goodwell

Julia Anne Isen, RN, BS, MSN, FNP-C
FNP-C Primary Care
University of California, San Francisco

Fiona Scott Johnson, RN, MSN, CCRN
Clinical Education Specialist
Memorial Health University Medical Center
Savannah, Ga.

Hope Siddons Knight, RN, BSN
Nursing Faculty
Redlands Community College
El Reno, Okla.

Megan McClintock, RN, BSN
Nursing Faculty
Redlands Community College
El Reno, Okla.

Aaron Pack, RN, BSN
Nursing Informatics Specialist
Redlands Community College
El Reno, Okla.

Noel C. Piano, RN, MS
Instructor/Coordinator
Lafayette School of Practical Nursing
Williamsburg, Va.
Adjunct Faculty
Thomas Nelson Community College
Hampton, Va.

Elizabeth (Libby) Richards, RN, MSN
Clinical Assistant Professor
Purdue University School of Nursing
West Lafayette, Ind.

Jennifer K. Sofie, APRN, MSN
Adjunct Assistant Professor & Nurse Practitioner
Montana State University
Bozeman

Leigh Ann Trujillo, RN, BSN
Nurse Educator
St. James Hospital and Health Centers
Olympia Fields, Ill.

Stacy E. Walz, BS, MT (ASCP)
Education Coordinator/Associate Lecturer
Clinical Laboratory Science Program
University of Wisconsin–Madison

Michele B. Zitzmann, MHS, MT(ASCP), CLS(NCA)
Associate Professor
Louisiana State University Health Sciences Center
School of Allied Health Professions
New Orleans

Not another boring foreword

If you're like me, you're too busy to wade through a foreword that uses pretentious terms and umpteen dull paragraphs to get to the point. So let's cut right to the chase! Here's why this book is so terrific:

☝ It will teach you all the important things you need to know about diagnostic tests. (And it will leave out all the fluff that wastes your time.)

✌ It will help you remember what you've learned.

✌ It will make you smile as it enhances your knowledge and skills.

Don't believe me? Try these recurring logos on for size:

 Now I get it!—Explains important aspects of a test in clear, easily understood terms

 Advice from the experts—Offers expert guidance on interpreting test results

 Stay on the ball—Alerts you to the factors that can interfere with test results

 Listen up—Discusses patient teaching points

 Memory jogger—Reinforces learning through easy-to-remember anecdotes and mnemonics.

See? I told you! And that's not all. Look for me and my friends in the margins throughout this book. We'll be there to explain key concepts, provide important care reminders, and offer reassurance. Oh, and if you don't mind, we'll be spicing up the pages with a bit of humor along the way, to teach and entertain in a way that no other resource can.

I hope you find this book helpful. Best of luck throughout your career!

Joy

Hematology and coagulation tests

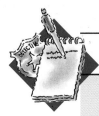

Just the facts

In this chapter, you'll learn:

♦ about hematology and coagulation tests

♦ the patient care associated with these tests

♦ factors that can interfere with test results

♦ what hematology and coagulation test results may indicate.

A look at hematology and coagulation tests

Hematology tests determine whether specific blood levels are higher or lower than normal and can be useful in diagnosing infection or such diseases as anemia and leukemia. Coagulation tests are performed for patients with bleeding disorders, thrombophilia, vascular injury, or trauma. They're also necessary to guide anticoagulant therapy.

Explain and reassure

The first step in preparing a patient for a hematology test is to explain the test. The patient should always know what's happening to him and why. Use simple, direct language and avoid jargon. If the patient is a child, an elderly person, or is otherwise unable to understand your instructions, you may also need to explain the test to a parent or caregiver.

Get to the point

Hematology and coagulation tests require a blood sample, and some patients may be a little uneasy about needles. Before taking

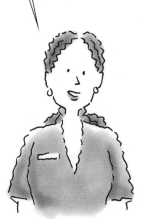

It's important to keep the patient informed of what's happening to him and why.

a blood sample, explain that some brief discomfort may accompany the needle puncture or tourniquet application.

Handle with care

Try to use a large-gauge needle when drawing the blood sample, and handle blood samples carefully to prevent the breakdown of red blood cells (RBCs), or *hemolysis*, which may interfere with test results. Observe standard precautions. Also, after taking a blood sample, check the venipuncture site for bleeding. If a hematoma develops at the venipuncture site, apply warm soaks.

Hematology tests

White blood cell count

The white blood cell (WBC) or *leukocyte* count measures the number of WBCs in a microliter of whole blood. This is done through the use of electronic devices. A WBC count can be useful in diagnosing infection and inflammation as well as in monitoring a patient's response to chemotherapy or radiation therapy. WBC counts can also help determine whether further tests are needed.

Counter culture

WBC counts can vary depending on a number of factors. On any given day, counts may vary by as much as 2,000 cells/µl (SI, 2 × 10^9/L) because of the effects of stress, strenuous exercise, or other factors. The count also can rise or fall significantly with certain diseases.

What it all means

The WBC count normally ranges from 4,000 to 10,000/µl (SI, 4 to 10 × 10^9/L). It's useful for diagnosing the severity of a disease process. However, the WBC differential gives more specific information about which type of WBC is being affected and is, therefore, more useful diagnostically.

The lowdown on levels

An elevated WBC count (leukocytosis) commonly signals infection, such as an abscess, meningitis, appendicitis, or tonsillitis. A high count may also indicate leukemia or tissue necrosis caused by burns, myocardial infarction (MI), or gangrene.

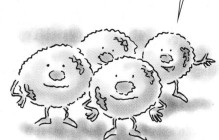

Hey gang! Looks like a normal-size crowd of us today.

A low WBC count (leukopenia) indicates bone marrow depression, which may result from viral infections or from toxic reactions, such as those following treatment with antineoplastics, ingestion of mercury or other heavy metals, or exposure to benzene or arsenicals. Leukopenia also accompanies influenza, typhoid fever, measles, infectious hepatitis, mononucleosis, and rubella.

What needs to be done

• Tell the patient that he should avoid strenuous exercise for 24 hours before the test to avoid altered readings and that he should also avoid ingesting a large meal before the test.
• Perform a venipuncture, and collect the sample in a 7-ml tube containing EDTA, or in a designated tube volume in accordance with laboratory protocol.
• Completely fill the sample collection tube, and invert it gently several times to adequately mix the sample and anticoagulant.

White blood cell differential

A WBC differential can provide more specific information about a patient's immune system. In a WBC differential, the laboratory classifies 100 or more WBCs in a stained film of blood according to five major types of leukocytes—neutrophils, eosinophils, basophils, lymphocytes, and monocytes—and determines the percentage of each type.

Relatively speaking

The differential count is the relative number of each type of WBC in the blood. Multiply the percentage value of each type by the total WBC count to obtain the absolute number of each type of WBC.

What it all means

The normal percentages of each WBC type in adults are:
• *neutrophils:* 54% to 75% (SI, 0.54 to 0.75)
• *eosinophils:* 1% to 4% (SI, 0.01 to 0.04)
• *basophils:* 0% to 1% (SI, 0 to 0.01)
• *monocytes:* 2% to 8% (SI, 0.02 to 0.08)
• *lymphocytes:* 25% to 40% (SI, 0.25 to 0.40).

The lowdown on levels

Elevated levels of WBCs are commonly associated with allergic reactions or the presence of infection. After the normal values for the patient have been determined, an assessment can be made.

Looking at the big picture

Keep in mind that to achieve an accurate diagnosis, differential test results must always be interpreted in relation to the total WBC count. Abnormal differential patterns suggest a range of disease states and other conditions. (See *How disease affects WBC differential values.*)

Danger signs

Some WBC differential findings indicate that immediate action is required. For instance, an absolute neutrophil count of 1,000/µl (SI, 1×10^9/L) or less requires neutropenic precautions, including protective isolation. (See *Drugs that influence the eosinophil count.*)

What needs to be done

• Tell the patient to avoid strenuous exercise before a WBC count to ensure accurate results.
• Perform a venipuncture, and collect the sample in a 7-ml tube containing EDTA, or in a designated tube volume in accordance with laboratory protocol.
• Completely fill the collection tube, and invert it gently several times to adequately mix the sample and anticoagulant.

Red blood cell count

RBCs are the main component of blood. The RBC count helps assess the blood's oxygen-carrying capacity and can be useful in diagnosing anemia and dehydration. An RBC count, also known as an *erythrocyte count*, is used to find the number of RBCs in a microliter (cubic milliliter) of whole blood. RBCs are commonly counted with electronic devices, which provide fast, accurate results. The RBC count itself provides no information about the size, shape, or concentration of hemoglobin (Hb) within the cells, but it may be used to calculate two erythrocyte indices: mean corpuscular volume and mean corpuscular Hb.

What it all means

Normal RBC values vary depending on a number of factors. In adult men, the RBC count ranges from 4.5 to 5.5 million/µl (SI, 4.5 to 5.5×10^{12}/L) of venous blood; in adult women, the count ranges from 4 to 5 million/µl (SI, 4 to 5×10^{12}/L) of venous blood; and in children, the count ranges from 4.6 to 4.8 million/µl (SI, 4.6 to 4.8×10^{12}/L) of venous blood. In full-term neonates, values

Drugs that influence the eosinophil count

Many drugs can affect the accuracy of the eosinophil count by increasing or decreasing it. Some of these drugs are listed below.

Increases count
• Anticonvulsants
• Gold compounds
• Isoniazid
• Penicillins
• Phenothiazines
• Rifampin
• Streptomycin
• Sulfonamides
• Tetracyclines

Decreases count
• Indomethacin
• Procainamide

Gently invert the test tube several times to make sure the contents are adequately mixed.

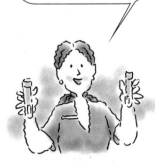

How disease affects WBC differential values

White blood cell (WBC) differential aids diagnosis because some disorders affect only one WBC type. Each cell type is listed here along with how it's affected by these disorders.

Cell type	How affected
Neutrophils	*Count increased by* • Infections: osteomyelitis, otitis media, septicemia, gonorrhea, endocarditis, chickenpox, herpes • Ischemic necrosis caused by myocardial infarction, burns, cancer • Metabolic disorders: diabetic acidosis, eclampsia, uremia, thyrotoxicosis • Stress response • Inflammatory diseases: rheumatic fever, rheumatoid arthritis, acute gout, vasculitis, myositis *Count decreased by* • Bone marrow depression caused by radiation or cytotoxic drugs • Infections: typhoid, hepatitis, influenza, measles, mumps, rubella, infectious mononucleosis • Hypersplenism: hepatic disease and storage diseases • Autoimmune diseases such as systemic lupus erythematosus • Deficiency of folic acid or vitamin B_{12}
Eosinophils	*Count increased by* • Allergic disorders: asthma, hay fever, food or drug sensitivity, serum sickness, angioneurotic edema • Parasitic infections: trichinosis, hookworm, roundworm, amebiasis • Skin diseases: eczema, pemphigus, psoriasis, dermatitis, herpes simplex • Neoplastic diseases: chronic myelocytic leukemia, Hodgkin's disease, metastasis *Count decreased by* • Stress response • Cushing's syndrome
Basophils	*Count increased by* • Chronic myelocytic leukemia, Hodgkin's disease, ulcerative colitis, chronic hypersensitivity states *Count decreased by* • Hyperthyroidism, ovulation, pregnancy, stress
Lymphocytes	*Count increased by* • Infections: tuberculosis, hepatitis, infectious mononucleosis, mumps, rubella, cytomegalovirus, pertussis • Thyrotoxicosis, hypoadrenalism, ulcerative colitis, immune diseases, lymphocytic leukemia *Count decreased by* • Severe debilitating illnesses, such as heart failure, renal failure, advanced tuberculosis • Defective lymphatic circulation, high levels of adrenal corticosteroids, immunodeficiency
Monocytes	*Count increased by* • Infections: subacute bacterial endocarditis, tuberculosis, hepatitis, malaria • Autoimmune diseases: systemic lupus erythematosus, rheumatoid arthritis • Carcinomas, monocytic leukemia, lymphomas

range from 4.4 to 5.8 million/µl (SI, 4.4 to 5.8 × 10^{12}/L) of capillary blood at birth, fall to 3 to 3.8 million/µl (SI, 3 to 3.8 × 10^{12}/L) at age 2 months, and increase slowly thereafter. Values are also generally higher in people living at high altitudes.

The lowdown on levels

An elevated RBC count may indicate absolute or relative polycythemia. A depressed count may indicate anemia, fluid overload, or hemorrhage lasting more than 24 hours. (See *RBC count interference.*)

What needs to be done

• For adults and older children, draw venous blood into a 7-ml tube containing EDTA, or in a designated tube volume in accordance with laboratory protocol. For younger children, collect capillary blood in a microcollection device.
• Completely fill the collection tube, and invert it gently several times to mix the sample and anticoagulant.

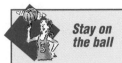

Stay on the ball

RBC count interference

The following factors may alter red blood cell (RBC) count results:
• high white blood cell count, which falsely elevates the RBC count in semiautomated and automated counters
• diseases that cause RBCs to clump, leading to a falsely decreased RBC count.

Hemoglobin

Hb, which transports oxygen, is the main component of an RBC. Each RBC contains about 250 million molecules of Hb; therefore, Hb concentration correlates closely with the RBC count. Hb level is a good indicator of anemia.

What it all means

Hb concentration varies depending on the patient's age and sex and on the type of blood sample drawn.

Through the ages

These values reflect normal Hb concentrations (in number of grams per deciliter):
• *neonates younger than age 1 week:* 17 to 22 (SI, 170 to 220 g/L)
• *neonates age 1 week:* 15 to 20 (SI, 150 to 200 g/L)
• *neonates age 1 month:* 11 to 15 (SI, 110 to 150 g/L)
• *children:* 11 to 13 (SI, 110 to 130 g/L)
• *adult men:* 14 to 17.4 (SI, 140 to 174 g/L)
• *men after middle age:* 12.4 to 14.9 (SI, 124 to 149 g/L)
• *women:* 12 to 16 (SI, 120 to 160 g/L)
• *women after middle age:* 11.7 to 13.8 (SI, 117 to 138 g/L).

The lowdown on levels

Low Hb concentration may indicate anemia, recent hemorrhage, or fluid retention, which can cause hemodilution; elevated Hb suggests hemoconcentration from polycythemia or dehydration. (See *Hb test interference*.)

What needs to be done

• For adults and older children, perform a venipuncture and collect the sample in a 7-ml tube containing EDTA, or in a designated tube volume in accordance with laboratory protocol. For younger children and infants, collect the sample by fingerstick or heelstick in a microcollection device containing EDTA.
• Completely fill the collection tube, and invert it gently several times to adequately mix the sample and anticoagulant.

Stay on the ball

Hb test interference

Very high white blood cell counts or red blood cells that resist lysis may falsely elevate hemoglobin (Hb) values.

Hematocrit

Hematocrit (HCT) levels reflect the proportion of blood occupied by RBCs. The HCT test is a common, reliable test that measures the percentage by volume of packed RBCs in a whole-blood sample. For example, an HCT of 40% (SI, 0.40) means that a 100-ml sample contains 40 ml of packed RBCs. The packing of RBCs is achieved by centrifugation of anticoagulated whole blood in a capillary tube, which tightly packs RBCs without causing hemolysis.

What it all means

HCT values vary depending on the patient's sex and age, the type of sample, and the laboratory performing the test.

These ranges represent normal HCT values for different age-groups:
• *neonates age 0 to 2 weeks:* 44% to 64% (SI, 0.44 to 0.64)
• *neonates age 2 to 8 weeks:* 39% to 59% (SI, 0.39 to 0.59)
• *infants age 2 to 6 months:* 35% to 49% (SI, 0.35 to 0.49)
• *infants age 6 months to 1 year:* 30% to 40% (SI, 0.3 to 0.4)
• *children age 1 to 6 years:* 30% to 40% (SI, 0.3 to 0.4)
• *children ages 6 to 16 years:* 32% to 42% (SI, 0.32 to 0.42)
• *adolescents age 16 to 18 years:* 34% to 44% (SI, 0.34 to 0.44)
• *adult men:* 42% to 52% (SI, 0.42 to 0.52)
• *adult women:* 36% to 48% (SI, 0.36 to 0.48).

The lowdown on levels

Low HCT suggests anemia, hemodilution, or massive blood loss; high HCT indicates polycythemia or hemoconcentration resulting from blood loss and dehydration. (See *HCT test interference*.)

Stay on the ball

HCT test interference

Hemoconcentration caused by tourniquet constriction for longer than 1 minute typically raises hematocrit (HCT) by 2.5% to 5% and may alter HCT test results.

What needs to be done

• For adults, perform a venipuncture and collect the sample in a 7-ml tube containing EDTA, or in a designated tube volume in accordance with laboratory protocol. For younger children and infants, collect the sample by fingerstick or heelstick in a microcollection device containing EDTA.
• Completely fill the collection tube, and invert it gently several times to adequately mix the sample and anticoagulant.
• Send the sample to the laboratory immediately.

Platelet count

Platelets, also called *thrombocytes*, are the smallest formed elements in the blood. Platelets promote coagulation by supplying phospholipids to the intrinsic clotting pathway, helping to form a hemostatic plug for vascular injuries.

The platelet count is one of the most important screening tests of platelet function. Accurate counts are vital for monitoring severe increases or decreases in the number of platelets in the blood. A platelet count that falls below 50,000/µl (SI, 50×10^9/L) can cause spontaneous bleeding; when the count drops below 5,000/µl (SI, 5×10^9/L), fatal central nervous system bleeding or massive GI hemorrhage is possible.

What it all means

A normal platelet count ranges from 140,000 to 400,000/µl (SI, 140 to 400×10^9/L) in adults and from 150,000 to 450,000/µl (SI, 150 to 450×10^9/L) in children.

The lowdown on levels

An increased platelet count, also called *thrombocytosis*, can result from hemorrhage, infectious disorders, cancers, iron deficiency anemia, or inflammatory disease as well as from recent surgery, pregnancy, or splenectomy. In such cases, the platelet count returns to normal after the patient recovers from the primary disorder. However, the count remains high in primary thrombocythemia, chronic idiopathic myelofibrosis, polycythemia vera, and chronic myelogenous leukemia.

A decreased platelet count, also called thrombocytopenia, can result from aplastic (undeveloped) or hypoplastic (underdeveloped) bone marrow; infiltrative bone marrow disease, such as leukemia or disseminated infection; ineffective platelet development caused by folic acid or vitamin B_{12} deficiency; pooling of platelets in an enlarged spleen; increased platelet destruction caused by drugs or immune disorders; disseminated intravascular

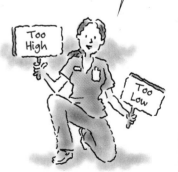

A platelet count that's too high or too low can indicate various disorders.

Too High

Too Low

coagulation (DIC); or mechanical injury to platelets. (See *Platelet count interference.*)

What needs to be done

• Perform a venipuncture, and collect the sample in a 7-ml tube containing EDTA, or in a designated tube volume in accordance with laboratory protocol.
• Completely fill the collection tube, and invert it gently several times to adequately mix the sample and anticoagulant.

Platelet aggregation

After vascular injury, platelets gather at the injury site and clump together to form an aggregate or plug that helps maintain hemostasis and promotes healing. The platelet aggregation test, an in vitro procedure, measures the rate at which the platelets in a plasma sample form a clump after the addition of an aggregating reagent, determining whether blood is clotting properly. The platelet aggregation test helps detect and distinguish between congenital and acquired platelet bleeding disorders.

What it all means

Normal platelet aggregation occurs in 3 to 5 minutes (SI, 3 to 5 minutes), but findings are temperature dependent and vary by laboratory. Aggregation curves obtained by using different reagents help to distinguish various qualitative platelet defects.

Abnormal findings may indicate congenital disorders, such as Glanzmann thrombasthenia, von Willebrand's disease, Bernard-Soulier syndrome, and storage pool disease, or acquired conditions, such as polycythemia vera, severe liver disease, uremia, autoimmune disorders, myeloproliferative disorders, and vasculitis. (See *Platelet aggregation test interference*, page 10.)

What needs to be done

• Instruct the patient to fast or to maintain a nonfat diet for 8 hours before the test because lipemia can affect the test results.
• Notify the laboratory and practitioner of medications the patient is taking that may affect test results; these medications may need to be restricted. Because the list of medications known to alter the results of this test is long and continually growing, the patient should be as close to drug-free as possible before the test.
• Perform a venipuncture, and collect the sample in a 4.5-ml siliconized tube.

Stay on the ball

Platelet count interference

• Acetazolamide, acetohexamide, antineoplastics, brompheniramine maleate, carbamazepine, chloramphenicol, ethacrynic acid, furosemide, gold salts, indomethacin, isoniazid, mephenytoin, oral diazoxide, phenytoin, salicylates, thiazide and thiazide-like diuretics, tricyclic antidepressants, and menstruation decrease platelet count.
• High altitudes, persistent cold temperatures, strenuous exercise, and excitement increase platelet count.

• Completely fill the collection tube, and invert it gently several times to adequately mix the sample and anticoagulant.
• Handle the sample gently to prevent hemolysis, and keep it between 71.6° F and 98.6° F (22° C and 37° C) to prevent aggregation.

Red cell indices

There are three main red cell indices, which are calculated through the use of other blood tests. Using the RBC count, HCT, and total Hb test, the red cell indices (also known as *erythrocyte indices*) provide important information about Hb concentration and weight and the size of an average RBC. The red cell indices include:
• mean corpuscular volume (MCV)
• mean corpuscular Hb (MCH)
• mean corpuscular Hb concentration (MCHC).

Eyes on the size

MCV, the ratio of HCT (packed cell volume) to the RBC count, expresses the average size of the erythrocytes and indicates whether they're undersized (microcytic), oversized (macrocytic), or normal (normocytic).

A weighty issue

MCH, the ratio of Hb weight to the RBC count, gives the weight of Hb in an average RBC.

Rating the ratio

MCHC, the ratio of Hb weight to HCT, defines the Hb concentration in 100 ml of packed RBCs. It helps distinguish normally colored (normochromic) RBCs from paler (hypochromic) RBCs.

What it all means

The range of normal red cell indices is:
• *MCV:* 84 to 99 mm^3 (SI, 84 to 99 fl)
• *MCH:* 26 to 32 pg (SI, 26 to 32 pg)
• *MCHC:* 30 to 36 g/dl (SI, 300 to 360 g/L).

The lowdown on levels

The red cell indices help to classify anemias. Low MCV and MCHC indicate microcytic, hypochromic anemias caused by iron deficiency anemia or thalassemia. A high MCV suggests macrocytic anemias caused by folic acid or vitamin B$_{12}$ deficiency, inherited

Stay on the ball

Platelet aggregation test interference

Aspirin, aspirin compounds, phenylbutazone, sulfinpyrazone, phenothiazines, anti-inflammatory drugs, antihistamines, and tricyclic antidepressants can decrease platelet aggregation values.

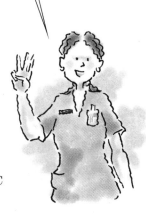

Each of the three main red cell indices "means" something different.

disorders of deoxyribonucleic acid synthesis, or reticulocytosis. (See *RBC indices interference.*)

Because MCV reflects the average volume of many cells, a value within the normal range can encompass RBCs of varying size, from microcytic to macrocytic.

What needs to be done

• Perform a venipuncture, and collect the sample in a 7-ml tube containing EDTA, or in a designated tube volume in accordance with laboratory protocol.
• Completely fill the collection tube, and invert it gently several times to adequately mix the sample and anticoagulant.

Stay on the ball

RBC indices interference

• Falsely elevated red blood cell (RBC) count, caused by a high white blood cell count in semi-automated and automated counters, invalidates mean corpuscular volume and mean corpuscular hemoglobin (MCH) results.
• Falsely elevated hemoglobin (Hb) values invalidate MCH and mean corpuscular Hb concentration (MCHC) results.
• Diseases that cause RBCs to clump together falsely decrease RBC count, invalidating MCHC and MCH results.

Reticulocyte count

Reticulocytes are nonnucleated, immature RBCs that remain in the peripheral blood for 24 to 48 hours while maturing. They're generally larger than mature RBCs. In the reticulocyte count test, reticulocytes in a whole blood sample are counted and expressed as a percentage of the total RBC count. Because the manual method of reticulocyte counting uses only a small sample, values may be imprecise and should be compared with the RBC count or HCT. The reticulocyte count is useful for evaluating anemia and is an index of effective erythropoiesis and bone marrow response to anemia. It's used to help distinguish between hypoproliferative and hyperproliferative anemias. It's also used to help assess blood loss, bone marrow response to anemia, and therapy for anemia. The patient with an abnormal reticulocyte count is monitored for trends or significant changes in repeated tests.

What it all means

Normal reticulocyte count is 0.5% to 2.5% (SI, 0.005 to 0.025) of the total RBC count. In infants, the normal reticulocyte count ranges from 2% to 6% (SI, 0.02 to 0.06) at birth, decreasing to adult levels in 1 to 2 weeks.

A low reticulocyte count indicates hypoproliferative bone marrow (hypoplastic anemia) or ineffective erythropoiesis (pernicious anemia). A high reticulocyte count indicates a bone marrow response to anemia caused by hemolysis or blood loss. The reticulocyte count may also increase after therapy for iron deficiency anemia or pernicious anemia. (See *Reticulocyte count test interference*, page 12.)

What needs to be done

• Perform a venipuncture, and collect the sample in a 3- or 4.5-ml tube containing EDTA.
• Completely fill the collection tube, and invert it gently several times to adequately mix the sample and anticoagulant.

Erythrocyte sedimentation rate

Erythrocyte sedimentation rate (ESR) measures the degree of erythrocyte, or RBC, settling during a specified time period. As the RBCs descend in the tube, they displace an equal volume of plasma upward, which slows the downward progress of other settling blood elements.

Early indicator

ESR is a sensitive but nonspecific test that's commonly the earliest indicator of disease when other chemical or physical signs are normal. ESR typically rises significantly in widespread inflammatory disorders caused by infection or autoimmune mechanisms; such elevations may be prolonged in localized inflammation and malignancy.

What it all means

Normal ESR ranges from 0 to 15 mm/hour (SI, 0 to 15 mm/hour) in males and from 0 to 20 mm/hour (SI, 0 to 20 mm/hour) in females. Rates gradually increase with age.

ESR rises in pregnancy, acute or chronic inflammation, tuberculosis, blood cell dyscrasias, rheumatic fever, rheumatoid arthritis, and some cancers. Anemia also tends to raise ESR because less upward displacement of plasma occurs to retard the relatively few sedimenting RBCs.

Polycythemia, sickle cell anemia, hyperviscosity (excessively thick blood), or low plasma fibrinogen or globulin levels tend to depress ESR.

> *Don't underestimate the importance of the ESR—even if all other signs are normal.*

What needs to be done

• Perform a venipuncture, and collect the sample in a 7-ml tube containing EDTA or in a 4.5-ml tube with sodium citrate added. (Check with the laboratory to determine preference.)

Stay on the ball

Reticulocyte count test interference

• Failure to use the proper anticoagulant, failure to adequately mix the sample, prolonged tourniquet constriction, recent blood transfusion, and hemolysis can interfere with test values.
• Azathioprine, chloramphenicol, dactinomycin, and methotrexate may cause a false-low value.
• Corticotropin, antimalarials, antipyretics, furazolidone (in infants), and levodopa can result in a false-high test result.
• Sulfonamides can cause a false-low or false-high result.

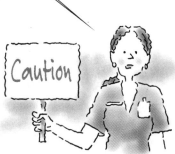

Caution

• Completely fill the collection tube, and invert it gently several times to adequately mix the sample and anticoagulant.
• Send the sample to the laboratory immediately after examining it for clots or clumps. The sample must be tested within 2 to 4 hours.

Methemoglobin

Methemoglobin (MetHb) is a variety of Hb formed when the iron in the heme portion of Hb is oxidized to a ferric state. When this oxidization occurs, the heme is incapable of combining with oxygen and transporting it to the tissues and the patient becomes cyanotic. Patients exposed to nitrites have an increased risk of becoming cyanotic.

What it all means

Normal MetHb levels fall between 0% and 1.5% (SI, 0 to 0.015) of total Hb.

The lowdown on levels

Increased MetHb levels may indicate acquired or hereditary methemoglobinemia or carbon monoxide (CO) poisoning. These levels can also be caused by certain drugs or substances.

Decreased MetHb levels may occur in pancreatitis. (See *MetHb test interference*.)

What needs to be done

• Obtain a patient history that includes the patient's hematologic status and any Hb disorders, conditions that produce nitrite, and exposure to sources of nitrites in drugs.
• Tell the patient to avoid such medications as benzocaine, nitrates, and sulfonamides.
• Perform a venipuncture, and collect a sample in a 7-ml heparinized tube, or in a designated tube volume in accordance with laboratory protocol.
• Completely fill the collection tube, and invert it gently several times.
• Place the collection tube on ice, and send it to the laboratory immediately.

Stay on the ball

MetHb test interference

These factors can increase methemoglobin (MetHb) levels:
• inorganic nitrate in the diet
• such drugs as aniline dyes, nitroglycerin, benzocaine, chlorates, lidocaine, nitrates, nitrites, sulfonamides, radiation, and primaquine.

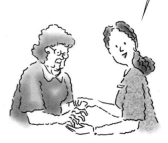

The accuracy of many tests depends on giving the patient good pretest instructions.

Carboxyhemoglobin

This test measures the level of carboxyhemoglobin in the blood and is useful in detecting CO poisoning. Exposure to CO occurs from smoke inhalation, exhaust fumes, fires, gas fumes (heaters and stoves), and petroleum fumes. Carboxyhemoglobin is formed when Hb combines with CO. CO bonds more rapidly with Hb than with oxygen, which leaves less Hb to combine with oxygen. When CO is attached to Hb, the Hb molecule alters and binds tighter to the oxygen present, resulting in a decreased ability of the oxygen to pass into the tissue. The decrease of oxygen availability results in hypoxemia. (See *CO levels and pulse oximetry.*)

What it all means

Normal carboxyhemoglobin findings are:
- *nonsmokers:* less than 2% of total Hb
- *light smokers:* 4% to 5% of total Hb
- *heavy smokers:* 6% to 8% of total Hb
- *neonates:* 10% to 12% of total Hb.

Abnormal findings indicate CO poisoning. At 10% to 20% of total Hb, the patient may be asymptomatic; at 20% to 30% of total Hb, the patient will have headache, nausea, vomiting, and possible loss of judgment; at 30% to 40% of total Hb, the patient will have tachycardia, hyperpnea, hypotension, and confusion; and at 50% to 60% of total Hb, the patient will have loss of consciousness. Values greater than 60% of the total Hb will cause seizures, respiratory arrest, and death.

What needs to be done

- Obtain a history from the patient for any possible CO exposure, and evaluate the patient for signs and symptoms of CO poisoning, such as headache, dizziness, malaise, and bright red mucous membranes.
- Draw blood as soon as possible after exposure.
- Perform a venipuncture, and collect 5 ml of blood in a tube containing EDTA.
- Immediately place the sample on ice and transport it to the laboratory.

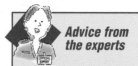

Advice from the experts

CO levels and pulse oximetry

When the patient has high levels of carbon monoxide (CO) in the blood, pulse oximetry studies may be normal despite the presence of hypoxia. This is because the study looks at the saturation of the hemoglobin, not what the hemoglobin is saturated with. Apply high concentrations of oxygen (O_2), as ordered, to help increase O_2 in the blood and displace the CO.

Sickle cell test

Sickle cells (Hb S) are severely deformed erythrocytes. The sickle cell test (also known as the *Hb S test*) helps identify sickle cell anemia. More than 50,000 Americans have sickle cell disease, and it's found almost exclusively in Blacks.

Spontaneous sickling

People who are homozygous for Hb S usually show abundant spontaneously sickled RBCs on a peripheral blood smear. People

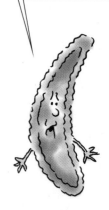

What do you mean I'm severely deformed?

who are heterozygous for Hb S alone or with another Hb deformity may have normal RBCs that can be easily changed to sickled forms by lowering oxygen tension. This sickling tendency can be identified by sealing a drop of blood between a glass slide and coverslip and adding a deoxygenating agent. The RBCs can then be observed under a microscope and compared to a central slide containing blood and saline solution. If the patient's Hb is of the S variation, the cells will assume the crescent (sickle) shape and the test is positive.

In another variation of the test, Hb solubility is determined by adding a blood sample to a reagent that lyses the RBCs, releasing the Hb. The reagent also contains a reducing agent to remove the oxygen from the Hb. Deoxygenated Hb S is insoluble and precipitates in the solution, causing turbidity.

May produce erroneous results

Although the sickle cell test is useful as a rapid screening procedure, it may produce erroneous results; consequently, Hb electrophoresis should be performed if sickle cell trait is strongly suspected.

What it all means

Results of this test are reported as positive or negative. A normal, or negative, test suggests the absence of Hb S. A positive test may indicate the presence of Hb S, but Hb electrophoresis is needed to distinguish between homozygous and heterozygous forms. (See *Sickle cell test interference.*)

What needs to be done

• Check the patient history for a blood transfusion within the past 3 months.
• Perform a venipuncture, and collect the sample in a 7-ml tube containing EDTA, or in a designated tube volume in accordance with laboratory protocol. For younger children, collect capillary blood in a microcollection device.
• Completely fill the collection tube, and invert it gently several times to adequately mix the sample and anticoagulant.

Stay on the ball

Sickle cell test interference

The following factors may produce false-negative results in a sickle cell test:
• hemoglobin concentration under 10%
• infants younger than age 6 months
• blood transfusion within the past 3 months.

If you study hard, you're "bound" to understand an iron assay test.

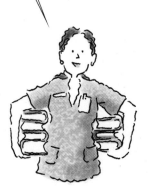

Iron and total iron-binding capacity

An iron assay is used to measure the amount of iron bound to transferrin in blood plasma. Total iron-binding capacity (TIBC) is a measure of the amount of iron that would appear in plasma if all the transferrin were saturated with iron. The percentage of saturation is obtained by dividing the serum iron result by the TIBC, which reveals the actual amount of saturated transferrin. Normally, transferrin is about 30% saturated.

What it all means

Reference values are:
- *serum iron:* 60 to 170 mcg/dl (SI, 10.7 to 30.4 µmol/L) for males; 50 to 130 mcg/dl (SI, 9 to 23.3 µmol/L) for females
- *TIBC:* 300 to 360 mcg/dl (SI, 54 to 64 µmol/L) for males and females
- *saturation:* 20% to 50% (SI, 0.2 to 0.5) for males and females.

The lowdown on levels

In iron deficiency, serum iron levels drop and TIBC increases to decrease the saturation. In cases of chronic inflammation, such as in rheumatoid arthritis, serum iron may be low in the presence of adequate body stores but TIBC may be unchanged or may drop to preserve normal saturation.

Iron overload may not alter serum levels until relatively late but, in general, serum iron increases and TIBC remains the same to increase the saturation. (See *Iron and TIBC test interference.*)

What needs to be done

- Check the patient history and withhold such drugs as chloramphenicol, corticotropin, iron supplements, and hormonal contraceptives, as ordered. If such medications must be continued, note this on the laboratory request.
- Perform a venipuncture, and collect the sample in a 7-ml clot-activator tube, or in a designated tube volume in accordance with laboratory protocol.
- As ordered, resume administration of any medications that were withheld for the test.

Stay on the ball

Iron and TIBC test interference

- Use of chloramphenicol and hormonal contraceptives can cause falsely elevated test results.
- Corticotropin can produce falsely low test results.
- Iron supplements can cause falsely elevated serum iron values but falsely low total iron-binding capacity (TIBC).

Ferritin

Ferritin, a major iron-storage protein found in reticuloendothelial cells (cells lining vascular and lymph vessels), normally appears in small quantities in serum. In healthy adults, serum ferritin levels are directly related to the amount of available iron stored in the body and can be measured accurately by immunologic methods. Unlike many other blood studies, the serum ferritin test isn't affected by moderate hemolysis of the sample or by the patient's use of drugs.

What it all means

Normal serum ferritin values vary with age and sex, as shown here:
- *men:* 20 to 300 ng/ml (SI, 20 to 300 µg/L)
- *women:* 20 to 120 ng/ml (SI, 20 to 120 µg/L)
- *ages 6 months to 15 years:* 7 to 140 ng/ml (SI, 7 to 140 µg/L)
- *ages 2 to 5 months:* 50 to 200 ng/ml (SI, 50 to 200 µg/L)
- *age 1 month:* 200 to 600 ng/ml (SI, 200 to 600 µg/L)
- *neonates:* 25 to 200 ng/ml (SI, 25 to 200 µg/L).

The lowdown on levels

High serum ferritin levels may indicate acute or chronic hepatic disease, iron overload, leukemia, acute or chronic infection or inflammation, Hodgkin's disease, or chronic hemolytic anemias; in these disorders, iron stores in bone marrow may be normal or significantly increased. Serum ferritin levels are characteristically normal or slightly elevated in a patient who has chronic renal disease.

Low serum ferritin levels indicate chronic iron deficiency. (See *Ferritin test interference.*)

What needs to be done

- Review the patient history for a recent transfusion.
- Perform a venipuncture, and collect the sample in a 10-ml tube without additives, or in a designated tube volume in accordance with laboratory protocol.

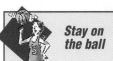

Stay on the ball

Ferritin test interference

A recent transfusion may elevate serum ferritin levels.

Coagulation tests

Bleeding time

The bleeding time test measures the duration of bleeding after a standardized skin incision. Bleeding time depends on the elasticity of the blood vessel wall and the number and function of platelets.

Not recommended for all

The bleeding time test usually isn't recommended for a patient whose platelet count is less than 75,000/µl (SI, 75×10^9/L). However, some patients with altered platelet morphology may have normal bleeding times despite low platelet counts.

What it all means

Normal bleeding time is 3 to 6 minutes (SI, 3 to 6 minutes) using the template method or Ivy's method, and 1 to 3 minutes (SI, 1 to 3 minutes) using Duke's method.

Bleeding overtime

Prolonged bleeding time may indicate the presence of disorders associated with thrombocytopenia, such as Hodgkin's disease; acute leukemia; DIC; hemolytic disease of the neonate; Schönlein-Henoch purpura; severe hepatic disease; or severe deficiency of factors I, II, V, VII, VIII, IX, or XI. Prolonged bleeding time in a person with a normal platelet count suggests a platelet function disorder and requires further investigation with clot retraction, prothrombin consumption, and platelet aggregation tests. (See *Bleeding time interference*.)

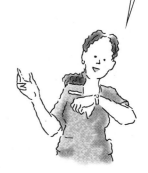

Coagulation tests are all about bleeding times.

What needs to be done

• Check for a recent history of drugs that prolong bleeding time. If the patient has taken such drugs, check with the laboratory for special instructions. If the test is being used to identify a suspected bleeding disorder, it should be postponed and the drugs discontinued as ordered; if it's being used preoperatively to assess hemostatic function, it should proceed as scheduled.
• Wrap a pressure cuff around the patient's upper arm and inflate it to 40 mm Hg. Select an area on the forearm that's free from superficial veins, and clean it with antiseptic. Let the skin dry completely before making the incisions. Apply the appropriate template lengthwise to the forearm. Use a lancet to make two incisions, each 1 mm deep and 9 mm long. Start the stopwatch. Without touching the cuts, gently blot the blood drops with filter paper every 30 seconds until bleeding stops in both cuts. Average the time of the two cuts, and record the results.
• If the bleeding doesn't diminish after 15 minutes, discontinue the test.
• For a patient with a bleeding tendency (such as hemophilia), maintain a pressure bandage over the incision for 24 to 48 hours to prevent further bleeding. If the template method was used, keep the edges of the cuts aligned to minimize scarring. Otherwise, a piece of gauze held in place by an adhesive bandage is sufficient. Check the test area frequently.
• As ordered, resume administration of medications discontinued before the test.

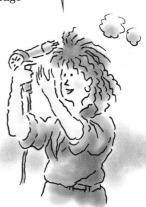

Be sure to let the skin dry completely before making any big decisions—I mean, incisions!

Activated partial thromboplastin time

The activated partial thromboplastin time (APTT) test evaluates all the clotting factors of the intrinsic and common pathways by measuring the time it takes a clot to form after adding calcium and phospholipid emulsion to a plasma sample. The partial thromboplastin time (PTT) and the APTT test for the same functions; however, the APTT is considered a more sensitive version of the PTT and is used to monitor a patient's response to heparin therapy.

What it all means

Normally, a fibrin clot forms 21 to 35 seconds (SI, 21 to 35 s) after the addition of reagents. For a patient on anticoagulant therapy, check with the attending practitioner to find out the desirable values for the therapy being delivered.

May signal deficiency

Prolonged APTT may indicate a deficiency of certain plasma clotting factors; the presence of heparin; or the presence of fibrin split products, fibrinolysins, or circulating anticoagulants that are antibodies to specific clotting factors.

What needs to be done

• Tell the patient receiving heparin therapy that this test may be repeated at regular intervals to assess his response to treatment.
• Perform a venipuncture, and collect the sample in a 7-ml tube with sodium citrate added, or in a designated tube volume in accordance with laboratory protocol.
• Completely fill the collection tube, invert it gently several times, and send it to the laboratory on ice.
• For a patient on anticoagulant therapy, additional pressure may be needed at the venipuncture site to control bleeding.

Stay on the ball

Bleeding time interference

Sulfonamides, thiazide diuretics, antineoplastics, anticoagulants, nonsteroidal anti-inflammatory drugs, aspirin and aspirin compounds, and some nonnarcotic analgesics may prolong bleeding time.

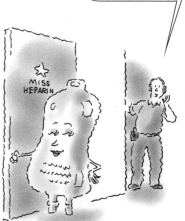

Miss Heparin? That fan with the prolonged APTT would like to speak to you.

Prothrombin time

Prothrombin, or *factor II*, is a plasma protein produced by the liver. The prothrombin time (PT) test measures the time required for a fibrin clot to form in a citrated plasma sample after the addition of calcium ions and tissue thromboplastin (factor III). It's an excellent screening procedure for overall evaluation of extrinsic and common pathways. PT is the test of choice for monitoring oral anticoagulant therapy.

What it all means

Normally, PT ranges from 10 to 14 seconds (SI, 10 to 14 s). In a patient receiving oral anticoagulant therapy, PT is usually maintained between 1 and 2.5 times the normal control value.

Prolonged PT

Prolonged PT may indicate hepatic disease or deficiencies in fibrinogen, prothrombin, vitamin K, or factors V, VII, or X (specific assays can pinpoint such deficiencies). Or, it may result from ongoing oral anticoagulant therapy. Prolonged PT that exceeds 2.5 times the control value is commonly associated with abnormal bleeding. (See *PT test interference*.)

What needs to be done

• Check the patient history for use of medications that may affect test results, such as vitamin K or antibiotics.
• Perform a venipuncture, and collect the sample in a 7-ml siliconized tube, or in a designated tube volume in accordance with laboratory protocol.
• Completely fill the collection tube, and invert it gently several times to adequately mix the sample and anticoagulant. If the tube isn't filled to the correct volume, an excess of citrate will appear in the sample.

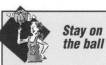

Stay on the ball

PT test interference

• Antihistamines, corticosteroids, digoxin, diuretics, glutethimide, progestin-estrogen combinations, pyrazinamide, vitamin K, and xanthines may shorten prothrombin time (PT).
• Alcohol overuse and administration of corticotropin, anabolic steroids, I.V. heparin, indomethacin, methimazole, phenylbutazone, phenytoin, propylthiouracil, quinidine, thyroid hormones, or vitamin A may prolong PT.

International Normalized Ratio

The International Normalized Ratio (INR) system is the best means of standardizing measurement of PT to monitor oral anticoagulant therapy.

What it all means

Normal INR for those receiving warfarin therapy is 2.0 to 3.0 (SI, 2.0 to 3.0). For those with mechanical prosthetic heart valves, an INR of 2.5 to 3.5 (SI, 2.5 to 3.5) is suggested.

Increased INR values may indicate DIC, cirrhosis, hepatitis, vitamin K deficiency, salicylate intoxication, uncontrolled oral anticoagulation, or massive blood transfusion.

What needs to be done

• Perform a venipuncture, and collect the sample in a 7-ml tube with sodium citrate added, or in a designated tube volume in accordance with laboratory protocol.
• Completely fill the collection tube; otherwise, excess citrate will appear in the sample.

- Gently invert the tube several times to thoroughly mix the sample and anticoagulant.
- Put the sample on ice, and send it to the laboratory promptly.

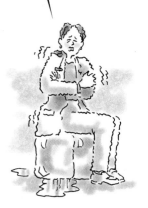

BRRRR! Don't forget to put the INR test sample on ice.

Activated clotting time

Activated clotting time, or *automated coagulation time*, measures the time it takes whole blood to clot. This test is commonly performed during procedures that require extracorporeal circulation (circulation occurring outside the body), such as cardiopulmonary bypass, ultrafiltration, hemodialysis, and extracorporeal membrane oxygenation (ECMO).

What it all means

In a patient who isn't receiving anticoagulants, normal activated clotting time is 107 ± 13 seconds (SI, 107 ± 13 s). During cardiopulmonary bypass, heparin is titrated to maintain an activated clotting time between 400 and 600 seconds (SI, 400 to 600 s). During ECMO, heparin is titrated to maintain an activated clotting time between 220 and 260 seconds (SI, 220 to 260 s).

What needs to be done

- Explain to the patient that the test requires a blood sample, which is usually drawn from an existing vascular access site; therefore, no venipuncture is necessary.
- Explain that two samples will be drawn. The first one will be discarded so that any heparin in the tubing doesn't interfere with the results.
- If the sample is drawn from a line with a continuous infusion, stop the infusion before drawing the sample.
- Withdraw 5 to 10 ml of blood from the line, and discard it.
- Withdraw a clean sample of blood into the special tube that contains celite, which was provided with the activated clotting time unit.
- Activate the activated clotting time unit, and wait for the signal to insert the tube.
- Flush the vascular access site according to your facility's protocol.

Plasma thrombin time

The plasma thrombin time test measures how quickly a clot forms when a standard amount of bovine thrombin is added to a platelet-poor plasma sample from the patient and is also added to a normal plasma control sample. After thrombin is added, the clotting time for each sample is compared with the other and recorded. Because thrombin rapidly converts fibrinogen to a fibrin clot, this test (also known as the *thrombin clotting time*) allows a quick but imprecise estimation of plasma fibrinogen levels, which are a function of clotting time.

What it all means

Normal thrombin times range from 10 to 15 seconds (SI, 10 to 15 s) and should be within 2 seconds of the control. Test results are usually reported with a normal control value.

Prolonged thrombin time

A prolonged thrombin time may indicate heparin therapy, hepatic disease, DIC, or fibrinogen defect or deficiency. Patients with prolonged thrombin times may require quantification of fibrinogen levels; in suspected DIC, the test for fibrin split products is also necessary. (See *Plasma thrombin time test interference.*)

What needs to be done

• If possible, withhold heparin therapy before the test as ordered. If heparin must be continued, note this on the laboratory request.
• Perform a venipuncture, and collect the sample in a 7-ml siliconized tube, or in a designated tube volume in accordance with laboratory protocol.
• Completely fill the collection tube, and invert it gently several times to adequately mix the sample and anticoagulant. If the tube isn't filled to the correct volume, excess citrate will appear in the sample.
• Send the sample to the laboratory immediately.

Plasma fibrinogen

The plasma fibrinogen test measures the plasma concentration of fibrinogen available for coagulation. Fibrinogen (factor I) isn't normally present in serum; it's converted to fibrin by thrombin during clotting. Because fibrin is a necessary part of a blood clot, fibrinogen deficiency can produce mild to severe bleeding disorders. When fibrinogen levels drop below 100 mg/dl (SI, 1 g/L), it becomes difficult to accurately interpret all coagulation tests that have a fibrin clot as an end point.

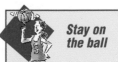

Stay on the ball

Plasma thrombin time test interference

Heparin, fibrinogen, or fibrin degradation products may prolong clotting time.

What it all means

Fibrinogen levels normally range from 200 to 400 mg/dl (SI, 2 to 4 g/L).

The lowdown on levels

Depressed fibrinogen levels may indicate congenital afibrinogenemia (absence of fibrinogen), hypofibrinogenemia (deficiency of fibrinogen), dysfibrinogenemia (abnormal fibrinogen), DIC, fibrinolysis, severe hepatic disease, bone marrow lesions, or cancer of the prostate, pancreas, or lung. Obstetric complications or trauma may also cause low levels.

Elevated levels may indicate cancer of the stomach, breast, or kidney or an inflammatory disorder, such as pneumonia or glomerulonephritis. (See *Plasma fibrinogen test interference*.)

What needs to be done

• Assess the patient for contraindications to this test, such as active bleeding or acute infection or illness. This test is also contraindicated in a patient who has received a blood transfusion within the past 4 weeks.
• Check the patient history for use of anticoagulants or hormonal contraceptives. Note such drugs on the laboratory request.
• If the patient is receiving heparin therapy, notify the laboratory; such therapy requires the use of a different reagent.
• Perform a venipuncture, and collect the sample in a 7-ml tube with sodium citrate added, or in a designated tube volume in accordance with laboratory protocol.
• Completely fill the collection tube, invert it gently several times, and send it to the laboratory immediately.

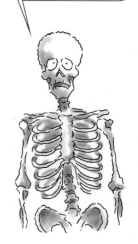

Depressed fibrinogen levels depress me, too. They can cause bone marrow lesions.

Plasminogen

Plasminogen testing is used to assess plasma plasminogen levels in a plasma sample. During fibrinolysis, plasmin dissolves fibrin clots to prevent excessive coagulation and impaired blood flow. Plasmin doesn't circulate in active form, however, so it can't be directly measured. Its circulating precursor, plasminogen, can be measured and used to evaluate the fibrinolytic system. This test is used to assess fibrinolysis in blood clotting and to detect congenital and acquired fibrinolytic disorders.

What it all means

Normal plasminogen levels range from 10 to 20 mg/dl (0.1 to 0.2 g/L) by immunologic methods. Diminished plasminogen levels can

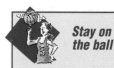

Stay on the ball

Plasma fibrinogen test interference

The following factors may alter plasma fibrinogen test results:
• fibrinogen levels that are elevated during the third trimester of pregnancy and in postoperative patients
• the transfusion of blood products within 4 weeks of the test.

result from DIC, tumors, preeclampsia, and eclampsia, which accelerate plasminogen conversion to plasmin and increase fibrinolysis. Some liver diseases prevent the formation of sufficient plasminogen, decreasing fibrinolysis. (See *Plasminogen test interference.*)

What needs to be done

• Notify the laboratory and the practitioner about medications the patient is taking that may affect test results; they may need to be restricted.
• Perform a venipuncture, and collect the sample in a 4.5-ml siliconized tube.
• Instruct the patient that he may resume medications discontinued before the test, as ordered.
• Collect the sample as quickly as possible to prevent stasis, which can slow blood flow, causing coagulation and plasminogen activation.
• To prevent hemolysis, avoid both excessive probing during venipuncture and rough handling of the sample.
• Invert the tube gently several times, and immediately send the sample to the laboratory. If testing must be delayed, plasma must be separated and frozen.

Fibrin split products

After a fibrin clot forms in response to vascular injury, the fibrinolytic system acts to break down the clot by converting plasminogen into the fibrin-dissolving enzyme plasmin. Plasmin breaks down fibrin and fibrinogen into fragments known as *fibrin split products* (FSP), or *fibrin degradation products*. An excess of these products in the circulation causes anticoagulant activity. This excess may lead to coagulation disorders, which may be due to fibrinogenolysis or such clotting excesses as DIC.

Reaction detected

FSP are detected by a reaction in which diluted serum left in a blood sample after clotting is mixed on a slide with latex particles that carry antibodies to some of the split products. Clumping of the latex particles occurs if FSP are present in the serum dilution.

What it all means

Serum normally contains less than 10 mcg/ml (SI, less than 10 mg/L) of FSP. A quantitative assay shows levels of less than 3 mcg/ml (SI, less than 3 mg/L).

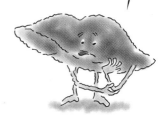

I thought liver disease was just my problem, but it turns out it decreases fibrinolysis, too.

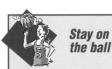

Stay on the ball

Plasminogen test interference

• Failure to use the proper collection tube, to adequately mix the sample and citrate, to send the sample to the laboratory immediately, or to have the sample separated and frozen
• Hemoconcentration due to prolonged tourniquet use before venipuncture (possible false-low)
• Hormonal contraceptives (possible slight increase)
• Thrombolytic drugs, such as streptokinase and urokinase (possible decrease)

Reasons for rising

FSP levels rise in primary fibrinolytic states because of increased levels of circulating profibrinolysin; they rise, in secondary states, because of DIC and subsequent fibrinolysis. Levels also increase in alcoholic cirrhosis, preeclampsia, abruptio placentae, heart disease, sunstroke, burns, intrauterine death, pulmonary embolus, deep vein thrombosis (transient increase), and MI (after 1 or 2 days). FSP levels usually exceed 100 mcg/ml (SI, greater than 100 mg/L) in active renal disease or kidney transplant rejection. (See *FSP test interference*.)

What needs to be done

• Check the patient history for use of medications (especially heparin) that may affect the accuracy of test results.
• Draw the sample before administering heparin, to help avoid false-positive test results.
• Perform a venipuncture, and draw 2 ml of blood into a plastic syringe. Transfer the sample to the tube provided by the laboratory. The tube contains a soybean trypsin inhibitor and bovine thrombin. Evacuated tubes are available in kits designed to provide a rapid semiquantitative analysis of FSP. Follow the manufacturer's directions for sample collection and handling.
• Gently invert the collection tube several times to adequately mix the contents. The blood clots within 2 seconds and must then be sent to the laboratory immediately to be incubated at 98.6° F (37° C) for 30 minutes before testing proceeds.

Stay on the ball

FSP test interference

• Pretest administration of heparin causes false-positive results.
• Fibrinolytic drugs, such as urokinase, streptokinase, and tissue plasminogen activator; and large doses of barbiturates increase FSP levels.

D-dimer

D-dimer is an asymmetrical carbon compound fragment formed after thrombin converts fibrinogen to fibrin, factor XIIIa stabilizes it into a clot, and plasma acts on the cross-linked, or clotted, fibrin. The test is specific for fibrinolysis because it confirms the presence of FSPs. The D-dimer test is used to determine whether the blood is clotting normally. It's used to diagnose DIC and to differentiate subarachnoid hemorrhage from a traumatic lumbar puncture in spinal fluid analysis.

What it all means

Normal D-dimer test results are negative or less than 250 mcg/L (SI, less than 250 µg/L). Increased D-dimer values may indicate DIC, pulmonary embolism, arterial or venous thrombosis, neoplastic disease, pregnancy (late and postpartum), surgery occurring up to 2 days before testing, subarachnoid hemorrhage (spinal fluid only), or secondary fibrinolysis. (See *D-dimer test interference*.)

What needs to be done

• Obtain the patient's history of hematologic diseases, recent surgery, and the results of other tests performed.
• Perform a venipuncture, and collect the sample in a 4.5-ml tube with sodium citrate added, or in a designated tube volume in accordance with laboratory protocol.
• Completely fill the collection tube, invert it gently several times, and send it to the laboratory immediately.
• For a patient with coagulation problems, you may need to apply additional pressure at the venipuncture site to control bleeding.

Stay on the ball

D-dimer test interference

High rheumatoid factor titers, increased CA 125 levels, estrogen therapy, and normal pregnancy can cause false-positive results.

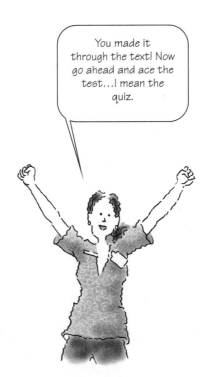

You made it through the text! Now go ahead and ace the test...I mean the quiz.

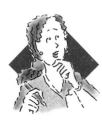

Quick quiz

1. ESR measures the degree of erythrocyte settling in a blood sample during a specified period. What's the significance of an elevated ESR?

    A.   An inflammatory disorder may be present.

    B.   It distinguishes between hypoproliferative and hyperproliferative anemias.

    C.   An infection is present.

    D   It indicates polycythemia.

Answer: A. An elevation in the patient's ESR may indicate the presence of an inflammatory disorder.

2. Which test provides information about the size and Hb weight of an average RBC?

    A.   HCT

    B.   Red cell indices

    C.   RBC count

    D.   Carboxyhemoglobin level

Answer: B. Red cell indices provide information about the size, Hb concentration, and Hb weight of an average RBC.

3. Which test provides the best means of standardizing measurement of PT to monitor oral anticoagulant therapy?

    A.   Platelet aggregation

    B.   Plasma thrombin time

    C.   INR

    D.   APTT

Answer: C. The INR is the best means of standardizing measurement of PT to monitor anticoagulant therapy.

4. Which action may interfere with results of FSP testing?

    A.   Pretest heparin administration

    B.   Filling the collection tube completely with blood

    C.   Failure to administer a fibrinolytic drug before testing

    D.   Administration of oxygen

Answer: A. Pretest heparin administration can result in falsely elevated FSP levels.

5. A patient's platelet count may decrease normally in what circumstance?

    A.   During strenuous exercise
    B.   During persistent cold temperatures
    C.   Just before menstruation
    D.   During stressful situations

Answer: C. The patient's platelet count may decrease normally just before menstruation.

Scoring

☆☆☆   If you answered all five questions correctly, super! Your knowledge is coagulating nicely.

☆☆   If you answered four questions correctly, great! You have a high "level" of understanding.

☆   If you answered fewer than four questions correctly, our diagnosis is test stress! Relax, and you'll ace the next test on tests.

Blood chemistry tests

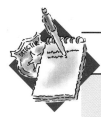

Just the facts

In this chapter, you'll learn:

♦ about blood chemistry tests

♦ patient care associated with these tests

♦ factors that can interfere with test results

♦ what blood chemistry test results may indicate.

A look at blood chemistry tests

Laboratory analysis of blood chemistry tests helps evaluate the body's respiratory and metabolic status. Arterial blood gas (ABG) values provide important information about the adequacy of gas exchange in the lungs, ventilatory function, blood pH, and acid-base balance. Electrolyte levels provide valuable data about the body's acid-base balance and fluid balance.

Takin' care of business

Before obtaining a sample for a blood chemistry test, make sure the patient understands the procedure. Explain the procedure's purpose, and tell the patient that he'll feel some pressure from the tourniquet (if one is used) and may feel brief discomfort from the needle puncture.

If possible, use a large-gauge needle when drawing the sample, and handle the sample gently to prevent hemolysis, which may interfere with test results. Observe standard precautions. Also, after taking a blood sample, check the venipuncture site for bleeding. If a hematoma develops at the site, apply warm soaks.

Running interference

A number of drugs can interfere with blood chemistry tests. Be sure to check the patient history and make notations as necessary.

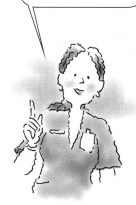

A number of drugs can interfere with blood chemistry tests, so know your patient's medication history.

Blood gases

Arterial blood gas analysis

ABG analysis evaluates gas exchange in the lungs by measuring the partial pressures of oxygen (PaO_2) and carbon dioxide ($PaCO_2$) as well as the pH of an arterial sample. PaO_2 measures the pressure exerted by the oxygen dissolved in the blood and evaluates the lungs' ability to oxygenate the blood. $PaCO_2$ measures the pressure exerted by carbon dioxide (CO_2) dissolved in the blood and reflects the adequacy of ventilation by the lungs. pH measures the blood's hydrogen ion concentration and is the best way to tell whether blood is too acidic or too alkaline. Bicarbonate (HCO_3^-) is a measure of the HCO_3^- ion concentration in the blood, which is regulated by the kidneys. Oxygen saturation (SaO_2) is the oxygen content of the blood expressed as a percentage of the oxygen capacity (the amount of oxygen the blood is capable of carrying if all of the hemoglobin [Hb] were fully saturated). Oxygen content (O_2CT) measures the actual amount of oxygen in the blood and isn't commonly used in blood gas evaluation.

What it all means

Normal ABG values fall within these ranges:
- *pH:* 7.35 to 7.45 (SI, 7.35 to 7.45)
- *$PaCO_2$:* 35 to 45 mm Hg (SI, 4.7 to 5.3 kPa)
- *PaO_2:* 80 to 100 mm Hg (SI, 10.6 to 13.3 kPa)
- *HCO_3^-:* 22 to 25 mEq/L (SI, 22 to 25 mmol/L)
- *SaO_2:* 94% to 100% (SI, 0.94 to 1.00)
- *O_2CT:* 15% to 23% (SI, 0.15 to 0.23).

The lowdown on levels

Low PaO_2, O_2CT, and SaO_2 levels in combination with a high $PaCO_2$ may occur with:
- respiratory muscle weakness or paralysis (as in Guillain-Barré syndrome or myasthenia gravis)
- respiratory center inhibition (from head injury, brain tumor, or drug abuse) or airway obstruction (possibly from a mucus plug or tumor)
- bronchiole obstruction associated with asthma or emphysema
- abnormal ventilation-perfusion ratio.

When inspired air contains insufficient oxygen, PaO_2, O_2CT, and SaO_2 also decrease but $PaCO_2$ may be normal. Such findings are common in:

- pneumothorax
- impaired diffusion between alveoli and blood (such as that caused by interstitial fibrosis)
- arteriovenous shunt that permits blood to bypass the lungs.

Low O_2CT with normal Pao_2, Sao_2 and, possibly, $Paco_2$ may result from severe anemia, decreased blood volume, and reduced oxygen-carrying capacity of Hb. (See *ABG analysis interference*.)

In addition to clarifying blood oxygen disorders, ABG values can provide considerable information about acid-base disorders.

What needs to be done

- Wait at least 20 minutes before drawing ABG measurements in the following situations:
  - after initiating, changing, or discontinuing oxygen therapy
  - after initiating or changing settings of mechanical ventilation
  - after extubation.
- Tell the patient which site—radial, brachial, or femoral artery—has been selected for the puncture.
- Instruct the patient to breathe normally during the test, and warn him that he may feel brief cramping or throbbing pain at the puncture site. (See *Obtaining an ABG sample*, page 32.)
- Include the following information on the laboratory request:
  - room air or amount of oxygen and method of delivery (for example, 40% aerosol face mask)
  - ventilator settings if on mechanical ventilation (fraction of inspired oxygen, tidal volume, mode, respiratory rate, positive-end expiratory pressure)
  - patient's temperature.
- Monitor vital signs and observe for signs of circulatory impairment, such as swelling, discoloration, pain, numbness, or tingling in the bandaged arm or leg.

Stay on the ball

ABG analysis interference

- Bicarbonate, ethacrynic acid, hydrocortisone, metolazone, prednisone, and thiazides may elevate partial pressure of carbon dioxide ($Paco_2$).
- Acetazolamide, methicillin, nitrofurantoin, and tetracycline may decrease $Paco_2$.
- Hypothermia may cause false-low partial pressure of oxygen (Pao_2) and $Paco_2$ levels.
- Fever may cause false-high Pao_2 and $Paco_2$ levels.

Total carbon dioxide

CO_2 is present in the body as an end product of metabolic processes as well as being present in small amounts in the air. When the pressure of CO_2 in the red cells exceeds 40 mm Hg (SI, 5.3 kPa), CO_2 flows out of the cells and dissolves in plasma. At this point, it combines with water to form carbonic acid, which in turn dissociates into hydrogen and HCO_3^- ions.

The total test measures the total concentration of all such forms of CO_2 in serum, plasma, or whole blood samples. Because about 90% of CO_2 in serum is in the form of HCO_3^-, this test is a close approximation of HCO_3^- levels. Total CO_2 content reflects

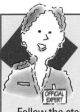

Advice from the experts

Obtaining an ABG sample

Follow the steps below to obtain a sample for an arterial blood gas (ABG) analysis:
• After Allen's test, perform a cutaneous arterial puncture (or if an arterial line is in place, draw blood from the arterial line).
• Use a heparinized blood gas syringe to draw the sample.
• Eliminate all air from the sample, place it on ice immediately, and transport it for analysis.
• Apply pressure to the puncture site for 3 to 5 minutes. If the patient is receiving anticoagulants or has a coagulopathy, hold the puncture site longer than 5 minutes, if necessary.
• Tape a gauze pad firmly over the puncture site. If the puncture site is on the arm, don't tape the entire circumference because this may restrict circulation.

Stay on the ball

Total CO_2 test interference

• Excessive use of corticotropin, cortisone, or thiazide diuretics or excessive ingestion of alkalis or licorice causes carbon dioxide (CO_2) levels to rise.
• Salicylates, paraldehyde, methicillin, dimercaprol, ammonium chloride, acetazolamide, or ingestion of ethylene glycol or methyl alcohol causes CO_2 levels to decrease.

the efficiency of the carbonic acid–HCO_3^- buffer system, which maintains acid-base balance and normal pH.

What it all means
Normal CO_2 levels range from 22 to 26 mEq/L (SI, 22 to 26 mmol/L).

Too much

High CO_2 levels may occur in metabolic alkalosis (caused by excessive ingestion or retention of base HCO_3^-), respiratory acidosis (from hypoventilation, for example, as in emphysema or pneumonia), primary aldosteronism, and Cushing's syndrome. CO_2 levels may also be elevated after excessive loss of acids, such as in severe vomiting and continuous gastric drainage.

Too little

Decreased CO_2 levels are common in metabolic acidosis (such as diabetic acidosis or renal tube acidosis caused by renal failure). Decreased total CO_2 levels in metabolic acidosis also result from loss of HCO_3^- (such as in severe diarrhea or intestinal drainage). Levels may also fall below normal in respiratory alkalosis (for example, from hyperventilation after trauma). (See *Total CO$_2$ test interference*.)

What needs to be done

• Perform a venipuncture. Because CO_2 content is usually measured along with electrolytes, a 7-ml clot-activator tube may be used, or use a designated tube volume in accordance with laboratory protocol. When this test is performed alone, a heparinized tube is appropriate.
• Fill the tube completely to prevent diffusion of CO_2 into the vacuum.

Electrolytes

Sodium

The serum sodium test measures serum levels of sodium, the major extracellular cation. Sodium affects body water distribution, maintains osmotic pressure of extracellular fluid, and helps promote neuromuscular function. It also helps maintain acid-base balance and influences chloride and potassium levels. Sodium is absorbed by the kidneys; a small amount is lost through the skin.

Relationship with water

Serum sodium levels are evaluated in relation to the amount of water in the body, which is affected by the cellular mechanics of sodium (decreased sodium levels promote water excretion, and increased levels promote retention). For example, a sodium deficit (hyponatremia) refers to a decreased level of sodium in relation to the body's water level.

What it all means

Normally, serum sodium levels range from 135 to 145 mEq/L (SI, 135 to 145 mmol/L).

Sodium imbalance can result from a loss or gain of sodium or from a change in water volume. Remember, serum sodium results must be interpreted in light of the patient's state of hydration.

When it's high

Elevated serum sodium levels (hypernatremia) may be caused by inadequate water intake; water loss that exceeds sodium loss, such as in diabetes insipidus, impaired renal function, prolonged hyperventilation and, occasionally, severe vomiting or diarrhea; and sodium retention such as in aldosteronism. Hypernatremia can also result from excessive sodium intake.

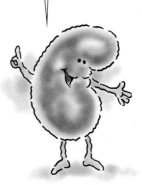

I let the skin have a little bit, but most sodium is mine, mine, mine!

When it's low

Abnormally low serum sodium levels (hyponatremia) may result from inadequate sodium intake or excessive sodium loss caused by profuse sweating, GI suctioning, diuretic therapy, diarrhea, vomiting, adrenal insufficiency, burns, or chronic renal insufficiency with acidosis. Urine sodium determinations are frequently more sensitive to early changes in sodium balance and should always be evaluated simultaneously with serum sodium findings. (See *Sodium test interference*.)

What needs to be done

• Perform a venipuncture, and collect the sample in a 7-ml clot-activator tube, or in a designated tube volume in accordance with laboratory protocol.

Stay on the ball

Sodium test interference

• Most diuretics, lithium, chlorpropamide, and vasopressin suppress serum sodium levels.
• Corticosteroids and antihypertensives (such as methyldopa, hydralazine, and reserpine) elevate serum sodium levels.

Potassium

Potassium is the major intracellular cation. The intracellular concentration of potassium is 150 to 160 mEq/L (SI, 150 to 160 mmol/L), and the extracellular concentration is 3.5 to 5 mEq/L (SI, 3.5 to 5 mmol/L). Evaluation of serum potassium measures the extracellular levels of this electrolyte.

Keeps cells neutral

Potassium is important in maintaining cellular electrical neutrality. The sodium-potassium active transport pump maintains the ratio of intracellular potassium to extracellular potassium that determines the resting membrane potential necessary for nerve impulse transmission. Disturbances in this ratio alter cardiac rhythms, transmission and conduction of nerve impulses, and muscle contraction.

What it all means

Normally, serum potassium levels range from 3.5 to 5 mEq/L (SI, 3.5 to 5 mmol/L).

A mess of potassium...

Hyperkalemia (elevated potassium level) occurs with:
• increased potassium intake
• shift in the concentration from intracellular to extracellular fluid
• decreased renal excretion
• infusion of stored whole blood
• penicillin G

> Careful! If I'm out of balance, I can cause some chaos.

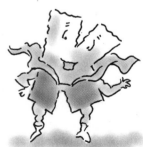

- replacement potassium
- acidosis
- insulin deficiency
- burns
- crushing injuries
- diabetic ketoacidosis
- extensive surgery
- myocardial infarction (MI)
- renal failure.

...or less of potassium?

Hypokalemia (decreased potassium level) occurs with depletion of total body potassium caused by shifts from extracellular fluid to intracellular fluid.

Depletion of total body potassium occurs with:
- diabetic ketoacidosis and insulin administration without potassium supplements
- GI and renal disorders
- vomiting
- diarrhea
- gastric suctioning
- diuretics
- excessive aldosterone secretion
- excessive licorice ingestion. (See *Potassium test interference.*)

What needs to be done

- Perform a venipuncture, and collect the sample in a 3- or 4-ml clot-activator tube, or in a designated tube volume in accordance with laboratory protocol.
- Draw the sample immediately after applying the tourniquet, because a delay may elevate the potassium level by allowing intracellular potassium to leak into the serum.
- Educate patients at risk for hypokalemia about increasing dietary intake of potassium-rich foods.

Stay on the ball

Potassium test interference

These factors may cause elevated potassium levels:
- hemolyzed specimen or rough handling of specimen
- excessive or rapid potassium infusion, spironolactone or penicillin G potassium therapy, or renal toxicity from administration of amphotericin B, methicillin, or tetracycline.

Magnesium

Magnesium is a commonly overlooked electrolyte vital to neuromuscular function. Magnesium activates many essential enzymes and affects the metabolism of nucleic acids and proteins. It also helps transport sodium and potassium across cell membranes and, through its effect on the secretion of parathyroid hormone, influences intracellular calcium levels.

Magnesium is measured to evaluate electrolyte status and assess neuromuscular or renal function. The serum magnesium test—a quantitative analysis—measures serum levels of magnesium, which is, after potassium, the most abundant intracellular cation.

An absorbing topic

Most magnesium is found in bone and in intracellular fluid; a small amount is found in extracellular fluid. Magnesium is absorbed by the small intestine and is excreted in the urine and feces.

What it all means

Normally, serum magnesium levels range from 1.3 to 2.1 mg/dl (SI, 0.65 to 1.05 mmol/L).

Renal failure

Elevated serum magnesium levels (hypermagnesemia) that aren't caused by magnesium administration or ingestion most commonly occur in renal failure, when the kidneys excrete inadequate amounts of magnesium. Adrenal insufficiency (Addison's disease) can also elevate serum magnesium levels.

Chronic alcoholism

Decreased serum magnesium levels (hypomagnesemia) most commonly result from chronic alcoholism. Other causes include malabsorption syndrome, diarrhea, faulty absorption after bowel resection, prolonged bowel or gastric aspiration, acute pancreatitis, primary aldosteronism, severe burns, hypercalcemic conditions (including hyperparathyroidism), and use of certain diuretics. (See *Magnesium test interference*.)

What needs to be done

• Tell the patient he shouldn't use magnesium salts, such as milk of magnesia or Epsom salts, for at least 3 days before the test.
• Perform a venipuncture (without a tourniquet, if possible), and collect the sample in a 3- or 4-ml clot-activator tube, or in a designated tube volume in accordance with laboratory protocol.
• Educate patients at risk for hypermagnesemia about antacids, laxatives, and mineral supplements that contain magnesium.

Phosphates

Phosphates are essential in the storage and utilization of energy, calcium regulation, red blood cell (RBC) function, acid-base balance, bone formation, and metabolism of carbohydrates, protein, and fat. Tests for phosphates measure serum levels of phosphates, the dominant cellular anions.

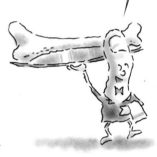

One order of magnesium coming right up!

Stay on the ball

Magnesium test interference

• Excessive use of antacids or cathartics or excessive infusion of magnesium sulfate raises magnesium levels.
• Prolonged I.V. infusions without magnesium suppress levels (excessive use of diuretics decreases magnesium levels).
• I.V. administration of calcium gluconate may falsely decrease serum magnesium levels.

Linked to calcium

The intestine absorbs a considerable amount of phosphates from dietary sources, but adequate levels of vitamin D are necessary for their absorption. The kidneys regulate phosphate excretion and retention. Because calcium and phosphates interact in a reciprocal relationship, urinary excretion of phosphates increases or decreases in inverse proportion to serum calcium levels.

Abnormal phosphate levels result more commonly from improper excretion than from abnormal ingestion or absorption from dietary sources.

What it all means

Normally, serum phosphate levels in adults range from 2.7 to 4.5 mg/dl (SI, 0.87 to 1.45 mmol/L). In children, the normal range is 4.5 to 6.7 mg/dl (SI, 1.45 to 1.78 mmol/L).

The lowdown on levels

Decreased phosphate levels (hypophosphatemia) may result from malnutrition, malabsorption syndromes, hyperparathyroidism, renal tubular acidosis, or treatment of diabetic acidosis. In children, low phosphate levels can suppress normal growth.

Elevated phosphate levels (hyperphosphatemia) may result from skeletal disease, healing fractures, hypoparathyroidism, acromegaly, diabetic acidosis, high intestinal obstruction, and renal failure. Elevated phosphate levels are rarely clinically significant; however, if prolonged, they can alter bone metabolism by causing abnormal calcium phosphate deposits. (See *Phosphate test interference*.)

What needs to be done

• Perform a venipuncture (without using a tourniquet, if possible), and collect the sample in a 3- or 4-ml clot-activator tube, or in a designated tube volume in accordance with laboratory protocol.

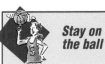

Stay on the ball

Phosphate test interference

The following factors may alter phosphate test results:
• extended I.V. infusion of dextrose 5% in water, the use of phosphate-binding antacids, and the use of acetazolamide, insulin, and epinephrine
• excessive vitamin D intake and the use of anabolic corticosteroids or androgens, which may elevate serum phosphate levels.

Calcium

Total calcium measurement is the most commonly performed test for evaluation of serum calcium levels. Approximately 1% of the total calcium in the body circulates in the blood. Of this 1%, about 50% is bound to plasma proteins and 40% is ionized, or free.

Calcium gets around

Evaluation of serum calcium levels measures the total amount of calcium circulating in the blood. Evaluation of ionized calcium levels measures the fraction of serum calcium that's in the ionized form, which is the most physiologically active form of serum calcium. The other 99% of the calcium in the body is stored in the bones and teeth.

Many laboratories don't have the equipment to measure ionized calcium levels. Because of this, serum albumin should be measured at the same time serum calcium is measured because the serum calcium level decreases 0.8 mg/dl for every 1-g decrease in the serum albumin level. The measured serum calcium is then adjusted upward by the amount of decrease in serum albumin. Ionized calcium is estimated to be about one-half of the adjusted calcium value.

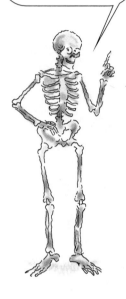

Need a place to store your calcium? I'm your guy!

What it all means

Normal calcium values are:
• *total calcium:* 8.2 to 10.2 mg/dl (SI, 2.05 to 2.54 mmol/L) in adults; 8.6 to 11.2 mg/dl (SI, 2.15 to 2.79 mmol/L) in children
• *ionized calcium:* 4.65 to 5.28 mg/dl (SI, 1.1 to 1.32 mmol/L).

Going overboard with calcium...

Hypercalcemia may occur in patients with hyperparathyroidism and parathyroid tumors (because of oversecretion of parathyroid hormone), Paget's disease of the bone, multiple myeloma, metastatic carcinoma, multiple fractures, or prolonged immobilization. Elevated serum calcium levels may also result from inadequate excretion of calcium, such as in adrenal insufficiency and renal disease; from excessive calcium ingestion; or from overuse of antacids such as calcium carbonate.

...or missing the calcium boat

Hypocalcemia may result from hypoparathyroidism, total parathyroidectomy, or malabsorption. Decreased serum levels of calcium may follow calcium loss in patients with Cushing's syndrome, renal failure, acute pancreatitis, or peritonitis. (See *Calcium test interference.*)

What needs to be done

• Perform a venipuncture (without using a tourniquet, if possible), and collect the sample in a 3- or 4-ml clot-activator tube, or in a designated tube volume in accordance with laboratory protocol.

Chloride

When interacting with sodium, chloride helps maintain the osmotic pressure of blood and therefore helps regulate blood volume

Stay on the ball

Calcium test interference

The following factors may alter calcium test results:
• excessive ingestion of vitamin D or its derivatives (dihydrotachysterol, calcitriol)
• use of androgens, calciferol-activated calcium salts, progestins-estrogens, or thiazide diuretics, which may elevate levels
• chronic laxative use
• excessive transfusions of citrated blood
• administration of acetazolamide, corticosteroids, or mithramycin.

Stay on the ball

Chloride test interference

• Ammonium chloride, cholestyramine, boric acid, oxyphenbutazone, phenylbutazone, or excessive I.V. infusion of sodium chloride may elevate serum chloride levels.
• Thiazide diuretics, ethacrynic acid, furosemide, bicarbonates, or prolonged I.V. infusion of dextrose 5% in water may decrease serum chloride levels.

and arterial pressure. Chloride levels also affect acid-base balance. Serum concentrations of this electrolyte are regulated by aldosterone secondarily to regulation of sodium. Chloride is absorbed from the intestines and is excreted primarily by the kidneys.

The serum chloride test—a quantitative analysis—measures serum levels of chloride, the major extracellular fluid anion.

What it all means

Normal serum chloride levels range from 100 to 108 mEq/L (SI, 100 to 108 mmol/L). Chloride levels relate inversely to those of HCO_3^- and thus reflect acid-base balance. Excessive loss of gastric juices or of other secretions containing chloride may cause hypochloremic metabolic alkalosis; excessive chloride retention or ingestion may lead to hyperchloremic metabolic acidosis.

The lowdown on levels

Elevated serum chloride levels (hyperchloremia) may result from HCO_3^- loss caused by diarrhea, severe dehydration, complete renal shutdown, head injury (producing neurogenic hyperventilation), or primary aldosteronism.

Low chloride levels (hypochloremia) are usually associated with low sodium and potassium levels. Possible underlying causes include prolonged vomiting, gastric suctioning, intestinal fistula, chronic renal failure, and Addison's disease. Heart failure or edema resulting in excess extracellular fluid can cause dilutional hypochloremia. (See *Chloride test interference*.)

What needs to be done

• Perform a venipuncture, and collect the sample in a 3- or 4-ml clot-activator tube, or in a designated tube volume in accordance with laboratory protocol.

Anion gap

The anion gap reflects anion-cation balance in the serum and helps distinguish types of metabolic acidosis without expensive, time-consuming measurement of all serum electrolytes. The anion gap test uses serum levels of routinely measured electrolytes—sodium, chloride, and HCO_3^-—for a quick calculation based on a simple physical principle: Total concentrations of cations and anions are normally equal, thereby maintaining electrical neutrality in serum.

Because sodium accounts for more than 90% of circulating cations, compared to chloride and HCO_3^-, which together account for 85% of the counterbalancing anions, the gap between measured cation and anion levels represents those anions not routinely measured, including sulfates, phosphates, proteins, and organic acids, such as ketone bodies and lactic acid.

What it all means

Normally, the anion gap ranges from 8 to 14 mEq/L (SI, 8 to 14 mmol/L). A normal anion gap doesn't rule out metabolic acidosis.

Normal anion gap acidosis

When acidosis results from loss of HCO_3^- in the urine or other body fluids, renal reabsorption of sodium promotes retention of chloride and the anion gap remains unchanged. Thus, metabolic acidosis associated with excessive chloride levels is known as *normal anion gap acidosis*.

High anion gap acidosis

When acidosis results from accumulation of metabolic acids, as with lactic acidosis, the anion gap increases above 14 mEq/L (14 mmol/L), with the increase being in unmeasured anions. Metabolic acidosis caused by such accumulation is known as *high anion gap acidosis*. (See *Understanding anion gap and metabolic acidosis*.)

Because the anion gap determines only total anion-cation balance, it doesn't necessarily reflect abnormal values for individual electrolytes. Further investigation and diagnostic tests are usually necessary to determine the specific cause of metabolic acidosis.

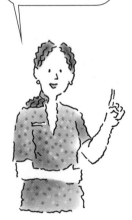

Mind the gap! The anion gap, that is.

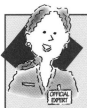

Advice from the experts

Understanding anion gap and metabolic acidosis

Metabolic acidosis with a normal anion gap (8 to 14 mEq/L [SI, 8 to 14 µmol/L]) occurs with bicarbonate loss, which may result from:
• hypokalemic acidosis associated with renal tubular acidosis, diarrhea, or ureteral diversions
• hyperkalemic acidosis caused by acidifying agents (for example, ammonium chloride or hydrochloric acid), hydronephrosis, or sickle cell nephropathy.

Metabolic acidosis with an increased anion gap (above 14 mEq/L [SI, greater than 14 mmol/L]) occurs with accumulation of organic acids, sulfates, or phosphates, which may result from:
• renal failure
• ketoacidosis associated with starvation, diabetes mellitus, or alcohol abuse
• lactic acidosis
• ingestion of toxins, such as salicylates, methanol, ethylene glycol (antifreeze), and paraldehyde.

Stay on the ball

Anion gap test interference

A range of medications and other substances can alter the anion gap.

Increases the gap
• Ammonium chloride
• Antihypertensives
• Bicarbonates
• Corticosteroids
• Ethacrynic acid
• Furosemide
• Prolonged infusion of dextrose 5% in water
• Salicylates
• Thiazide diuretics

Decreases the gap
• Chlorothiazide diuretics
• Chlorpropamide
• Cortisone
• Diuretics
• Excessive ingestion of alkalis or licorice
• Lithium
• Vasopressin

A decreased anion gap (less than 8 mEq/L) is rare but may occur in hypermagnesemia and in paraproteinemic states, such as multiple myeloma and Waldenström's macroglobulinemia. (See *Anion gap test interference*.)

What needs to be done

• Perform a venipuncture, and collect the sample in a 3- or 4-ml clot-activator tube, or in a designated tube volume in accordance with laboratory protocol.
• As ordered, instruct the patient to resume the use of any drugs discontinued for the test.

Proteins and protein metabolites

Blood urea nitrogen

Urea is the chief end product of protein metabolism. Formed in the liver from ammonia and excreted by the kidneys, urea constitutes 40% to 50% of the blood's nonprotein nitrogen. Because the level of reabsorption of urea in the renal tubules is directly related to the rate of urine flow through the kidneys, the blood urea nitrogen (BUN) level is a less reliable indicator of uremia than is the

Stay on the ball

BUN test interference

• Chloramphenicol and streptomycin can depress blood urea nitrogen (BUN) levels.
• Nephrotoxic drugs, such as allopurinol, aminoglycosides, amphotericin B, methicillin, and nonsteroidal anti-inflammatory and thiazide drugs can elevate BUN levels.

serum creatine level. The BUN test measures the nitrogen fraction of urea.

What it all means

BUN values normally range from 8 to 20 mg/dl (SI, 2.9 to 7.5 mmol/L), with slightly higher values in elderly patients. Elevated BUN levels occur in renal disease, reduced renal blood flow (such as with dehydration), urinary tract obstruction, and increased protein catabolism (such as occurs in burns).

Depressed BUN levels occur in severe hepatic damage, malnutrition, and overhydration. (See *BUN test interference*.)

What needs to be done

• Tell the patient to avoid a diet high in meat.
• Perform a venipuncture, and collect the sample in a 3- or 4-ml clot-activator tube, or in a designated tube volume in accordance with laboratory protocol.

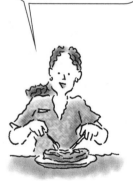

It's a good thing that I'm not having a BUN test because I'm sure enjoying this steak.

Creatinine

As a quantitative analysis of serum creatinine levels, the serum creatinine test provides a more sensitive measure of renal damage than do BUN levels because renal impairment is virtually the only cause of creatinine elevation. The creatinine level is an approximation of the glomerular filtration rate. Because creatinine levels normally remain constant, elevated levels usually indicate diminished renal function.

Stay on the ball

Creatinine test interference

• Ascorbic acid, barbiturates, cephalosporins, cimetidine, cisplatin, gentamicin, and diuretics may raise serum creatinine levels.
• Sulfobromophthalein or phenolsulfonphthalein given within the previous 24 hours can elevate creatinine levels.
• Exceptionally large muscle mass, such as in athletes, may cause above-average creatinine levels, even with normal renal function.

What it all means

Serum creatinine levels in males normally range from 0.8 to 1.2 mg/dl (SI, 62 to 115 µmol/L); in females, from 0.6 to 0.9 mg/dl (SI, 53 to 97 µmol/L). Elevated serum creatinine levels generally indicate renal disease that has seriously damaged 50% or more of the nephrons. They may also be associated with gigantism and acromegaly. (See *Creatinine test interference*.)

What needs to be done

• Perform a venipuncture, and collect the sample in a 3- or 4-ml clot-activator tube, or in a designated tube volume in accordance with laboratory protocol.

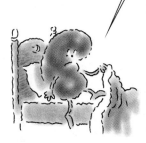

That elevated creatinine level has really wiped me out.

Uric acid

Used primarily to detect gout, the uric acid test measures serum levels of uric acid—the major end metabolite of purine. Purine is a nitrogen-containing compound produced in the digestion of certain dietary proteins.

What it all means

Uric acid concentrations in males normally range from 3.4 to 7 mg/dl (SI, 202 to 416 µmol/L); in females, from 2.3 to 6 mg/dl (SI, 143 to 357 µmol/L).

The lowdown on levels

Increased serum uric acid levels may indicate gout or impaired renal function (levels don't correlate with the severity of disease, however). Levels may also rise in heart failure; glycogen storage disease, such as type I and von Gierke's disease; infections; he-

Stay on the ball

Uric acid test interference

• Aspirin, alcohol use, caffeine, epinephrine, a high-purine diet, stress, loop diuretics, ethambutol, pyrazinamide, strenuous exercise, and thiazides may raise levels.
• Acetaminophen, ascorbic acid, and levodopa may cause false elevations.
• Allopurinol, azathioprine, clofibrate, corticosteroids, estrogen, glucose, guaifenesin, and warfarin may decrease levels.

molytic or sickle cell anemia; polycythemia; neoplasms; and psoriasis.

Depressed uric acid levels may indicate defective tubular absorption (such as in Fanconi syndrome and Wilson's disease) or acute hepatic atrophy. (See *Uric acid test interference*.)

What needs to be done

• Tell the patient that he must fast for 8 hours before the test.
• Perform a venipuncture, and collect the sample in a 3- or 4-ml clot-activator tube, or in a designated tube volume in accordance with laboratory protocol.

Albumin

Albumin is the most abundant protein, composing almost 54% of plasma proteins. It helps maintain hydrostatic pressure in the capillary system. (See *Fluid movement through capillary walls*.)

This test measures the amount of albumin in serum. It's used to help determine whether a patient has liver or kidney disease, and to determine whether or not the body is absorbing protein.

What it all means

Normal albumin levels will differ according to age:
• *adult:* 3.4 to 5.4 g/dl (SI, 34 to 54 g/L)
• *child:* 4 to 5.8 g/dl (SI, 40 to 58 g/L)
• *infant:* 4.4 to 5.4 g/dl (SI, 44 to 54 g/L)
• *neonate:* 2.9 to 5.4 g/dl (SI, 29 to 54 g/L).

Drink up! There's no need for fluid restriction when testing for albumin.

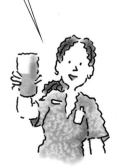

Fluid movement through capillary walls

The movement of fluids through capillaries—a process called *capillary filtration*—results from blood pushing against the walls of the capillary. This pressure, called *hydrostatic* or *fluid-pushing pressure,* forces fluids and solutes through the capillary wall.

When the hydrostatic pressure inside a capillary is greater than the pressure in the surrounding interstitial space, fluids and solutes inside the capillaries are forced out into the interstitial space, as shown here. When the pressure inside the capillary is less than the pressure outside, fluids and solutes move back into it.

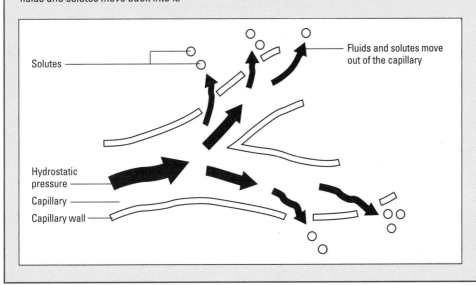

Solutes

Fluids and solutes move out of the capillary

Hydrostatic pressure

Capillary

Capillary wall

The lowdown on levels

A decreased level (hypoalbuminemia) may indicate cirrhosis, acute liver failure, severe burns, severe malnutrition, and ulcerative colitis. An elevated level (hyperalbuminemia) may indicate dehydration, severe vomiting, and severe diarrhea.

What needs to be done

• Tell the patient that there's no need for fluid restriction.
• Certain medications can increase albumin measurements; the patient may need to stop these drugs prior to the test. (See *Albumin test interference*.)
• Perform a venipuncture, and collect 5 to 10 ml in a red-top tube, or in a designated tube volume in accordance with laboratory protocol.
• Apply direct pressure to the venipuncture site until bleeding stops.

• Encourage the patient to eat a diet high in protein, if not contraindicated.

Prealbumin

Prealbumin is a protein produced primarily in the liver. It has a short half-life (2 days), which makes it a good indicator of nutritional status.

What it all means

Normal prealbumin levels are 19 to 38 mg/dl (SI, 190 to 380 mg/L). Decreased values are seen in malnutrition and liver disease, which impair protein synthesis. Values of 10 to 15 mg/dl (SI, 100 to 150 mg/L) indicate mild protein depletion. Values of 5 to 10 mg/dl (SI, 50 to 100 mg/L) indicate moderate protein depletion. Values of 0 to 5 mg/dl (SI, 0 to 50 mg/L) indicate severe protein depletion.

What needs to be done

• Withhold food and fluid from the patient for 4 hours before the test.
• Perform a venipuncture, and collect the sample in a 3- or 4-ml clot-activator tube, or in a designated tube volume in accordance with laboratory protocol.
• Apply direct pressure to the venipuncture site until the bleeding stops.
• Handle the sample gently to prevent hemolysis.

Protein electrophoresis

Protein electrophoresis measures serum albumin and globulins, the major blood proteins, by separating the proteins into five distinct fractions: albumin, $alpha_1$, $alpha_2$, beta, and gamma proteins.

What it all means

Normal protein values are:
• *total serum protein:* 6.4 to 8.3 g/dl (SI, 64 to 83 g/L)
• *albumin:* 3.5 to 5 g/dl (SI, 35 to 50 g/L)
• *$alpha_1$-globulin:* 0.1 to 0.3 g/dl (SI, 1 to 3 g/L)
• *$alpha_2$-globulin:* 0.6 to 1 g/dl (SI, 6 to 10 g/L)
• *beta globulin:* 0.7 to 1.1 g/dl (SI, 7 to 11 g/L)
• *gamma globulin:* 0.8 to 1.6 g/dl (SI, 8 to 16 g/L). (See *Clinical implications of abnormal protein levels* and *Protein electrophoresis interference,* page 48.)

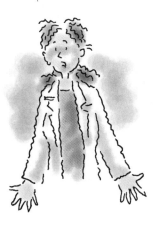

Studying tests to be tested on tests is making me a little testy.

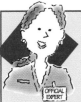

Advice from the experts

Clinical implications of abnormal protein levels

Abnormal levels of albumin or globulins occur in many pathologic states, including those listed here.

Increased levels

Total proteins
- Chronic inflammatory disease (such as rheumatoid arthritis or early-stage Laënnec's cirrhosis)
- Dehydration
- Diabetic acidosis
- Diarrhea
- Fulminating and chronic infections
- Monocytic leukemia
- Multiple myeloma
- Vomiting

Albumin
- Dehydration
- Multiple myeloma

Globulins
- Chronic syphilis
- Collagen diseases
- Diabetes mellitus
- Hodgkin's disease
- Multiple myeloma
- Rheumatoid arthritis
- Subacute bacterial endocarditis
- Systemic lupus erythematosus
- Tuberculosis

Decreased levels

Total proteins
- Benzene and carbon tetrachloride poisoning
- Blood dyscrasias
- Essential hypertension
- GI disease
- Heart failure
- Hemorrhage
- Hepatic dysfunction
- Hodgkin's disease
- Hyperthyroidism
- Malabsorption
- Malnutrition
- Nephrosis
- Severe burns
- Surgical and traumatic shock
- Toxemia of pregnancy
- Uncontrolled diabetes mellitus

Albumin
- Acute cholecystitis
- Collagen diseases
- Diarrhea
- Essential hypertension
- Hepatic disease
- Hodgkin's disease
- Hyperthyroidism
- Hypogammaglobulinemia
- Malnutrition
- Metastatic cancer
- Nephritis, nephrosis
- Peptic ulcer
- Plasma loss from burns
- Rheumatoid arthritis
- Sarcoidosis
- Systemic lupus erythematosus

Globulins
- Variable levels in neoplastic and renal diseases, hepatic dysfunction, and blood dyscrasias

Stay on the ball

Protein electrophoresis interference

- Pretest administration of a contrast agent falsely elevates protein test results.
- Cytotoxic drug use may lower serum albumin levels.
- Pregnancy may lower serum albumin levels.

What needs to be done

- This test must be performed on a serum sample to avoid measuring the fibrinogen fraction. (The fibrinogen fraction, if present, would be indistinguishable from certain monoclonal gammopathies.)
- Perform a venipuncture, and collect the sample in a 7-ml clot-activator tube, or in a designated tube volume in accordance with laboratory protocol.

Haptoglobin

The haptoglobin test measures serum levels of haptoglobin, a glycoprotein produced in the liver. Haptoglobin binds with free Hb and prevents its accumulation in plasma, permitting clearance by reticuloendothelial cells and conserving body iron.

Hb circulates inside erythrocytes (RBCs); when aged erythrocytes die, they release free Hb into plasma. Certain anemias, bacterial toxins, mechanical disruptions (from a prosthetic heart valve, for example), or antibodies can increase intravascular hemolysis (the breakdown of RBCs and the release of Hb). In acute intravascular hemolysis, haptoglobin levels fall rapidly; low levels may last for 5 to 7 days until the liver synthesizes more glycoprotein.

What it all means

Serum haptoglobin concentrations, measured in terms of the protein's Hb-binding capacity, normally range from 40 to 180 mg/dl (SI, 0.4 to 1.8 g/L). Nephelometric procedures yield lower results. Markedly depressed serum haptoglobin levels are characteristic in acute and chronic hemolysis, severe hepatocellular disease, infectious mononucleosis, and transfusion reactions. Hepatocellular disease inhibits the synthesis of haptoglobin. In hemolytic transfusion reactions, haptoglobin levels begin falling after 6 to 8 hours and drop to 40% of pretransfusion levels after 24 hours.

The lowdown on levels

Although haptoglobin is absent in 90% of neonates, levels usually rise to normal by age 4 months. However, in about 1% of the population—including 4% of blacks—haptoglobin is permanently absent; this disorder is known as *congenital ahaptoglobinemia*.

Markedly elevated serum haptoglobin levels occur in diseases marked by chronic inflammatory reactions or tissue destruction, such as rheumatoid arthritis and malignant neoplasms. (See *Haptoglobin test interference*.)

What needs to be done

• Perform a venipuncture, and collect the sample in a 7-ml clot-activator tube, or in a designated tube volume in accordance with laboratory protocol.

Stay on the ball

Haptoglobin test interference

• Corticosteroids and androgens can elevate haptoglobin levels.
• Hormonal contraceptives, chlorpromazine, diphenhydramine, indomethacin, isoniazid, and quinidine decrease haptoglobin levels.

Transferrin

Transferrin (also known as *siderophilin*), a glycoprotein formed in the liver, transports circulating iron obtained from dietary sources and from the breakdown of RBCs by reticuloendothelial cells.

The transferrin test measures serum transferrin levels to evaluate iron metabolism.

Taking it to the bone

Most of this iron is transported to bone marrow for use in Hb synthesis; some is converted to hemosiderin and ferritin and is stored in the liver, spleen, and bone marrow. Inadequate transferrin levels may lead to impaired Hb synthesis and, possibly, anemia. Transferrin is normally about 30% saturated with iron. Serum iron levels are usually obtained simultaneously.

What it all means

Normal serum transferrin values range from 200 to 400 mg/dl (SI, 2 to 4 g/L). Depressed serum transferrin levels may indicate inadequate production caused by hepatic damage or excessive protein loss from renal disease. They may also result from acute or chronic infection or from cancer. Elevated serum transferrin levels may indicate severe iron deficiency. (See *Transferrin test interference*.)

Stay on the ball

Transferrin test interference

Late pregnancy or hormonal contraceptives may raise transferrin

What needs to be done

Perform a venipuncture, and collect the sample in a 4-ml clot-activator tube, or in a designated tube volume in accordance with laboratory protocol.

Folic acid

The folic acid test is a quantitative analysis of serum folic acid levels (also called *pteroylglutamic acid*, *folacin*, or *folate*) by radio-isotope assay of competitive binding. It's commonly performed concomitantly with measurement of serum vitamin B_{12} levels. Like vitamin B_{12}, folic acid is a water-soluble vitamin that influences hematopoiesis, deoxyribonucleic acid synthesis, and overall body growth.

Normally, diet supplies folic acid in organ meats, such as liver or kidneys; yeast; fruits; leafy vegetables; fortified breads and cereals; eggs; and milk. Inadequate dietary intake may cause a deficiency, especially during pregnancy. Because of folic acid's vital role in hematopoiesis, the usual indication for this test is a suspected hematologic abnormality. This test is used to aid in the differential diagnosis of megaloblastic anemia, which may result from folic acid or vitamin B_{12} deficiency. It also helps to assess folate stores in pregnancy.

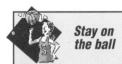

Folic acid! Get your folic acid here!

What it all means

Normally, serum folic acid values are 1.8 to 20 ng/ml (SI, 4 to 45.3 nmol/L).

The lowdown on levels

Low serum levels may indicate hematologic abnormalities, such as anemia (especially megaloblastic anemia), leukopenia, and thrombocytopenia. The Schilling test is usually performed to rule out vitamin B_{12} deficiency, which also causes megaloblastic anemia. Decreased folic acid levels can also result from hypermetabolic states (such as hyperthyroidism), inadequate dietary intake, small-bowel malabsorption syndrome, hepatic or renal diseases, chronic alcoholism, or pregnancy.

Serum levels greater than normal may indicate excessive dietary intake of folic acid or folic acid supplements. Even when taken in large doses, this vitamin is nontoxic. (See *Folic acid test interference*.)

What needs to be done

• Instruct the patient to fast the night before the test.

Stay on the ball

Folic acid test interference

• Alcohol; anticonvulsants such as primidone; antineoplastics; antimalarials; hormonal contraceptives; phenytoin; and pyrimethamine may decrease values.

• Check the patient's history for drugs that may affect test results, such as phenytoin or pyrimethamine.
• Perform a venipuncture, and collect the sample in a 4.5-ml tube without additives, or in a designated tube volume in accordance with laboratory protocol.
• Apply direct pressure to the venipuncture site until bleeding stops.
• Instruct the patient to resume his usual diet.
• Protect the sample from light, and send it to the laboratory immediately.

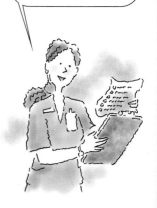

Always check the patient's history for drugs that could affect test results.

Phenylalanine

The phenylalanine test (also known as the *Guthrie test*) is a screening method that detects elevated levels of serum phenylalanine, which is a naturally occurring amino acid essential to growth and nitrogen balance.

Metabolic upset

Elevated levels of phenylalanine may indicate phenylketonuria (PKU), a metabolic disorder inherited as an autosomal recessive trait. An infant with PKU usually has normal phenylalanine levels at birth but, after he begins feeding with breast milk or formula (both contain phenylalanine), levels gradually rise because of a deficiency of the liver enzyme that converts phenylalanine to tyrosine. The resulting accumulation of phenylalanine, phenylpyruvic acid, and other metabolites hinders normal development of central nervous system (CNS) cells, causing mental retardation.

Day 3 for accuracy

To ensure accurate results, the test must be performed after 3 (or, preferably, 4) full days of breast milk or formula feeding. (In some states, a preliminary test is done 25 hours after birth.)

What it all means

In the laboratory, the sample is added to a culture medium containing a phenylalanine-dependent strain of *Bacillus subtilis* and an antagonist to phenylalanine. A negative test, in which the presence of the phenylalanine antagonist inhibits growth of *B. subtilis* around the blood on the filter paper, indicates normal phenylalanine levels (less than 2 mg/dl [SI, less than 121 µmol/L]) and no appreciable danger of PKU.

Danger ahead

Growth of *B. subtilis* on the filter paper indicates that serum phenylalanine levels are high enough to overcome the antagonist

Confirming PKU

After the Guthrie test detects the possible presence of phenylketonuria (PKU), serum phenylalanine and tyrosine levels are measured to confirm the diagnosis. Phenylalanine hydroxylase is the enzyme that converts phenylalanine to tyrosine. If this enzyme is absent, increasing phenylalanine levels with concomitant decreasing tyrosine levels indicate PKU.

Samples are obtained by venipuncture (femoral or external jugular). Serum phenylalanine levels greater than 4 mg/dl (SI, greater than 242 µmol/L) and low tyrosine levels—with urinary excretion of phenylpyruvic acid—confirm PKU.

(greater than or equal to 2 mg/dl [SI, greater than or equal to 121 µmol/L]). Such a positive test suggests the possibility of PKU. Diagnosis requires exact serum phenylalanine measurement and urine testing. (See *Confirming PKU.*) A positive test may also result from hepatic disease, galactosemia (an inherited autosomal-recessive disorder of galactose metabolism), or delayed development of certain enzyme systems.

What needs to be done

• Perform a heelstick, and collect three drops of blood—one in each circle—on the filter paper.
• Note the infant's name and birth date and the date of the first breast milk or formula feeding on the laboratory request, and send the sample to the laboratory immediately.
• Reassure the parents of a child who may have PKU that early detection and continuous treatment with a low-phenylalanine diet can prevent permanent mental retardation.

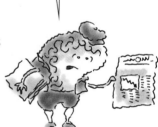

Good news! Early detection of PKU can prevent permanent mental retardation.

Plasma ammonia

The plasma ammonia test measures plasma levels of ammonia, a nonprotein nitrogen compound that helps maintain acid-base balance. Most ammonia is absorbed from the intestinal tract, where it's produced by bacterial action on protein; a smaller amount of ammonia is produced in the kidneys from hydrolysis of glutamine. Normally, the body uses the nitrogen fraction of ammonia to rebuild amino acids and then converts the ammonia to urea in the liver for excretion by the kidneys. In such diseases as cirrhosis of the liver, ammonia can bypass the liver and accumulate in the blood. Therefore, measurement of plasma ammonia levels may help indicate the severity of hepatocellular damage.

What it all means

Normally, plasma ammonia levels are 15 to 56 mcg/dl (SI, 9 to 33 µmol/L). Elevated plasma ammonia levels are common in patients with severe hepatic disease, such as cirrhosis and acute hepatic necrosis, and may lead to hepatic coma. Elevated levels are also possible in patients with Reye's syndrome, severe heart failure, GI hemorrhage, and erythroblastosis fetalis (a type of hemolytic anemia in neonates). (See *Plasma ammonia test interference.*)

What needs to be done

• Tell the patient that an overnight fast before the test is required because plasma ammonia levels may vary with protein intake.
• Notify the laboratory before performing the venipuncture so that preliminary preparations can begin.
• Perform a venipuncture, and collect the sample in a 10-ml heparinized tube, or in a designated tube volume in accordance with laboratory protocol.
• Make sure bleeding has stopped before removing pressure from the venipuncture site.
• Handle the sample gently, pack it in ice, and send it to the laboratory immediately. *Don't* use a chilled container.
• Watch for signs of impending or established hepatic coma if plasma ammonia levels are high.

Plasma ammonia test interference

• Acetazolamide, thiazides, ammonium salts, and furosemide as well as total parenteral nutrition or a portacaval shunt raise ammonia levels.
• Lactulose, neomycin, and kanamycin depress ammonia levels.

Lead

Blood lead levels is a test that measures the amount of lead in the blood. Lead is present in the environment and is absorbed through the respiratory and GI tracts; it's also transmitted through the placenta to the fetus. Although low levels of lead in adults aren't thought to be harmful, low levels in infants and children can lead to toxicity with presenting deficits in intellectual or cognitive development over time.

Screening for lead levels may be done in industrial workers or children prone to toxicity (such as those living in urban areas). It's also useful in monitoring improvement of those with increased serum lead levels or lead toxicity.

Low blood lead levels in infants and children can lead to toxicity and resulting deficits in intellectual and cognitive development.

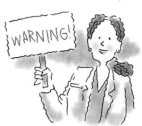

WARNING!

What it all means

Normally, serum lead levels are 0 to 10 mcg/dl (SI, of 0 to 0.48 µmol/L). In adults, workers exposed to lead should have blood lead levels below 40 mcg/dl (SI, less than 1.9 μmol/L). Levels greater than 40 mcg/dl (SI, greater than 1.9 μmol/L) are reported to the state occupational agency. Treatment by chelation therapy is recommended if the level exceeds 60 mcg/dl (SI, greater than 2.9 μmol/L).

Danger ahead with children

Children with levels of 10 to 14 mcg/dl (SI, 0.48 to 0.68 μmol/L) should be screened frequently. Children with levels less than 10 mcg/dl (SI, less than 0.48 μmol/L) but greater than zero are at risk for reduced IQ, hearing, and growth. Levels of 15 to 19 mcg/dl (SI, 0.72 to 0.92 μmol/L) require nutritional and educational intervention. Levels of 20 to 44 mcg/dl (SI, 0.97 to 2.1 μmol/L) require environmental evaluation and, possibly, chelation therapy. Children with levels greater than 20 mcg/dl (SI, greater than 0.97 μmol/L) may exhibit impaired nerve function; in those with levels greater than 30 mcg/dl (SI, greater than 1.45 μmol/L), reduced vitamin D metabolism occurs; in those with levels greater than 40 mcg/dl (SI, greater than 1.93 μmol/L), damage to blood-forming systems occurs.

Children with levels of 45 to 69 mcg/dl (SI, 2.17 to 3.33 μmol/L) require environmental intervention and chelation therapy. Children with levels greater than 50 mcg/dl (SI, greater than 2.41 μmol/L) may experience severe stomach cramps; in those with levels greater than 60 mcg/dl (SI, greater than 2.90 μmol/L), severe anemia occurs. Levels greater than 69 mcg/dl (SI, greater than 3.33 μmol/L) require emergency treatment. Children with levels greater than 80 mcg/dl (SI, greater than 3.86 μmol/L) experience severe brain damage; levels greater than 125 mcg/dl (SI, greater than 6.04 μmol/L) result in death.

> Children with high levels of lead need environmental intervention.

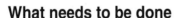

What needs to be done
• Tell the patient that fasting is unnecessary.
• Obtain the sample by a fingerstick using lead-free heparinized capillary tubes or by performing a venipuncture. Collect the sample in a 3-ml trace element–free tube, or in a designated tube volume in accordance with laboratory protocol.
• Make sure bleeding has stopped before removing pressure from the site.
• Refrigerate the sample.

Cardiac enzymes and proteins

Creatine kinase

Creatine kinase (CK) is an enzyme that catalyzes the creatine-creatinine metabolic pathway in muscle cells and brain tissue. Because CK has an important role in energy production, its levels reflect normal tissue catabolism; above-normal serum levels indicate trauma to cells with high CK content.

A triad of isoenzymes

CK may be separated into three isoenzymes with distinct molecular structures: CK-BB (CK_1), found primarily in brain tissue; CK-MB (CK_2), found primarily in cardiac muscle (a small amount also appears in skeletal muscle); and CK-MM (CK_3), found mainly in skeletal muscle.

Getting specific

Total serum CK levels were once widely used to detect acute MI, but elevated levels caused by skeletal muscle damage reduce the test's specificity for this disorder. Fractionation and measurement of CK isoenzymes has replaced total CK assay to accurately localize the site of increased tissue destruction. In addition, subunits of CK-MM and CK-MB, called *isoforms*, can be assayed to increase the sensitivity of the test.

What it all means

Total CK values normally range from 55 to 170 units/L (SI, 0.94 to 2.89 µkat/L) for men and from 30 to 135 units/L (SI, 0.51 to 2.3 µkat/L) for women. CK levels may be significantly higher in very muscular people. Infants up to age 1 year have levels two to four times higher than adults, possibly reflecting birth trauma and striated muscle development. The normal ranges for isoenzyme levels are as follows: CK-BB, undetectable; CK-MB, less than 5% (SI, less than 0.05); CK-MM, 90% to 100% (SI, 0.90 to 1.00).

Detectable CK-BB

CK-MM constitutes over 99% (SI, over 0.99) of total CK normally present in serum. Detectable CK-BB levels may indicate brain tissue injury, certain widespread malignant tumors, severe shock, or renal failure. However, such elevations don't confirm a specific diagnosis.

High CK-MB

CK-MB levels greater than 5% of total CK indicate MI, especially if the lactate dehydrogenase 1 and 2 (LD_1-LD_2) isoenzyme ratio is greater than 1 (flipped LD). In acute MI and after cardiac surgery, CK-MB levels begin to rise in 2 to 4 hours, peak in 12 to 24 hours, and usually return to normal in 24 to 48 hours; persistent elevations or increasing levels indicate ongoing myocardial damage.

Total CK follows roughly the same pattern but rises slightly later. CK-MB levels don't rise in heart failure or during angina pectoris not accompanied by myocardial cell necrosis, although not all researchers agree about this.

Serious skeletal muscle injury that occurs in certain muscular dystrophies, polymyositis, and severe myoglobinuria may produce mildly elevated CK-MB levels because a small amount of this isoenzyme is present in some skeletal muscles.

Rising CK-MM

Rising CK-MM values follow skeletal muscle damage from trauma, such as surgery and I.M. injections, or from diseases, such as dermatomyositis and muscular dystrophy (values may be 50 to 100 times normal). A moderate rise in CK-MM levels develops in patients with hypothyroidism; sharp elevations occur with muscular activity caused by agitation such as an acute psychotic episode.

Total CK

Total CK levels may be elevated in patients with severe hypokalemia, carbon monoxide poisoning, malignant hyperthermia, or alcoholic cardiomyopathy; in those who have recently had a seizure; and, occasionally, in those who have suffered pulmonary or cerebral infarctions. (See *CK test interference.*)

What needs to be done

- If the patient is being evaluated for skeletal muscle disorders, advise him to avoid exercising for 24 hours before the test.
- Advise the patient that he must not take the following before the test: alcohol, aminocaproic acid, lithium, clofibrate, codeine, dexamethasone, digoxin, lithium, morphine, succinylcholine, furosemide, glutethimide, halothane, heroin, imipramine, meperidine, and phenobarbital. If these substances must be continued, note this on the laboratory request.
- Obtain the sample as scheduled. Because timing is important to the diagnosis, be sure to record the date and time the sample was drawn and the number of hours that elapsed since the onset of chest pain.

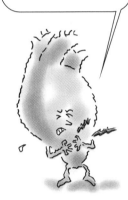

Oh, MI! CK-MB levels greater than 5% of total CK indicate—you guessed it—myocardial infarction.

Stay on the ball

CK test interference

The following factors may raise total creatine kinase (CK) values:
- halothane and succinylcholine, alcohol, lithium, and large doses of aminocaproic acid
- I.M. injections, cardioversion, invasive diagnostic procedures, recent vigorous exercise or muscle massage, and severe coughing and trauma
- surgery through skeletal muscle.

• Draw the sample before giving an I.M. injection, or wait at least 1 hour after the injection, because muscle trauma raises total CK levels.
• Perform a venipuncture, and collect the sample in a 4-ml tube without additives, or in a designated tube volume in accordance with laboratory protocol.
• Send the sample to the laboratory immediately because CK activity diminishes significantly after 2 hours at room temperature.
• Resume medications discontinued before the test, as ordered.

Troponin I and cardiac troponin T

Cardiac troponin I (cTn1) and cardiac troponin T (cTnT) are proteins in the striated cells, part of the calcium-binding complex of the thin myofilaments of myocardial tissue.

Troponins mark the spot

Troponins are extremely specific markers of cardiac damage. When injury occurs to the myocardial tissue, these proteins are released into the bloodstream, increasing from normally undetectable blood levels to levels of more than 50 mcg/L (SI, 50 µg/L). Elevations in troponin levels can be seen within 1 hour of MI and will persist for 1 week or longer, making this a useful diagnostic tool.

What it all means

Laboratories may give varying results, with some calling a cardiac troponin test positive if it shows any detectable levels and others giving a range for abnormal results.

Normally, cTn1 levels are less than 0.35 mcg/L (SI, less than 0.35 µg/L). cTnT levels are less than 0.1 mcg/L (SI, less than 0.1 µg/L). Troponin levels rise rapidly, are detectable within 4 to 6 hours of myocardial cell injury, and peak within 12 to 24 hours.

A hurtin' heart

Levels of cTn1 greater than 2 mcg/L (SI, greater than 2 µg/L) are suggestive of cardiac injury. Results of a qualitative cTnT rapid immunoassay that are greater than 0.1 mcg/L (SI, greater than 0.1 µg/L) are considered positive for cardiac injury. (See *Cardiac troponin test interference.*)

What needs to be done

• Tell the patient that this test helps assess myocardial injury and that multiple samples may be drawn to detect fluctuations in serum levels.

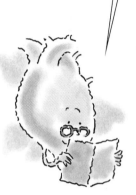

Hmmm. This information on cardiac markers is quite interesting.

Stay on the ball

Cardiac troponin test interference

These factors may increase cardiac troponin levels:
• chronic muscle or renal disease
• cardiotoxic drugs such as doxorubicin.

• Obtain each specimen on schedule, and note the date and collection time on each.
• Perform a venipuncture, and collect the sample in a 7-ml clot-activator tube, or in a designated tube volume in accordance with laboratory protocol.

Myoglobin

Myoglobin, which is normally found in skeletal and cardiac muscle, functions as an oxygen-binding muscle protein. It's released into the bloodstream in ischemia, trauma, and inflammation of the muscle.

What it all means

Normal myoglobin values are 5 to 70 ng/ml (SI, 5 to 70 mcg/L). In addition to occurring in MI, increased myoglobin levels may occur in acute alcohol intoxication, dermatomyositis, hypothermia (with prolonged shivering), muscular dystrophy, polymyositis, rhabdomyelitis, severe burn injuries, trauma, severe renal failure, and systemic lupus erythematosus. (See *Myoglobin test interference*.)

What needs to be done

• Expect to collect blood samples 4 to 8 hours after the onset of an acute MI.
• Tell the patient that the results of this test need to be correlated with other tests for a definitive diagnosis.
• Perform a venipuncture, and collect the sample in a 4-ml tube with no additives, or in a designated tube volume in accordance with laboratory protocol.
• Send the sample to the laboratory immediately.

Stay on the ball

Myoglobin test interference

The following factors may alter myoglobin test results:
• radioactive scans performed within 1 week of the test
• recent angina, cardioversion, or improper timing of the test, which may increase levels
• I.M. injection, which may cause a false-positive result.

B-type natriuretic peptide

B-type natriuretic peptide (BNP) is a neurohormone produced predominantly by the heart ventricle. BNP is released from the heart in response to blood volume expansion or pressure overload. Plasma BNP increases with the severity of heart failure. Studies have demonstrated that the heart is the major source of circulating BNP. It's an excellent hormonal marker of ventricular systolic and diastolic dysfunction. This test is used to help diagnose and determine the severity of heart failure.

What it all means

The normal value is less than 100 pg/ml. Blood concentrations greater than 100 pg/ml are an accurate predictor of heart failure. The level of BNP in the blood is related to the severity of heart failure—the higher the level, the worse the symptoms of heart failure. (See *Linking BNP levels to heart failure symptom severity* and *BNP test interference.*)

What needs to be done

• Perform a venipuncture, and collect the sample in a 3.5-ml tube containing EDTA, or in a designated tube volume in accordance with laboratory protocol.
• Apply direct pressure to the venipuncture site until bleeding stops.

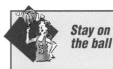

Stay on the ball

BNP test interference

Natrecor may cause increased levels.

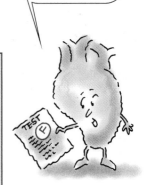

It must be those high BNP levels that made me fail.

Linking BNP levels to heart failure symptom severity

The following chart shows B-type natriuretic peptide (BNP) levels and their correlation with symptoms of heart failure. The higher the level of BNP, the more severe the symptoms are.

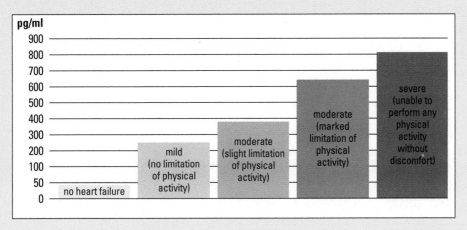

pg/ml

- no heart failure
- mild (no limitation of physical activity)
- moderate (slight limitation of physical activity)
- moderate (marked limitation of physical activity)
- severe (unable to perform any physical activity without discomfort)

C-reactive protein

C-reactive protein (CRP) is an abnormal protein that appears in the blood during an inflammatory process. This nonspecific protein is mainly synthesized in the liver and is found in many body fluids (pleural, peritoneal, pericardial, and synovial). It's absent from the blood of healthy people.

CRP appears in the blood 18 to 24 hours after the onset of tissue damage with levels that increase up to 1,000-fold and then decline rapidly when the inflammatory process regresses. CRP has been found to rise before increases in antibody titers and erythrocyte sedimentation rate (ESR) levels occur. It also decreases sooner than ESR levels. (See *Hs-CRP*.)

This test is used to:
• evaluate the inflammatory disease course and severity in conditions, including tissue necrosis (MI, malignancy, rheumatoid arthritis)
• monitor acute inflammatory phases of rheumatoid arthritis and rheumatic fever so that early treatment can be initiated
• monitor the patient's response to treatment or determine whether the acute phase is declining
• help interpret the ESR

Hs-CRP

A more sensitive C-reactive protein (CRP) test, the high-sensitivity C-reactive protein (hs-CRP) assay, can determine a person's risk of heart disease. Although a high CRP level is usually considered a positive risk factor for heart disease, it isn't known whether it actually plays a role in causing cardiovascular problems. The hs-CRP usually is evaluated with other cardiovascular risk profile testing, such as cholesterol and triglycerides.

Hs-CRP values of less than 1 mg/d (SI, < 10 mg/L) indicate a low risk of developing cardiovascular disease; levels between 1 and 3 mg/dl (SI, 10 to 30 mg/L) indicate an average risk; and high risk is higher than 3 mg/dl (SI, 30 mg/L). A patient with high hs-CRP results is four times more likely to have a heart attack than a patient with CRP values at the low end of the normal range.

Because the hs-CRP and CRP tests measure the same molecule, people with chronic inflammatory diseases (such as arthritis) shouldn't have hs-CRP levels measured. CRP levels in these individuals are typically high, and therefore the hs-CRP test will also be elevated.

• monitor the wound healing process of internal incisions, burns, and organ transplantation.

What it all means

CRP usually isn't present in the blood. In adults, results may be reported as less than 0.8 mg/dl (SI, less than 8 mg/L). An elevated CRP level may be present in rheumatoid arthritis, rheumatic fever, complications of diabetes, obesity, MI, cancer (active and widespread), acute bacterial and viral infections, inflammatory bowel disease, Hodgkin's disease, and systemic lupus erythematosus, and in postoperative patients (declining after the fourth day). (See *CRP test interference.*)

What needs to be done

• Inform the patient that he needs to restrict all fluids except for water for 8 to 12 hours before the test.
• Notify the laboratory and practitioner about medications the patient is taking that may affect test results; they may need to be restricted.
• Perform a venipuncture, and collect the sample in a 5-ml clot-activator tube, or in a designated tube volume in accordance with laboratory protocol.
• Instruct the patient that he may resume his usual diet and medications discontinued before the test, as ordered.
• Keep the blood sample away from heat.

Carbohydrates

Fasting plasma glucose

Commonly used to screen for diabetes mellitus, the fasting plasma glucose test, also known as the *fasting blood sugar test*, measures plasma glucose levels following a 12- to 14-hour fast.

What it all means

The normal range for fasting plasma glucose varies according to the laboratory procedure. Generally, normal values after at least an 8-hour fast are 70 to 110 mg of true glucose per deciliter (SI, 3.9 to 6.1 mmol/L) of blood.

Stay on the ball

CRP test interference

• Any recent illness, tissue injury, infection, or general inflammation will raise the amount of C-reactive protein (CRP) and give a falsely elevated estimate of risk. You should collect a blood sample at least 2 weeks after the resolution of an inflammatory disease process.
• Steroids, salicylates, nonsteroidal anti-inflammatory drugs, or statins may cause a false normal level.
• Hormonal contraceptives may cause a false increase.
• Pregnancy (third trimester) and intrauterine contraceptive devices may cause an increase.

Confirming diabetes

A fasting plasma glucose level of 126 mg/dl (SI, 7 mmol/L) or higher (also known as *hyperglycemia*) obtained on two or more occasions confirms provisional diabetes mellitus. An impaired blood glucose level is 125 mg/dl (SI, 6.9 mmol/L).

Boosting levels

Increased fasting plasma glucose levels can also result from pancreatitis, recent acute illness (such as MI), Cushing's syndrome, acromegaly (a metabolic condition characterized by enlargement and elongation of facial bones and extremities), and pheochromocytoma (a tumor of the adrenal medulla). Hyperglycemia may also stem from hyperlipoproteinemia (especially type III, IV, or V), chronic hepatic disease, nephrotic syndrome, brain tumor, sepsis, or gastrectomy with dumping syndrome and is typical in eclampsia, anoxia, and seizure disorders.

Depressed levels

Depressed plasma glucose levels can result from hyperinsulinism, insulinoma, von Gierke's disease (glycogen storage disease), functional or reactive hypoglycemia, myxedema, adrenal insufficiency, congenital adrenal hyperplasia, hypopituitarism, malabsorption syndrome, and some cases of hepatic insufficiency.

Fast action needed

When using fasting plasma glucose tests to monitor drug or diet therapy in patients with diabetes mellitus, you may obtain results that require immediate action. Most patients develop symptoms when blood glucose is between 50 and 60 mg/dl (SI, 2.8 to 3 mmol/L). Symptoms include fatigue, malaise, nervousness, mood changes, irritability, trembling, tension, headache, hunger, cold sweats, rapid heart rate, and palpitations. Without immediate reversal of the hypoglycemia with parenteral or I.V. glucose, the blood glucose level will continue to fall. Evidence of progressive CNS disturbance includes blurry or double vision, inability to concentrate, confusion, motor weakness, hemiplegia, seizures, loss of consciousness, irreversible brain damage, and death.

Plasma glucose levels higher than 300 mg/dl (15 mmol/L) can also lead to an urgent situation. Treatment with appropriate insulin dosages can correct the hyperglycemia. (See *Fasting plasma glucose test interference.*)

What needs to be done

• Tell the patient he must fast for 12 to 14 hours before the test.

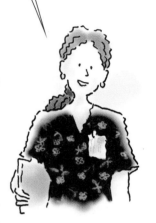

The fasting blood sugar test is commonly used to screen for diabetes mellitus.

Stay on the ball

Fasting plasma glucose test interference

These factors may increase plasma glucose levels:
• acetaminophen, which may cause false-positive findings
• recent illness, infection, or pregnancy
• chlorthalidone, thiazide diuretics, furosemide, triamterene, hormonal contraceptives (estrogen-progestogen combination), benzodiazepines, phenytoin, phenothiazines, lithium, epinephrine, arginine, phenolphthalein, dextrothyroxine, dizoxide, large doses of nicotinic acid, corticosteroids, and recent I.V. glucose infusions as well as ethacrynic acid (which may also cause hyperglycemia or, in large doses, hypoglycemia in patients with uremia).
      These factors may decrease plasma glucose levels:
• beta-adrenergic blockers, ethanol, clofibrate, insulin, oral antidiabetic agents, and monoamine oxidase inhibitors
• strenuous exercise.

• Advise the patient to avoid drugs that affect test results, as ordered. Advise the patient with diabetes that he'll receive his medication after the test.
• Instruct the patient to report the symptoms of hypoglycemia (weakness, restlessness, nervousness, hunger, and sweating).
• Perform a venipuncture, and collect the sample in a 5-ml clot-activator tube, or in a designated tube volume in accordance with laboratory protocol.
• Specify on the laboratory request the time the patient last ate, the sample collection time, and the time he received the last pretest dose of insulin or oral antidiabetic drug (if applicable).
• Send the sample to the laboratory immediately because blood glucose levels decrease when the sample is left at room temperature. If transport is delayed, refrigerate the sample.
• Provide a balanced meal or a snack. As ordered, resume administration of medications withheld before the test.

Oral glucose tolerance

The oral glucose tolerance test (OGTT) is the most sensitive method of evaluating borderline cases of diabetes mellitus in selected patients. Plasma and urine glucose levels are monitored for

3 hours after a challenge dose of glucose to assess insulin secretion and the body's ability to metabolize glucose.

What it all means

Normal plasma glucose levels peak at 160 to 180 mg/dl (SI, 8.8 to 9.9 mmol/L) within 30 minutes to 1 hour after administration of an oral glucose test dose, and return to fasting levels or lower in 2 to 3 hours. Urine glucose tests remain negative throughout.

Intolerant...

Depressed glucose tolerance, in which levels peak sharply before falling slowly to fasting levels, may confirm diabetes or may result from Cushing's disease, hemochromatosis (a rare disease of iron metabolism), pheochromocytomas, or CNS lesions.

...or too tolerant

Increased glucose tolerance, in which levels may peak at less than normal, may indicate insulinoma, malabsorption syndrome, Addison's disease, hypothyroidism, or hypopituitarism. (See *OGTT interference.*)

What needs to be done

• Tell the patient that he must maintain a high-carbohydrate diet for 3 days and then fast for 10 to 16 hours before the test.
• Advise the patient not to smoke, drink coffee or alcohol, or exercise strenuously for 8 hours before or during the test.
• Tell the patient that the test usually requires five blood samples and five urine specimens. Have him bring a book or other quiet diversion; the procedure usually takes 3 hours but can last as long as 6 hours.
• Remind the patient that the symptoms of hypoglycemia (weakness, restlessness, nervousness, hunger, and sweating) should be reported immediately.
• Between 7 a.m. and 9 a.m., draw a fasting blood sample in a 7-ml clot-activator tube, or in a designated tube volume in accordance with laboratory protocol. Collect a urine specimen at the same time if your facility includes this as part of the test. After collecting these samples, administer the test load of oral glucose and record the time of ingestion. Encourage the patient to drink the entire glucose solution within 5 minutes.
• Using 7-ml clot-activator tubes, draw blood samples in 30-minute, 1-hour, 2-hour, and 3-hour intervals after giving the loading dose. Collect urine specimens at the same intervals. Tell the patient to lie down if he feels faint from the numerous venipunc-

Stay on the ball

OGTT interference

The following factors may alter oral glucose tolerance test (OGTT) results.

• Carbohydrate deprivation before the test can produce an abnormal increase followed by a delayed decrease.
• Chlorthalidone, thiazide diuretics, furosemide, triamterene, hormonal contraceptives, benzodiazepines, phenytoin, phenothiazines, lithium, epinephrine, caffeine, large doses of nicotinic acid, corticosteroids, and recent I.V. glucose infusions may increase levels.
• Beta-adrenergic blockers, amphetamines, ethanol, insulin, oral antidiabetic drugs, and monoamine oxidase inhibitors may decrease levels.
• Recent infection, fever, pregnancy, or acute illness (such as myocardial infarction) may elevate levels.

tures. Encourage him to drink water throughout the test to promote adequate urine excretion.

• Send blood samples and urine specimens to the laboratory immediately, or refrigerate them. Specify when the patient last ate and the blood and urine collection times. As appropriate, record the time the patient received his last pretest dose of insulin or oral antidiabetic drug.

• If the patient develops severe hypoglycemia, notify the doctor. Draw a blood sample, record the time on the laboratory request, and discontinue the test. Have the patient drink a glass of orange juice or administer glucose I.V. to reverse the reaction.

• Provide a balanced meal or a snack, but observe for a hypoglycemic reaction.

• As ordered, resume administration of medications withheld for the test.

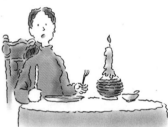

Feast, then famine. An OGTT patient will be on a high-carbohydrate diet for 3 days and then fast for 10 to 16 hours before the test.

Glycosylated hemoglobin

The glycosylated Hb test (also known as the *total fasting Hb* or *glycohemoglobin test*) helps monitor the effectiveness of diabetes therapy. Glycosylated Hb levels reflect the average blood glucose level during the preceding 2 to 3 months. This test requires only one venipuncture every 6 to 8 weeks and can therefore be used for evaluating long-term effectiveness of diabetes therapy.

What it all means

Glycosylated Hb values are reported as a percentage of the total Hb within an RBC. Because Hb A_{1c} is present in a larger quantity than the other minor Hbs, it's commonly measured and reported separately. Hb A_{1a} and Hb A_{1b} account for about 1.6% and 0.8%, respectively; Hb A_{1c} accounts for approximately 5%; and total glycosylated Hb accounts for 4% to 7%.

Under control

Hb A_{1c} values are normally 4% to 8%.

Out of control

In diabetes, the patient has good control of blood glucose levels when the Hb A_{1c} value is less than 8%. A value greater than 10% indicates poor control. (See *Glycosylated Hb test interference*.)

What needs to be done

• Perform a venipuncture, and collect the sample in a 5-ml tube containing EDTA, or in a designated tube volume in accordance with laboratory protocol.

Stay on the ball

Glycosylated Hb test interference

• Hemolytic anemia, chronic blood loss, or abnormal hemoglobins (S, C, or D) may lower results.

• Hyperglycemia, thalassemia, or chronic renal failure; dialysis; a recent splenectomy; or elevated triglyceride or Hb F levels may elevate results.

• Fill the collection tube completely, and invert it gently several times to adequately mix the sample and anticoagulant.
• Schedule the patient for an appointment in 6 to 8 weeks for appropriate follow-up testing.

Oral lactose tolerance test

The oral lactose tolerance test measures plasma glucose levels after ingestion of a challenge dose of lactose. It's used to screen for lactose intolerance caused by lactase deficiency. Absence or deficiency of lactase causes undigested lactose to remain in the intestinal tract, producing abdominal cramps and watery diarrhea.

Congenital or secondary?

Congenital lactase deficiency is rare; lactose intolerance is usually acquired as lactase levels decline with age.

What it all means

Normally, plasma glucose levels rise more than 20 mg/dl (SI, more than 1.1 mmol/L) over fasting levels within 15 to 60 minutes after ingestion of the lactose-loading dose. A rise in plasma glucose of less than 20 mg/dl (SI, less than 1.1 mmol/L) indicates lactose intolerance. Accompanying signs and symptoms provoked by the test also suggest but don't confirm the diagnosis because such symptoms may develop in patients with normal lactase activity after a loading dose of lactose. Small-bowel biopsy with lactase assay may be done to confirm the diagnosis. (See *Oral lactose tolerance test interference.*)

What needs to be done

• Tell the patient to fast and avoid strenuous activity for 8 hours before the test.
• After the patient has fasted for 8 hours, perform a venipuncture and collect a blood sample in a 7-ml tube with sodium fluoride and potassium oxalate added.
• Administer the loading dose of lactose (for an adult, 50 g of lactose dissolved in 400 ml of water; for a child, 50 g/m^2 of body surface area). Record the time of ingestion.
• Watch for symptoms of lactose intolerance (abdominal cramps, nausea, bloating, flatulence, and watery diarrhea) caused by the loading dose.
• Draw blood samples at 30-minute, 1-hour, and 2-hour intervals after giving the loading dose, using 4-ml tubes with sodium fluoride and potassium oxalate added, or a designated tube volume in accordance with laboratory protocol.

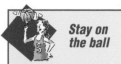

Stay on the ball

Oral lactose tolerance test interference

These factors may alter oral lactose tolerance test results:
• delayed emptying of stomach contents, which may depress glucose levels
• thiazide diuretics, hormonal contraceptives, benzodiazepines, propranolol, and insulin
• glycolysis, which may cause false-negative results.

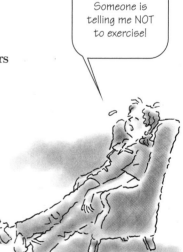

Finally! Someone is telling me NOT to exercise!

• Send blood samples to the laboratory immediately, or refrigerate them if transport is delayed. Note the collection time on the laboratory request.
• As ordered, instruct the patient to resume diet, activity, and medications withheld before the test.

Lactic acid and pyruvic acid

Lactic acid is an intermediate product of carbohydrate metabolism and is normally metabolized by the liver. It's present in blood as lactate ion and is derived primarily from muscle cells and RBCs. Blood lactate concentration depends on the body's production rate and metabolism rate; lactate levels may rise significantly during exercise.

Deficient or adequate oxygen?

Together, lactate and pyruvate form a reversible reaction that's regulated by oxygen supply. When oxygen levels are deficient, pyruvate converts to lactate; when they're adequate, lactate converts to pyruvate.

Lactic acidosis?

When the hepatic system fails to metabolize lactate sufficiently, or when excess pyruvate converts to lactate because of tissue hypoxia and circulatory collapse, lactic acidosis may result. Measurement of blood lactate levels is recommended for all patients with symptoms of lactic acidosis such as Kussmaul's respirations.

What it all means

Blood lactate values range from 0.93 to 1.65 mEq/L (SI, 0.93 to 1.6 mmol/L); pyruvate levels range from 0.08 to 0.16 mEq/L (SI, 0.08 to 0.16 mmol/L). Normally, the lactate-pyruvate ratio is less than 10:1.

When lactate levels are high

Elevated blood lactate levels associated with hypoxia may result from strenuous muscle exercise, shock, hemorrhage, septicemia, MI, pulmonary embolism, or cardiac arrest. When no reason for diminished tissue perfusion is apparent, increased lactate levels may result from systemic disorders (such as diabetes mellitus, leukemias, lymphomas, hepatic disease, and renal failure) or from enzymatic defects (such as in von Gierke's disease and fructose 1,6-diphosphatase deficiency).

Lactic acidosis

Lactic acidosis can follow ingestion of large doses of acetaminophen or ethanol, as well as I.V. infusion of epinephrine, glucagon, fructose, or sorbitol.

What needs to be done

• Tell the patient that he must abstain from food overnight and rest for at least 1 hour before the tests.
• Because venostasis may raise blood lactate levels, it's best to avoid using a tourniquet; if you do use one, release it at least 2 minutes before collecting the sample, so the blood can circulate. Tell the patient that he must not clench his fist during the venipuncture.
• Perform a venipuncture, and collect the sample in a 5-ml tube with sodium fluoride and potassium oxalate added, or in a designated tube volume in accordance with laboratory protocol.
• Because lactate and pyruvate are extremely unstable, place the sample container in an ice-filled cup and send it to the laboratory immediately.
• As ordered, instruct the patient to resume his normal diet.

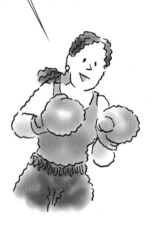

Patients should stay fist-free during lactic acid and pyruvic acid tests.

Pancreatic enzymes

Amylase

Amylase (alpha-amylase or AML) is an enzyme that helps the body digest starch and glycogen in the mouth, stomach, and intestine. In cases of suspected acute pancreatic disease, measurement of serum or urine amylase is the most important laboratory test. Alpha-amylase is synthesized primarily in the pancreas and the salivary glands and secreted into the GI tract.

What it all means

Serum amylase levels for adults age 18 and older normally range from 25 to 85 units/L (SI, 0.39 to 1.45 µkat/L). After the onset of acute pancreatitis, serum amylase levels begin to rise in 2 hours, peak at 12 to 48 hours, and return to normal in 3 to 4 days. Determination of urine levels should follow normal serum amylase results to rule out pancreatitis.

Stay on the ball

Amylase test interference

Elevate levels
• Aminosalicylic acid, azathioprine, bethanechol, chloride salts, cholinergics, corticosteroids, ethacrynic acid, ethyl alcohol, fluoride salts, furosemide, indomethacin, mercaptopurine, opioids, pancreozymin, rifampin, hormonal contraceptives, sulfasalazine, and thiazide diuretics
• Recent trauma to the salivary glands, pancreatic surgery, perforated ulcer or intestine, abscess, and spasm of the sphincter of Oddi

Decrease levels
• Citrates
• Oxalates

Elevations and depressions

Moderate serum elevations may accompany pancreatic injury from perforated peptic ulcer, pancreatic cancer, acute salivary gland disease, impaired renal function, or obstruction of the common bile duct, the pancreatic duct, or the ampulla of Vater. Levels may be slightly elevated in a patient who's asymptomatic or who has an unusual response to therapy. Depressed amylase levels can occur in patients with chronic pancreatitis, pancreatic cancer, cirrhosis, hepatitis, and toxemia of pregnancy. (See *Amylase test interference.*)

What needs to be done

• Tell the patient that he must abstain from alcohol for 24 hours before the test.
• If the patient has severe abdominal pain, draw the sample before diagnostic or therapeutic intervention. For accurate results, obtaining an early sample is important.
• Perform a venipuncture, and collect the sample in a 4-ml clot-activator tube, or in a designated tube volume in accordance with laboratory protocol.
• Handle the sample gently to prevent hemolysis.
• As ordered, resume administration of drugs that were discontinued before the test.

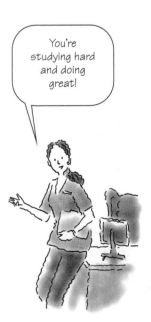

You're studying hard and doing great!

Lipase

Lipase is produced in the pancreas and secreted into the duodenum, where it converts triglycerides and other fats into fatty acids and glycerol. Destruction of pancreatic cells, which occurs in acute pancreatitis, releases large amounts of lipase into the blood. Also, obstruction of the pancreatic duct prevents the enzymes from reaching their destination, and large amounts of lipase are diverted to the bloodstream. The lipase test measures serum lipase levels; it's most useful when performed with a serum or urine amylase test.

What it all means

Serum lipase levels normally are less than 160 units/L (SI, less than 2.72 µkat/L).

Obstruction ahead

High lipase levels lasting up to 14 days suggest acute pancreatitis or pancreatic duct obstruction. Lipase levels may also increase in other pancreatic injuries, such as perforated peptic ulcer with chemical pancreatitis caused by gastric juices, and in patients with a high intestinal obstruction, pancreatic cancer, or renal disease with impaired excretion. (See *Lipase test interference*.)

What needs to be done

- Tell the patient that he must fast overnight before the test.
- Instruct the patient to avoid taking cholinergics, codeine, meperidine, and morphine before the test, as ordered. If any of these drugs must be continued, note this on the laboratory request.
- Perform a venipuncture, and collect the sample in a 4-ml clot-activator tube, or in a designated tube volume in accordance with laboratory protocol.
- As ordered, resume administration of drugs discontinued before the test.

Stay on the ball

Lipase test interference

Cholinergics, codeine, meperidine, and morphine can cause spasm of the sphincter of Oddi, producing false-positive results.

Hepatic enzymes

Aspartate aminotransferase

Aspartate aminotransferase (AST) is one of two enzymes that catalyze the conversion of the nitrogenous portion of an amino acid to an amino acid residue. This enzyme is essential to energy production in the Krebs cycle (tricarboxylic acid or citric acid cycle). AST is found in the cytoplasm and mitochondria of many cells, primarily in the liver, heart, skeletal muscles, kidneys, and pancreas and, to a lesser extent, in RBCs. It's released into serum in proportion to cellular damage. The change in AST values over time is a reliable monitoring mechanism.

What it all means

AST levels range from 14 to 20 units/L (SI, 0.23 to 0.33 µkat/L) in men and from 10 to 36 units/L (SI, 0.17 to 0.60 µkat/L) in women. Values for children are 9 to 80 units/L (SI, 0.15 to 1.3 µkat/L) and for neonates, 47 to 150 units/L (SI, 0.78 to 2.5 µkat/L).

AST levels fluctuate in response to the extent of cellular necrosis and therefore may be temporarily and slightly elevated early in the disease process and extremely elevated during the most acute phase. Depending on when during the course of the disease the initial sample was drawn, AST levels can rise, indicating increasing disease severity and tissue damage, or fall, indicating disease resolution and tissue repair. Thus, the relative change in AST values serves as a reliable monitoring mechanism.

The lowdown on levels

Very high AST levels (more than 20 times normal) may indicate acute viral hepatitis, severe skeletal muscle trauma, extensive surgery, drug-induced hepatic injury, or severe passive liver congestion.

High levels (ranging from 10 to 20 times normal) may indicate severe MI, severe infectious mononucleosis, or alcoholic cirrhosis. They also occur during the initial or resolving stages of conditions listed above that cause very high elevations.

Moderate to high levels (ranging from 5 to 10 times normal) may indicate Duchenne's muscular dystrophy, dermatomyositis, or chronic hepatitis. They also occur during initial and resolving stages of diseases that cause high elevations.

Low to moderate levels (ranging from 2 to 5 times normal) may indicate hemolytic anemia, metastatic hepatic tumors, acute pancreatitis, pulmonary emboli, alcohol withdrawal syndrome, or fatty liver. AST levels also rise slightly after the first few days of biliary duct obstruction. (See *AST test interference.*)

What needs to be done

• Tell the patient that the test usually requires three venipunctures—one at admission and one each day for the next 2 days.

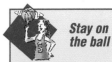

Stay on the ball

AST test interference

• Chlorpropamide, opiates, methyldopa, erythromycin, sulfonamides, pyridoxine, dicumarol, and antituberculosis agents as well as large doses of acetaminophen, salicylates, or vitamin A may elevate aspartate aminotransferase (AST) levels.

• Strenuous exercise and muscle trauma associated with I.M. injections raise AST levels.

• Tell the patient that he must refrain from taking morphine, codeine, meperidine, chlorpropamide, methyldopa, phenazopyridine, and antituberculosis drugs (such as isoniazid and pyrazinamide), as ordered. If any of these medications must be continued, note this on the laboratory request.
• To avoid missing peak AST levels, draw serum samples at the same time each day.
• Perform a venipuncture, and collect the sample in a 4-ml clot-activator tube, or in a designated tube volume in accordance with laboratory protocol.
• As ordered, resume medications discontinued before the test.

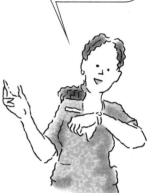

Timing is critical when drawing serum samples for AST levels.

Alanine aminotransferase

Alanine aminotransferase (ALT) is one of two enzymes that catalyze a reversible amino group transfer reaction in the Krebs cycle. This enzyme is necessary for tissue energy production. ALT is found primarily in the liver—with lesser amounts in the kidneys, heart, and skeletal muscles—and is a relatively specific indicator of acute hepatocellular damage.

What it all means

Normally, serum ALT levels range from 10 to 35 units/L (SI, 0.17 to 0.60 µkat/L) in adults; for neonates, ALT levels are 13 to 45 units/L (SI, 0.22 to 0.77 µkat/L).

Highs and lows

Very high ALT levels (up to 50 times normal) suggest viral or severe drug-induced hepatitis or another hepatic disease with extensive necrosis. In these cases, AST levels are also elevated but usually to a lesser degree. Moderate to high levels may indicate infectious mononucleosis, chronic hepatitis, intrahepatic cholestasis (arrest of bile secretion) or cholecystitis, early or improving acute viral hepatitis, or severe hepatic congestion associated with heart failure.

Slight to moderate ALT elevations, usually with higher increases in AST levels, may appear in any condition that produces acute hepatocellular injury, such as active cirrhosis and drug-induced or alcoholic hepatitis. Marginal elevations occasionally occur in association with acute MI, reflecting secondary hepatic congestion or the release of small amounts of ALT from myocardial tissue. (See *ALT test interference.*)

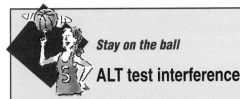

Stay on the ball

ALT test interference

Falsely elevated alanine aminotransferase (ALT) levels can result from barbiturates, griseofulvin, isoniazid, nitrofurantoin, methyldopa, phenothiazines, phenytoin, salicylates, tetracycline, chlorpromazine, or para-aminosalicylic acid.

What needs to be done

• Tell the patient that he should avoid hepatotoxic or cholestatic drugs, such as methotrexate, chlorpromazine, salicylates, and opioids, before the test. If they must be continued, note this on the laboratory request.

• Perform a venipuncture, and collect the sample in a 4-ml tube without additives, or in a designated tube volume in accordance with laboratory protocol.

• Be aware that ALT activity is stable in serum for up to 3 days at room temperature.

• As ordered, resume administration of drugs that were withheld before the test.

Alkaline phosphatase

An enzyme most active at a pH of about 10, alkaline phosphatase (ALP) influences bone calcification and lipid and metabolite transport. Total serum levels reflect the combined activity of several ALP isoenzymes found in the liver, bones, kidneys, intestinal lining, and placenta.

Bone and liver ALP are always present in adult serum, with liver ALP making up the largest amount—except during the third trimester of pregnancy, when about half of all ALP originates from the placenta. The intestinal variant of this enzyme can be a normal component, or it can be an abnormal finding associated with hepatic disease.

What it all means

Total ALP levels normally range from 45 to 115 International Units/ml (SI, 45 to 115 units/L).

Although significant ALP elevations are possible with diseases that affect many organs, they usually indicate skeletal disease or

Stay on the ball

ALP test interference

These factors may alter alkaline phosphatase (ALP) levels:
• drugs that influence liver function or cause cholestasis, such as barbiturates, chlorpropamide, hormonal contraceptives, isoniazid, methyldopa, phenothiazines, phenytoin, and rifampin, which can cause a mild increase
• healing long-bone fractures and third-trimester pregnancy, which raise ALP levels
• halothane sensitivity, which may increase ALP levels sharply
• clofibrate, which decreases ALP levels.

extrahepatic or intrahepatic biliary obstruction causing cholestasis. Many acute hepatic diseases cause ALP elevations before they result in any change in serum bilirubin levels. A moderate rise in ALP levels may reflect acute biliary obstruction from hepatocellular inflammation, inactive cirrhosis, mononucleosis, or viral hepatitis. Moderate increases are also seen in osteomalacia (increased softness of bones) and deficiency-induced rickets.

Climbing the ALPs

Sharp ALP level elevations may result from complete biliary obstruction by malignant or infectious infiltrations or fibrosis. Such markedly high levels are most common in Paget's disease and, occasionally, in biliary obstruction, extensive bone metastasis, or hyperparathyroidism. Metastatic bone tumors resulting from pancreatic cancer raise ALP levels without a concomitant rise in serum alanine aminotransferase levels.

A rare low

In rare cases, low ALP levels are associated with hypophosphatasia or with protein or magnesium deficiency. (See *ALP test interference*.)

What needs to be done

• Tell the patient that he must fast for at least 8 hours before the test because fat intake stimulates intestinal ALP secretion.
• Perform a venipuncture, and collect the sample in a 4-ml clot-activator tube, or in a designated tube volume in accordance with laboratory protocol.

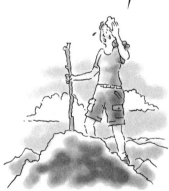

I didn't know learning about ALP elevations would be such hard work!

- Send the sample to the laboratory immediately because ALP activity increases at room temperature in association with a pH rise.
- Tell the patient he may resume a normal diet after the test.

Gamma glutamyl transferase

Gamma glutamyl transferase (GGT), also known as *gamma glutamyl transpeptidase*, participates in the transfer of amino acids across cellular membranes and, possibly, in glutathione metabolism.

A well-traveled enzyme

Highest concentrations of GGT exist in the renal tubules, where amino acids are reabsorbed from glomerular filtrate, but this enzyme also appears in the liver, biliary tract epithelium, pancreas, lymphocytes, brain, and testes.

What it all means

Normal serum GGT levels range as follows:
- *men*: age 16 and older, 6 to 38 units/L (SI, 0.10 to 0.63 µkat/L)
- *women:* between ages 16 and 45, 4 to 27 units/L (SI, 0.08 to 0.46 µkat/L); age 45 and older, 6 to 37 units/L (SI, 0.10 to 0.63 µkat/L)
- *children:* 3 to 30 units/L (SI, 0.05 to 0.51 µkat/L).

Liver levels

Serum GGT levels rise in any acute hepatic disease as enzyme production increases in response to hepatocellular injury. Moderate increases occur in acute pancreatitis, renal disease, prostatic metastasis, in some patients with epilepsy or brain tumors, and postoperatively. Levels also increase after alcohol ingestion and in chronic alcoholism, even without evidence of hepatic injury. Elevations occur in patients with obstructive jaundice or metastatic liver disease. GGT may increase within 5 to 10 days after acute MI, either as a result of tissue granulation and healing or as an indication of the effects of cardiac insufficiency on the liver. (See *GGT test interference*.)

What needs to be done

- Tell the patient that he doesn't need to restrict food or fluids.
- Perform a venipuncture, and collect the sample in a 4-ml tube without additives, or in a designated tube volume in accordance with laboratory protocol.

Stay on the ball

GGT test interference

Clofibrate and hormonal contraceptives decrease serum gamma glutamyl transferase (GGT) levels. Aminoglycosides, barbiturates, phenytoin, and glutethimide increase serum GGT levels.

Special enzymes

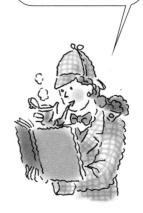

Hmmm…it appears I've been misled. These acid phosphatase levels aren't what they seem.

Acid phosphatase

Acid phosphatases are a group of phosphatase enzymes most active at a pH of about 5. These enzymes appear in the prostate gland and semen and, to a lesser extent, in the liver, spleen, RBCs, bone marrow, and platelets. Prostatic and erythrocytic enzymes are the major isoenzymes in this group and can be isolated in the laboratory.

What it all means

Total serum acid phosphatase levels depend on the assay method; they generally range from 0 to 3.7 units/L (SI, 0 to 3.7 U/L).

Moderate and misleading levels

Misleading results may occur if ALP levels are high, because acid phosphatase and ALP enzymes are very similar and differ mainly in the optimum pH ranges. Some ALP isoenzymes may react at a lower pH and thus be detected as acid phosphatase.

Acid phosphatase levels rise moderately in patients with prostatic infarction or Gaucher's disease (congenital disease of lipid metabolism), in some patients with Paget's disease, and occasionally in association with other conditions such as multiple myeloma.

Dangerously high levels

High levels of acid phosphatase in the prostate usually indicate a tumor that has spread beyond the prostatic capsule. If the tumor has metastasized to bone, high acid phosphatase levels are accompanied by high ALP levels, reflecting increased osteoblastic activity. (See *Acid phosphatase test interference*.)

What needs to be done

• Don't draw the sample within 48 hours of prostate manipulation (rectal examination).
• Withhold fluorides, phosphates, and clofibrate before the test as ordered. If any of these drugs must be continued, be sure to note this on the laboratory request.
• Perform a venipuncture, and collect the sample in a 4-ml tube without additives, or in a designated tube volume in accordance with laboratory protocol. The sample should be iced for delivery to the laboratory. Some laboratories ask for a heparinized tube so

Stay on the ball

Acid phosphatase test interference

These factors may alter acid phosphatase test results:
• fluorides, phosphates, and oxalates, which may cause false-low test results; clofibrate, which may cause false-high results
• prostate massage, catheterization, or rectal examination within 48 hours of the test.

they won't have to wait for the sample to clot. If the sample can't be analyzed in less than 30 minutes, it should be frozen.
• Send the sample to the laboratory immediately. Acid phosphatase levels drop by 50% within 1 hour if the sample remains at room temperature without a preservative or if it isn't packed in ice.

Prostate-specific antigen

Measurement of prostate-specific antigen (PSA) helps track the course of this disease and evaluates response to treatment.

What it all means

Normal PSA values are:
• *ages 40 to 50:* 2.0 to 2.8 ng/ml (SI, 2 to 2.8 µg/L)
• *ages 51 to 60:* 2.9 to 3.8 ng/ml (SI, 2.9 to 3.8 µg/L)
• *ages 61 to 70:* 4.0 to 5.3 ng/ml (SI, 4 to 5.3 µg/L)
• *age 71 and older:* 5.6 to 7.2 ng/ml (SI, 5.6 to 7.2 µg/L).

About 80% of patients with prostate cancer have pretreatment PSA values greater than 4 ng/ml (SI, 4 µg/L). This percentage is higher in advanced stages and lower in early stages.

Not a solo act

However, PSA results alone shouldn't be considered diagnostic for prostate cancer because approximately 20% of patients with benign prostatic hyperplasia also have levels over 4 ng/ml. Further testing, including tissue biopsy and digital rectal examination, is needed to confirm a diagnosis of cancer. (See *PSA test interference.*)

What needs to be done

• Collect the sample either before a digital rectal examination or at least 48 hours after one to avoid falsely elevated PSA levels.
• Perform a venipuncture, and collect the sample in a 7-ml clot-activator tube, or in a designated tube volume in accordance with laboratory protocol.
• Put the sample on ice, and send it to the laboratory immediately.

> *Stay on the ball*
>
> **PSA test interference**
>
> Excessive doses of chemotherapeutic drugs, such as cyclophosphamide, diethylstilbestrol, and methotrexate, may alter prostate-specific antigen (PSA) test results.

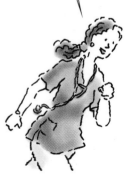

> I've got to get this sample to the lab in a hurry!

Plasma renin activity

Renin is released into the renal veins in response to sodium depletion and blood loss. Renin secretion from the kidneys is the first stage of the renin-angiotensin-aldosterone cycle, which controls the body's sodium-potassium balance, fluid volume, and blood pressure. The plasma renin activity (PRA) test is a screening procedure for renovascular hypertension but doesn't confirm it.

What it all means

PRA and aldosterone levels decrease with age. In a sodium-depleted, upright peripheral vein, normal levels are:
- *ages 18 to 39:* 2.9 to 24 ng/ml/hour (mean, 10.8 ng/ml/hour)
- *age 40 and older:* 2.9 to 10.8 ng/ml.hour (mean, 5.9 ng/ml/hour).
  In a sodium-replete, upright peripheral vein, normal levels are:
- *ages 18 to 39:* less than or equal to 0.6 to 4.3 ng/ml/hour (mean, 1.9 ng/ml/hour)
- *age 40 and older:* less than or equal to 0.6 to 3 ng/ml/hour (mean, 1 ng/ml/hour).

Decreased renin levels may come from hypovolemia associated with a high-sodium diet. But I didn't mean to cause trouble, I swear!

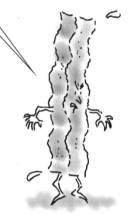

When renin is up...

Elevated renin levels may occur in essential hypertension (this is uncommon), malignant and renovascular hypertension, cirrhosis, hypokalemia, hypovolemia caused by hemorrhage, renin-producing renal tumors (Bartter syndrome), and adrenal hypofunction (Addison's disease). High renin levels may also be found in chronic renal failure with parenchymal disease, end-stage renal disease, and transplant rejection.

...and when it's down

Decreased renin levels may indicate hypervolemia associated with a high-sodium diet, salt-retaining steroids, primary aldosteronism, Cushing's syndrome, licorice ingestion syndrome, or essential hypertension with low renin levels.

High aldosterone

High serum and urine aldosterone levels with low plasma renin activity help identify primary aldosteronism. In the sodium-depleted renin test, low plasma renin confirms this diagnosis and differentiates it from secondary aldosteronism (characterized by increased renin). (See *PRA test interference.*)

What needs to be done

- Collect the sample in the morning, if possible.
- Instruct the patient to discontinue use of diuretics, antihypertensives, vasodilators, hormonal contraceptives, and licorice as ordered by the practitioner, and maintain a normal sodium diet (3 g/day) during this period.

Stay on the ball

PRA test interference

These factors may alter plasma renin activity (PRA) test results:
- salt-retaining corticosteroid therapy and antidiuretic therapy, which decrease the level
- salt intake, hormonal contraceptives and diuretic therapy, antihypertensives, or vasodilators, which increase the level
- radioisotope use within several days before the test.

• Explain to the patient that, for the sodium-depleted plasma renin test, he'll receive furosemide (or, if he has angina or cerebrovascular insufficiency, chlorothiazide) and will follow a specific low-sodium diet for 3 days.

• Make sure the patient avoids radioactive treatments for several days before the test.

• If a recumbent sample is ordered, tell the patient to remain in bed at least 2 hours before the sample is obtained because posture influences renin secretion.

• If an upright sample is ordered, have the patient stand or sit upright for 2 hours before the test is performed.

• If renal vein catheterization is ordered, have the patient sign an informed consent form and explain that the procedure will be done in the radiography department under local anesthetic.

For a peripheral vein sample

• Perform a venipuncture, and collect the sample in a 4-ml tube that contains EDTA, or in a designated tube volume in accordance with laboratory protocol.

• Note on the laboratory slip whether the patient was fasting and whether he was in an upright or supine position during sample collection.

For a renal vein catheterization

• A catheter is advanced to the kidneys through the femoral vein under fluoroscopic control, and samples are obtained from both renal veins and the vena cava.

• After renal vein catheterization, apply pressure to the catheterization site for 10 to 20 minutes to prevent extravasation.

• Monitor vital signs, and check the catheterization site every 30 minutes for 2 hours and then every hour for 4 hours to ensure that the bleeding has stopped. Check distal pulse for signs of thrombus formation and arterial occlusion (cyanosis, loss of pulse, and coolness of skin).

For both methods

• Because renin is unstable, draw the sample into a chilled syringe and collection tube, place it on ice, and send it to the laboratory immediately.

• Completely fill the collection tube, and invert it gently several times to mix the sample and the anticoagulant adequately.

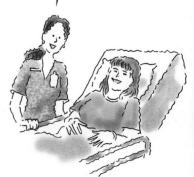

Up or down? It's important to note whether the patient was in an upright or supine position during peripheral vein sample collection.

Cholinesterase

The cholinesterase test measures the amounts of two similar enzymes that hydrolyze acetylcholine: acetylcholinesterase (or *true cholinesterase*) and pseudocholinesterase (also known as *serum cholinesterase*).

Acetylcholinesterase is present in nerve tissue, the spleen, RBCs, and the gray matter of the brain. It inactivates acetylcholine at nerve junctions and helps transmit impulses across nerve endings to muscle fibers.

Is something bugging you?

The cholinesterase test has a number of purposes, one of which is to assess for overexposure to insecticides that contain organophosphates.

What it all means

Pseudocholinesterase levels range from 204 to 532 International Units/dl (SI, 2.04 to 5.32 kU/L). Acetylcholinesterase levels are 30 to 40 units/g Hb.

How low can you go?

Pseudocholinesterase levels are usually normal in early extrahepatic obstruction and decreased in hepatocellular damage, such as hepatitis or cirrhosis. Levels also decline in acute infections, chronic malnutrition, anemia, MI, obstructive jaundice, and metastasis.

Very low pseudocholinesterase levels suggest a congenital deficiency or organophosphate insecticide poisoning; levels near zero necessitate emergency treatment. (See *Cholinesterase test interference*.)

Increased acetylcholinesterase levels may occur in sickle-cell and hemolytic anemias. Decreased acetylcholinesterase levels may indicate megaloblastic anemia or organic phosphate poisoning.

What needs to be done

• Perform a venipuncture, and collect the sample in a 7-ml red-top tube, or in a designated tube volume in accordance with laboratory protocol.
• If the sample can't be sent to the laboratory within 6 hours after being drawn, refrigerate it.
• Resume administration of medications discontinued before the test, as ordered.

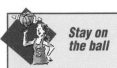

Stay on the ball

Cholinesterase test interference

Cyclophosphamide, echothiophate iodide, monoamine oxidase inhibitors, succinylcholine, neostigmine, quinidine, chloroquine, caffeine, theophylline, epinephrine, ether, barbiturates, atropine, morphine, codeine, phenothiazines, vitamin K, and folic acid can falsely depress levels.

Glucose-6-phosphate dehydrogenase

Glucose-6-phosphate dehydrogenase (G6PD), an enzyme found in most body cells, is part of a pathway that metabolizes glucose. The G6PD test, which measures serum G6PD levels, tests for deficiency of this enzyme. G6PD deficiency is a hereditary, sex-linked condition carried on the female X chromosome (with clinical disease found mostly in males) that impairs the stability of the RBC membrane and makes RBCs susceptible to destruction by strong oxidizing agents.

What it all means

Serum G6PD values vary with the measurement method used but usually range from 4.3 to 11.8 units/g (SI, 0.28 to 0.76 milliunits/mmol) of Hb). They may also be reported simply as normal or abnormal.

Fluorescent spot testing or staining for Heinz bodies or erythrocytes can test for G6PD deficiency. If results are positive, the kinetic quantitative assay for G6PD may be performed. Electrophoretic techniques assess genetic variants of deficiencies (which may cause lifelong, mild, or asymptomatic anemia). Some variants are symptomatic only when the patient experiences stress or illness or is exposed to drugs or agents that elicit hemolytic episodes. (See *G6PD test interference*.)

What needs to be done

- Perform a venipuncture, and collect the sample in a 4-ml tube containing EDTA, or in a designated tube volume in accordance with laboratory protocol.
- Completely fill the collection tube, and invert it gently several times to mix the sample and anticoagulant.
- If the sample can't be sent to the laboratory immediately, refrigerate it.

Stay on the ball

G6PD test interference

These factors may alter G6PD test results:
- Aspirin, sulfonamides, nitrofurantoin, vitamin K derivative, primaquine, and fava beans decrease G6PD enzyme activity and precipitate hemolytic episodes.
- Performing the test after a hemolytic episode or a blood transfusion can cause false-negative results.

It's all in the family; G6PD deficiency is a hereditary condition.

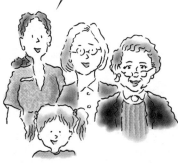

Pyruvate kinase

The erythrocyte enzyme pyruvate kinase (PK) takes part in the anaerobic metabolism of glucose. Abnormally low PK levels are inherited as an autosomal recessive trait and may result in an erythrocyte membrane defect associated with congenital hemolytic anemia.

Although PK deficiency is fairly uncommon, it's the most prevalent congenital hemolytic anemia after G6PD deficiency. PK assay confirms PK deficiency when RBC enzyme deficiency is the suspected cause of anemia.

What it all means

In a routine assay, serum PK levels range from 9 to 22 units/g of Hb; in the low substrate assay, they range from 1.7 to 6.8 units/g of Hb.

Low serum PK levels confirm a diagnosis of PK deficiency and allow differentiation between PK-deficient hemolytic anemia and other inherited disorders. (See *PK test interference.*)

What needs to be done

• Perform a venipuncture, and collect the sample in a 4-ml tube containing EDTA, or in a designated tube volume in accordance with laboratory protocol.
• Completely fill the collection tube, and invert it gently several times to mix the sample and anticoagulant.
• Refrigerate the sample if it can't be sent to the laboratory immediately.

Stay on the ball

PK test interference

These factors may alter pyruvate kinase (PK) test results:
• failure to notify the laboratory of a recent blood transfusion
• removal of white blood cells (WBCs) from the sample by the laboratory to prevent false results. (PK levels in WBCs remain normal in hemolytic anemia.)

Angiotensin-converting enzyme

The angiotensin-converting enzyme (ACE) test measures serum levels of ACE, an enzyme found in high concentrations in lung capillaries and in lesser concentrations in blood vessels and kidney tissue. Its primary function is to help regulate arterial pressure by converting angiotensin I to angiotensin II, a powerful vasoconstrictor.

What it all means

Normal serum ACE values for patients age 20 and older range from 8 to 52 units/L (SI, 0.14 to 0.88 µkat/L).

The lowdown on levels

Elevated serum ACE levels may indicate sarcoidosis (a disease characterized by granular tumors that affect any organ or tissue), Gaucher's disease, or Hansen's disease (leprosy), but results must be correlated with the patient's clinical condition. In some patients, elevated ACE levels may result from hyperthyroidism, diabetic retinopathy, or liver disease.

Serum ACE levels decline as the patient responds to steroid or prednisone therapy for sarcoidosis.

What needs to be done

• If the patient is younger than age 20, ask the doctor about postponing the test because ACE levels vary in a patient younger than age 20.

Remember to correlate high serum ACE levels with the patient's existing clinical condition.

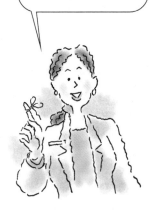

- Instruct the patient to fast for 12 hours before the test.
- Avoid using a collection tube with EDTA because this can decrease ACE levels, altering test results.
- Perform a venipuncture, and collect the sample in a 7-ml clot-activator tube, or in a designated tube volume in accordance with laboratory protocol.
- Note the patient's age on the laboratory request; send the sample to the laboratory immediately, or freeze it and place it on dry ice until the test can be done.

Lipids and lipoproteins

Triglycerides

Serum triglyceride testing provides quantitative analysis of triglycerides, the main storage form of lipids, which constitute about 95% of fatty tissue. Although not in itself diagnostic, serum triglyceride analysis permits early identification of hyperlipidemia (characteristic in nephrotic syndrome and other conditions) and determination of the risk of coronary artery disease (CAD).

What it all means

Triglyceride values are age- and sex-related. Some controversy exists over the most appropriate normal ranges. Nonetheless, serum values of 40 to 180 mg/dl (SI, 0.44 to 2.01 mmol/L) for adult males and 10 to 190 mg/dl (SI, 0.11 to 2.21 mmol/L) for adult females are widely accepted.

Increased or decreased serum triglyceride levels merely suggest a clinical abnormality; additional tests are required for a definitive diagnosis. For example, measurement of cholesterol may also be necessary, because cholesterol and triglyceride levels vary independently. High levels of triglyceride and cholesterol reflect an increased risk of CAD.

Increased levels: Mild, moderate, and severe

A mild to moderate increase in serum triglyceride levels may indicate biliary obstruction, diabetes, nephrotic syndrome, endocrine disorders, or overconsumption of alcohol. Markedly increased levels without an identifiable cause reflect congenital hyperlipoproteinemia and necessitate lipoprotein phenotyping to confirm the diagnosis.

Decreased levels

Decreased serum levels are rare, occurring mainly in malnutrition or abetalipoproteinemia (a rare inherited disease characterized by defective apoprotein B synthesis). In the latter, serum is virtually devoid of beta lipoproteins and triglycerides because the body lacks the capacity to transport preformed triglycerides from the epithelial cells of the intestinal mucosa or from the liver. (See *Triglyceride test interference.*)

What needs to be done

• Be sure to inform the practitioner if the patient has an acute illness, infection, fever, or other acute problem that might interfere with the laboratory result.
• Because triglycerides are highly affected by a fat-containing meal, with levels rising and peaking 4 hours after ingesting a meal, tell the patient that he should abstain from food for 10 to 14 hours before the test and from alcohol for 24 hours but that he may drink water.
• Have the patient sit down for 5 minutes before drawing the blood.
• Perform a venipuncture, collect a sample in a 4-ml tube containing EDTA, or in a designated tube volume in accordance with laboratory protocol, and send the sample to the laboratory immediately.

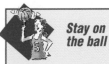

Stay on the ball

Triglyceride test interference

• Alcohol ingestion within 24 hours of the test may cause elevated triglyceride levels.
• Long-term use of corticosteroids increases triglyceride levels, as do hormonal contraceptives, estrogen, ethyl alcohol, furosemide, and miconazole. (Cholestyramine and colestipol hydrochloride either raise or have no effect on triglycerides.)
• Clofibrate, dextrothyroxine, gemfibrozil, and niacin lower triglyceride levels.

Total cholesterol

The total serum cholesterol test measures the circulating levels of free cholesterol and cholesterol esters; it reflects the level of the two forms in which this biochemical compound appears in the body.

What it all means

Total cholesterol levels vary with age and sex. Total cholesterol values for adults and children are:
• *adults:* desirable: less than 205 mg/dl (SI, less than 5.30 mmol/L) for women and less than 190 mg/dl (SI, less than 4.90 mmol/L)
• *children ages 12 to 18:* desirable: less than 170 mg/dl (SI, less than 4.4 mmol/L); high: greater than 200 mg/dl (SI, greater than 5.15 mmol/L).

Keep the risk in context

The cholesterol level needs to be evaluated in the context of the entire risk factor analysis for each patient. If the level is abnormal, a second cholesterol test should be completed 1 week later to verify the results. Marked fluctuations can occur from day to day. A decision to begin treatment will be based on the number of risk factors and a patient's prior cardiovascular history. (See *VAP cholesterol test*.)

Danger signs

An elevated serum cholesterol level (hypercholesterolemia) may indicate an increased risk of CAD as well as impending hepatitis, lipid disorders, bile duct blockage, nephrotic syndrome, obstructive jaundice, pancreatitis, and hypothyroidism. Hypercholesterolemia associated with increased intake of fats and cholesterol-rich foods requires dietary changes and, possibly, medication to slow absorption of cholesterol.

A low serum cholesterol level (hypocholesterolemia) is commonly associated with malnutrition, cellular necrosis of the liver, or hyperthyroidism.

Getting to the heart of the matter

Abnormal cholesterol levels commonly require further testing to pinpoint the causative disorder, depending on the type of abnormality and the presence of overt signs. Abnormal levels associated with cardiovascular diseases, for example, may require lipoprotein phenotyping. (See *Total cholesterol test interference*.)

What needs to be done

• Fasting isn't necessary for isolated cholesterol checks or screening, but it's required if the check is part of a lipid profile. If fasting is required, instruct the patient to abstain from food and drink for 12 hours before the test.

Stay on the ball

Total cholesterol test interference

These factors may alter total cholesterol test results:

• cholestyramine, clofibrate, colestipol, dextrothyroxine, haloperidol, neomycin, niacin, and chlortetracycline, which lower cholesterol levels; epinephrine, chlorpromazine, trifluoperazine, hormonal contraceptives, and trimethadione, which raise cholesterol levels; androgens, which may have a variable effect on cholesterol levels
• certain vitamins (such as vitamin E) that may cause false elevations.

VAP cholesterol test

The VAP (Vertical Auto Profile) cholesterol test is a new cholesterol test that improves testing for risk of coronary heart disease and management. It measures patients at risk as well as new emerging lipid risk factors (total cholesterol, low-density lipoprotein, high-density lipoprotein, very-low-density lipoprotein, and cholesterol subclasses).

The VAP enables specific treatment initiatives to be geared toward the patient. Because lipoprotein response to treatment can vary, additional information provided by the VAP can help determine the most appropriate therapy, such as drug choice and the intensity of risk-reduction therapy.

• Perform a venipuncture, and collect the sample in a 4-ml tube containing EDTA, or in a designated tube volume in accordance with laboratory protocol. The patient should be in a sitting position for 5 minutes before the blood is drawn.
• Fingersticks can also be used for initial screening when using an automated analyzer. Document any drugs the patient is taking.
• Send the sample to the laboratory immediately.

Lipoprotein-cholesterol fractionation

Lipoprotein fractionation tests are used to isolate and measure the types of cholesterol in serum, low-density lipoproteins (LDLs), and high-density lipoproteins (HDLs). The HDL level is inversely related to the risk of CAD; the higher the HDL level, the lower the incidence of CAD. Conversely, the higher the LDL level, the higher the incidence of CAD.

What it all means

LDL cholesterol

For individuals who don't have CAD, desirable levels are less than 130 mg/dl (SI, less than 3.36 mmol/L) and borderline high levels are greater than 160 mg/dl (SI, greater than 3.30 mmol/L). According to the American College of Cardiology, optimal LDL levels are less than 100 mg/dl (SI, less than 2.6 mmol/L), with levels of 160 mg/dl or more considered high (SI, greater than 3.30 mmol/L).

HDL cholesterol

In males, these values range from 37 to 70 mg/dl (SI, 0.96 to 1.8 mmol/L); in females, from 40 to 85 mg/dl (SI, 1.03 to 2.2 mmol/L). The American College of Cardiology recommends an HDL level of 40 mg/dl or higher in females. HDL levels greater than 60 mg/dl are optional.

The lowdown on levels

Decreased LDL levels can occur during acute stress (illness, burns, MI), inflammatory joint disease, chronic pulmonary disease, and myeloma. Decreased HDL levels are commonly seen in patients with hypertriglyceridemia. The HDL level may increase if the elevated triglyceride level is treated.

High LDL levels increase the risk of CAD. Elevated HDL levels generally reflect a healthy state, but they can also indicate chronic hepatitis, early-stage primary biliary cirrhosis, or alcohol consumption. Rarely, a sharp rise (to as high as 100 mg/dl [SI, 2.58 mmol/L]) indicates a second type of HDL (alpha-HDL) that may signal CAD. (See *Lipoprotein-cholesterol fractionation test interference.*)

What needs to be done

• Tell the patient to maintain a normal diet for 2 weeks before the test.
• Tell the patient to abstain from alcohol for 24 hours before the test and to fast and avoid exercise for 12 to 14 hours before the test.
• As ordered, tell the patient to discontinue use of thyroid hormone, hormonal contraceptives, and antilipemic agents until after the test because they alter test results.
• Perform a venipuncture, and collect the sample in a 7-ml tube containing EDTA, or in a designated tube volume in accordance with laboratory protocol.
• Send the sample to the laboratory immediately to avoid spontaneous redistribution among the lipoproteins. If the sample can't be transported immediately, refrigerate it but don't allow it to freeze.

Lipoprotein electrophoresis

Lipoprotein electrophoresis, also known as *lipoprotein phenotyping* and *lipid fractionalization*, is used to determine levels of four major lipoproteins: chylomicrons, very-low-density lipoproteins (VLDLs), LDLs, and HDLs. Classification of patients by the pattern of their lipoprotein levels identifies hyperlipoproteinemias and hypolipoproteinemias.

What it all means

Normal results aren't applicable for this test. The types of hyperlipoproteinemias or hypolipoproteinemias are identified by their characteristic electrophoretic patterns. The laboratory reports the type of lipoproteinemia present. Familial lipoprotein disorders are classified as either hyperlipoproteinemias or hypolipoproteinemias. (See *Classifying familial hyperlipoproteinemias*, page 88.)

Six types

The hyperlipoproteinemias break down into six types—I, IIa, IIb, III, IV, and V. Types IIa, IIb, and IV are relatively common. In contrast, all hypolipoproteinemias are rare; they include hypobetalipoproteinemia, abetalipoproteinemia (Bassen-Kornzweig syndrome), and alpha lipoprotein deficiency (Tangier disease). (See *Lipoprotein electrophoresis interference*, page 89.)

Stay on the ball

Lipoprotein-cholesterol fractionation test interference

• Antilipemic medications, such as clofibrate, cholestyramine, colestipol, niacin, and gemfibrozil, lower values.
• Hormonal contraceptives, disulfiram, alcohol, miconazole, and high doses of phenothiazines increase values.
• Estrogens, bilirubin, hemoglobin, salicylates, iodine, vitamins A and D, and concurrent illness may alter test results.

Classifying familial hyperlipoproteinemias

Type	Causes and incidence	Laboratory findings
I	• Deficient lipoprotein lipase, resulting in increased chylomicrons • May be induced by alcoholism • Incidence: rare	• Increased chylomicron, total cholesterol, and triglyceride levels • Normal or slightly increased very-low-density lipoprotein (VLDL) levels • Normal or decreased low-density lipoprotein (LDL) levels and high-density lipoprotein levels • Cholesterol-triglyceride ratio under 0.2
IIa	• Deficient cell receptor, resulting in increased LDL levels and excessive cholesterol synthesis • May be induced by hypothyroidism • Incidence: common	• Increased LDL levels • Normal VLDL levels • Cholesterol-triglyceride ratio over 2.0
IIb	• Deficient cell receptor, resulting in increased LDL levels and excessive cholesterol synthesis • May be induced by dysgammaglobulinemia, hypothyroidism, uncontrolled diabetes mellitus, or nephrotic syndrome • Incidence: common	• Increased LDL, VLDL, total cholesterol, and triglyceride levels
III	• Unknown cause, resulting in deficient VLDL-to-LDL conversion • May be induced by hypothyroidism, uncontrolled diabetes mellitus, or paraproteinemia • Incidence: rare	• Increased total cholesterol, VLDL, and triglyceride levels • Normal or decreased LDL levels • Cholesterol-triglyceride ratio of VLDL over 0.4 • Broad beta band observed on electrophoresis
IV	• Unknown cause, resulting in decreased levels of lipoprotein lipase • May be induced by uncontrolled diabetes mellitus, alcoholism, pregnancy, steroid or estrogen therapy, dysgammaglobulinemia, or hyperthyroidism • Incidence: common	• Increased VLDL and triglyceride levels • Normal LDL • Cholesterol-triglyceride ratio of VLDL under 0.25
V	• Unknown cause, resulting in defective triglyceride clearance • May be induced by alcoholism, dysgammaglobulinemia, uncontrolled diabetes mellitus, nephrotic syndrome, pancreatitis, or steroid therapy • Incidence: rare	• Increased VLDL total cholesterol and triglyceride levels • Chylomicrons present • Cholesterol-triglyceride ratio under 0.6

What needs to be done

• Check the patient's drug history for use of heparin. Notify the laboratory if the patient is hospitalized for any other condition that might significantly alter lipoprotein metabolism, such as diabetes mellitus, nephrosis, or hypothyroidism.
• As ordered, withhold antilipemics, such as cholestyramine, for about 2 weeks before the test.
• Instruct the patient to abstain from alcohol for 24 hours before the test, eat a low-fat meal the night before the test, and then begin fasting at midnight.
• Perform a venipuncture, and collect the sample in a 4-ml tube containing EDTA, or in a designated tube volume in accordance with laboratory protocol.
• When drawing multiple samples, collect the sample for lipoprotein electrophoresis first, if possible, because venous obstruction by the tourniquet for 2 minutes (while other blood samples are being drawn) can affect test results.
• Fill the collection tube completely, and invert it gently several times to mix the sample and the anticoagulant adequately.

Stay on the ball

Lipoprotein electrophoresis interference

These factors may alter lipoprotein electrophoresis results:
• failure to observe dietary and alcohol restrictions or recent use of antilipemics, which lower lipid levels
• administration of heparin (which activates the enzyme lipase, producing fatty acids from triglycerides) or collection of the sample in a heparinized tube, which may falsely elevate values.

Other chemistry tests

Bilirubin

The serum bilirubin test measures serum levels of bilirubin. The main pigment in bile, bilirubin is the major product of Hb catabolism. Serum bilirubin values are especially significant in neonates because excessive unconjugated bilirubin can accumulate in the brain, causing irreversible damage.

What it all means

In adults, indirect serum bilirubin measures 1.1 mg/dl (SI, 19 µmol/L) or less; direct serum bilirubin measures less than 0.5 mg/dl (SI, less than 6.8 µmol/L). In neonates, total serum bilirubin measures 2 to 12 mg/dl (SI, 34 to 205 µmol/L).

Abnormal indirect level

Elevated indirect serum bilirubin levels commonly indicate hepatic damage in which the cells can no longer conjugate bilirubin. Consequently, indirect bilirubin reenters the bloodstream. High levels of indirect bilirubin are also common in patients with severe hemolytic anemia, when excessive indirect bilirubin overwhelms the liver's conjugating mechanism. If hemolysis continues, both direct and indirect bilirubin may rise. Other causes of elevated indirect bilirubin levels include congenital enzyme deficiency, such as Gilbert disease or Crigler-Najjar syndrome.

Abnormal direct level

Elevated direct serum bilirubin levels usually indicate biliary obstruction, in which direct bilirubin, blocked from its normal pathway from the liver into the biliary tree, overflows into the bloodstream. If the obstruction continues, both direct and indirect bilirubin eventually may be elevated because of hepatic damage. In severe chronic hepatic damage, direct bilirubin concentrations may return to normal or near-normal levels but elevated indirect bilirubin levels persist. (See *Bilirubin test interference.*)

All about jaundice

In neonates, total bilirubin levels that reach or exceed 15 mg/dl (SI, 257 µmol/L) indicate the need for an exchange transfusion. Notify the practitioner immediately of the results so prompt action can be taken.

What needs to be done

• Instruct the adult patient to fast for at least 4 hours before the test, although he may drink fluids. (Fasting isn't necessary for neonates.)
• If the patient is an adult, perform a venipuncture and collect the sample in a 3- or 4-ml clot-activator tube, or in a designated tube volume in accordance with laboratory protocol.
• If the patient is a neonate, perform a heelstick and fill the microcapillary tube to the designated level with blood.
• Protect the sample from strong sunlight and ultraviolet light because bilirubin breaks down when exposed to light.
• Send the sample to the laboratory immediately.

Stay on the ball

Bilirubin test interference

These factors may decrease bilirubin levels:
• exposure of the specimen to sunlight or high-intensity artificial light for 1 hour or more
• air bubbles and shaking of the specimen
• high-fat meal
• contrast media administered in the prior 24 hours.
    Prolonged fasting and anorexia may increase bilirubin levels.

Are you ready to see what you've learned about blood chemistry tests? You'll be quizzed soon, so get ready!

Homocysteine

Homocysteine, a sulfur-containing amino acid, is a transmethylation product of methionine. It's an intermediate in the synthesis of cysteine, which is produced by the enzymatic or acid hydrolysis of proteins. The test is useful for the biochemical diagnosis of inborn errors of methionine, folate, and vitamins B_6 and B_{12} metabolism.

What it all means

Normal total homocysteine levels are 0.54 to 2.30 mg/L (SI, 4 to 17 µmol/L) for fasting specimens.

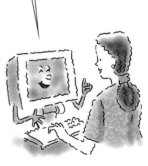

The lowdown on levels

Low homocysteine levels are associated with inborn or acquired folate or cobalamin deficiency and inborn vitamins B_6 or B_{12} deficiency.

Elevated homocysteine levels are associated with a higher incidence of atherosclerotic vascular disease. In patients with type 2 diabetes mellitus, studies have shown that homocysteine levels increase with even a modest deterioration in renal function. (See *Homocysteine test interference*.)

What needs to be done

• Perform a venipuncture, and collect the sample in a 5-ml tube containing EDTA, or in a designated tube volume in accordance with laboratory protocol.
• Send the sample to the laboratory immediately to be frozen in a plastic vial on dry ice.

Stay on the ball

Homocysteine test interference

• Penicillamine reduces homocysteine levels.
• Nitrous oxide, methotrexate deficiency, and 6-azauridine increase homocysteine levels.

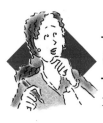

Quick quiz

1. Which therapy may suppress serum potassium levels?
   A.   Penicillin G therapy
   B.   Spironolactone therapy
   C.   Insulin and glucose administration
   D.   Blood administration

Answer: C. Insulin and glucose administration, diuretic therapy, or I.V. infusions without potassium suppress serum potassium levels.

2. A patient's serum sodium level is 130 mEq/L (SI, 130 mmol/L). You should interpret that result as:
   A.   below normal.
   B.   normal.
   C.   above normal.
   D.   exceedingly above normal.

Answer: A. Normally, serum sodium levels range from 135 to 145 mEq/L (SI, 135 to 145 mmol/L).

3. Chloride levels relate inversely to which of the following?

    A.   Bicarbonate

    B.   Magnesium

    C.   Potassium

    D.   Carbon dioxide

Answer: A. Chloride levels relate inversely to those of bicarbonate and thus reflect acid-base balance.

4. Which action may cause a false decrease in serum bilirubin levels?

    A.   Exposing the blood sample to room temperature

    B.   Exposing the blood sample to direct sunlight

    C.   Sulfonamide therapy

    D.   Freezing the sample

Answer: B. Exposing the sample to direct sunlight or ultraviolet light may depress the bilirubin serum level.

Scoring

⭐⭐⭐   If you answered all four questions correctly, fantastic! Your knowledge shows excellent bloodlines.

⭐⭐   If you answered three questions correctly, good job! You're more persistent than a bloodhound.

⭐   If you answered fewer than three questions correctly, take heart! You can always try again.

Hormone tests

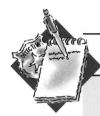

Just the facts

In this chapter, you'll learn:

♦ about hormone tests and how they're performed

♦ the patient care associated with hormone tests

♦ factors that can interfere with these tests

♦ what hormone test results may indicate.

A look at hormone tests

Hormones are substances that control activities of various tissues throughout the body. They act by altering the rate of synthesis and secretion of enzymes or other hormones, affecting the rate of enzymatic chemical reactions and altering cell membrane permeability. Each hormone is important to the overall functioning of the body.

Taking care of business

When performing hormone tests, make sure that the patient is comfortable and that he understands the test to be performed. Use clear, simple language and avoid jargon. Inform him that the needle puncture might cause some brief discomfort and that he may feel brief pressure from the tourniquet.

After the test is over

Be sure to label blood samples clearly, and handle them gently to prevent hemolysis. Also, check the venipuncture site for bleeding and, if a hematoma develops, apply warm soaks. If the hematoma is large, check circulation in the extremity distal to the venipuncture site.

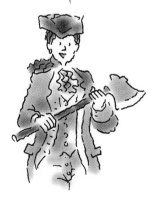

I cannot tell a lie: The needle may hurt a little.

Pituitary hormones

Corticotropin

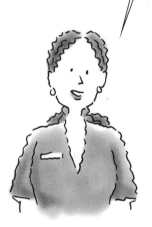

The corticotropin test helps diagnose adrenal dysfunction.

Corticotropin stimulates the adrenal cortex to secrete cortisol and, to a lesser degree, androgens and aldosterone. It increases the uptake of amino acids by muscle cells, promotes breakdown of fats, stimulates the pancreas to secrete insulin, and may contribute to the release of growth hormone. Corticotropin levels vary throughout the day; they typically peak between 6 a.m. and 8 a.m. and decline between 6 p.m. and 11 p.m.

The corticotropin test measures the plasma levels of corticotropin (also known as *adrenocorticotropic hormone,* or *ACTH*). The test may be ordered for patients with signs of adrenal hypofunction (insufficiency) or hyperfunction (also known as *Cushing's syndrome*).

What it all means

Baseline values at less than 120 pg/ml (SI, less than 26.4 pmol/L at 6 a.m. to 8 a.m.); these values may vary, however, depending on the laboratory.

The lowdown on levels

A higher-than-normal corticotropin level may indicate Addison's disease. In suspected Cushing's syndrome, an elevated corticotropin level suggests Cushing's disease. When corticotropin levels are moderately elevated, pituitary-dependent adrenal hyperplasia and nonadrenal tumors, such as oat cell carcinoma of the lungs, are suggested.

A low-normal corticotropin level suggests secondary adrenal hypofunction resulting from pituitary or hypothalamic dysfunction and implies adrenal hyperfunction due to adrenocortical tumor or hyperplasia. (See *Corticotropin test interference.*)

What needs to be done

• Withhold interfering medications for 48 hours or longer before the test. If they must be continued, note this on the laboratory slip.
• Provide a low-carbohydrate diet for 2 days before the test.
• The patient must fast and limit his physical activity for 10 to 12 hours before the test.

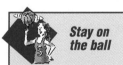

Stay on the ball

Corticotropin test interference

• Corticosteroids, dexamethasone, ethanol, and lithium carbonate can lower levels.
• Estrogens, calcium gluconate, and levodopa can increase levels.

- For a patient with suspected adrenal hypofunction, perform the venipuncture for a baseline level between 6 a.m. and 8 a.m. (peak secretion).
- For a patient with suspected Cushing's syndrome, perform the venipuncture between 6 p.m. and 11 p.m. (low secretion).
- Collect the sample in a plastic tube or in a tube with EDTA.
- Make sure the tube is full because excess anticoagulant will affect the results.
- Pack the sample in ice, and send it to the laboratory immediately to ensure reliable test results. A temperature of 39.2° F (4° C) is necessary to retard enzyme activity.

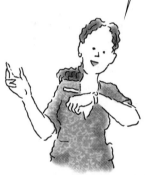

The rapid corticotropin test provides faster results to help identify primary and secondary adrenal hypofunction.

Rapid corticotropin

The rapid corticotropin test, also known as the *rapid ACTH test* or *cosyntropin test*, is gradually replacing the 8-hour corticotropin stimulation test as the most effective diagnostic tool for evaluating adrenal hypofunction. It provides faster results and causes fewer allergic reactions than the 8-hour test.

Back to baselines

This test requires baseline cortisol levels to evaluate the effect of cosyntropin administration on cortisol secretion. When morning cortisol levels are clearly high, adrenal hypofunction is ruled out and further testing isn't necessary.

What it all means

Normally, cortisol levels rise after 30 or 60 minutes to a peak of 18 mcg/dl (SI, 500 mmol/L) or more after the cosyntropin injection. Generally, a doubled baseline cortisol value indicates a normal response and eliminates the possibility of adrenal hypofunction or insufficiency.

Hypofunction junction

In patients with primary adrenal hypofunction (Addison's disease), cortisol levels remain low. If test results show below-normal increases in cortisol levels, stimulation of the adrenal cortex may be required for a longer period to determine whether the patient has primary or secondary adrenal hypofunction. (See *Rapid corticotropin test interference.*)

What needs to be done

- The patient may be required to fast for 10 to 12 hours before the test and must be relaxed and resting quietly for 30 minutes before the test. Tell the patient that the test will take at least 1 hour.

Stay on the ball

Rapid corticotropin test interference

- Estrogens and amphetamines increase levels.
- Lithium carbonate decreases levels.
- Radioactive scan within 1 week before the test may alter results.

- Draw 5 ml of blood for a baseline value in a 5-ml heparinized tube labeled "preinjection," or a tube volume in accordance with laboratory policy, and send it to the laboratory.
- Inject 250 mcg (0.25 mg) of cosyntropin I.V. (directly, over 2 minutes).
- Draw another 5 ml (or a tube volume in accordance with laboratory policy) of blood at 30 and 60 minutes after the cosyntropin injection in 5-ml heparinized tubes labeled with the exact draw time and "30 minutes postinjection" and "60 minutes postinjection," respectively. Send the samples to the laboratory immediately.
- Observe the patient for signs of allergic reaction to cosyntropin, such as hives, itching, and tachycardia.
- Tell the patient to resume his usual diet, activities, and medications as ordered.

Human growth hormone

Human growth hormone (hGH), also known as *growth hormone* and *somatotropin*, is a protein secreted by the anterior pituitary and is the primary regulator of human growth.

The hGH test, a quantitative analysis of plasma hGH levels, is usually performed as part of an anterior pituitary stimulation or suppression test. Such testing is crucial because clinical manifestations of an hGH deficiency can rarely be reversed by therapy.

What it all means

Normal hGH levels for men range from undetectable to 5 ng/ml (SI, 5 µg/L). Normal levels for women range from undetectable to 10 ng/ml (SI, 10 µg/L). Estrogen causes levels in women to be higher than levels in men. Children generally have higher hGH levels; these levels may range from undetectable to 16 ng/ml (SI, 16 µg/L).

The lowdown on levels

Increased hGH levels may indicate a pituitary or hypothalamic tumor (frequently an adenoma), which causes gigantism in children and acromegaly in adults and adolescents.

Patients with diabetes mellitus sometimes have elevated hGH levels without acromegaly. Suppression testing is necessary to confirm the diagnosis.

Pituitary infarction, metastatic disease, and tumors may reduce hGH levels. Dwarfism may be caused by low hGH levels, but confirmation of the diagnosis requires stimulation testing with arginine or insulin. (See *Growth hormone test interference.*)

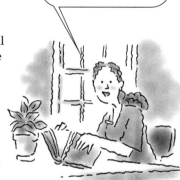

The hGH test helps diagnose dwarfism and pituitary or hypothalamic tumors and helps monitor hGH therapy.

Stay on the ball

Growth hormone test interference

- Amphetamines, arginine, beta blockers, bromocriptine, dopamine, estrogens, glucagon, histamine, insulin, levodopa, methyldopa, nicotinic acid, and pituitary-based steroids may increase levels.
- Phenothiazines and corticosteroids may reduce levels.

What needs to be done

- Withhold all medications that affect hGH levels, such as pituitary-based steroids, as ordered. If these medications must be continued, note this on the laboratory request.
- Tell the patient to fast and limit physical activity for 10 to 12 hours before the test.
- Make sure the patient is relaxed and recumbent for 30 minutes before the test because stress and physical activity elevate hGH levels.
- Tell the patient that another sample may have to be drawn the following day for comparison and that the laboratory requires at least 2 days for analysis.
- Between 6 a.m. and 8 a.m. on 2 consecutive days, or as ordered, draw venous blood into a 7-ml clot-activator tube, or a tube volume in accordance with laboratory policy, and send it to the laboratory.

Growth hormone suppression

Growth hormone suppression, also known as the *glucose loading test*, evaluates excessive baseline levels of hGH from the anterior pituitary by measuring the secretory response to a loading dose of glucose.

Secretion suppression

Normally, hGH raises plasma glucose and fatty acid concentrations; in response, insulin secretion increases to counteract these effects. A glucose load should suppress hGH secretion. In a patient with excessive hGH levels, the failure to suppress hGH indicates anterior pituitary dysfunction and confirms a diagnosis of acromegaly or gigantism.

The hGH suppression test helps assess elevated hGH levels and can confirm gigantism and acromegaly.

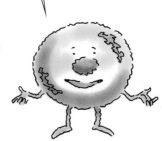

What it all means

Normally, glucose suppresses hGH to levels ranging from undetectable to 3 ng/ml (SI, 3 µg/L) in 30 minutes to 2 hours. In a patient with active acromegaly, elevated baseline levels of hGH levels (5 ng/ml [SI, 5 µg/L]) aren't suppressed after glucose loading. In children, rebound stimulation may occur after 2 to 5 hours.

Suspicion and repetition

When the hGH levels are unchanged or increased in response to glucose loading, hGH hypersecretion is indicated and may confirm suspected acromegaly or gigantism. This response may be verified by repeating the test after a 1-day rest. (See *Growth hormone suppression test interference.*)

What needs to be done

• Withhold all steroids—including estrogens and progestogens—and other pituitary-based hormones. If these or other medications must be continued, note this on the laboratory request.
• Tell the patient to fast for 10 to 12 hours before the test and that two blood samples will be drawn.
• Make sure the patient is relaxed and recumbent for 30 minutes before the test to prevent a false-high reading.
• Tell the patient that he may experience nausea after drinking the glucose solution and may feel some discomfort from the needle punctures. Tell him that the test takes about 1 hour.
• Between 6 a.m. and 8 a.m., draw 6 ml of venous blood (basal sample) into a 7-ml clot-activator tube or a tube volume in accordance with laboratory policy. Label the tube, and send it to the laboratory immediately.
• Administer 100 g of glucose solution by mouth. To prevent nausea, advise the patient to drink the glucose slowly.
• About 1 hour later, draw venous blood into a second 7-ml clot-activator tube, label the tube, and send it to the laboratory immediately.

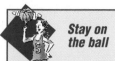

Stay on the ball

Growth hormone suppression test interference

• Amphetamines, arginine, estrogens, glucagon, levodopa, and niacin cause possible increased human growth hormone (hGH) secretion.
• Phenothiazines (chlorpromazine) and corticosteroids reduce hGH secretion.

Insulin tolerance

The insulin tolerance test measures serum levels of hGH and corticotropin after administration of a loading dose of insulin. It's more reliable than direct measurement of hGH and corticotropin. Normally, insulin-induced hypoglycemia stimulates hGH and corticotropin secretion. When stimulation fails, anterior pituitary or adrenal hypofunction is indicated and helps confirm an hGH or corticotropin insufficiency.

No-tolerance patients

Because the insulin tolerance test stimulates an adrenergic response, it isn't recommended for patients with cardiovascular or cerebrovascular disorders, epilepsy, or low basal plasma cortisol levels.

What it all means

Normally, blood glucose falls to 50% of the fasting level 20 to 30 minutes after insulin administration. This stimulates an increase of 10 to 20 ng/dl (SI, 10 to 20 µg/L) over baseline values in hGH and corticotropin, with peak levels occurring 60 to 90 minutes after insulin administration.

Reading responses

An increase in hGH levels of less than 10 ng/dl above baseline suggests hGH deficiency. However, a definitive diagnosis requires a supplementary stimulation test such as the arginine test. Additional testing is necessary to determine the site of the abnormality.

An increase in corticotropin levels of less than 10 ng/dl (SI, 10 µg/L) above baseline suggests adrenal insufficiency. The metyrapone or corticotropin stimulation test then confirms the diagnosis and determines whether insufficiency is primary or secondary. (See *Insulin tolerance test interference*.)

What needs to be done

- Instruct the patient to fast and restrict physical activity for 10 to 12 hours before the test.
- Tell the patient that he must remain relaxed and recumbent for 90 minutes before the test to prevent falsely elevated readings.
- Tell the patient that this test requires I.V. infusion of insulin and the collection of multiple blood samples.
- Warn the patient that he may experience an increased heart rate, diaphoresis, hunger, and anxiety after administration of insulin; these are transient, but if they become severe, the test will be discontinued.
- Between 6 a.m. and 8 a.m., collect three 5-ml samples of venous baseline samples, or a tube volume in accordance with laboratory policy—one in a tube with sodium fluoride and potassium oxalate for blood glucose (laboratory requirements may vary) and two in heparinized tubes for hGH and corticotropin.
- Next, administer an I.V. bolus of U-100 regular insulin (0.15 unit/kg or as ordered) over 1 to 2 minutes.
- Using an indwelling venous catheter, draw additional blood samples (as described previously) at 15, 30, 45, 60, 90, and 120 minutes after administration of insulin.

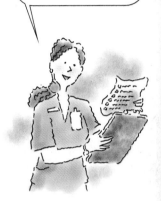

The insulin tolerance test helps diagnose hGH or corticotropin deficiency, pituitary dysfunction, and adrenal hypofunction.

Stay on the ball

Insulin tolerance test interference

- Corticosteroids and pituitary-based drugs elevate human growth hormone (hGH) levels; beta-adrenergic blockers and glucocorticoids depress hGH levels.
- Glucocorticoids, estrogens, calcium gluconate, amphetamines, methamphetamines, spironolactone, and ethanol depress corticotropin levels.

- Label the tubes appropriately, note the collection time on the laboratory request, and send samples to the laboratory immediately.
- Have concentrated glucose solution available in case the patient has a severe hypoglycemic reaction to insulin.

Serum follicle-stimulating hormone

A test of gonadal function that's performed more commonly in females than in males, the serum follicle-stimulating hormone (FSH) test is vital to infertility studies. To make a definitive diagnosis, FSH is typically combined with other hormone testing, such as luteinizing hormone (LH), estrogen, or progesterone. This test can also help diagnose precocious puberty in girls (before age 9) and in boys (before age 10), as well as aid in diagnosing hypogonadism.

Flirtin' with follicles

In females, FSH spurs development of primary ovarian follicles into graafian follicles for ovulation. Secretion varies daily, and it fluctuates during the menstrual cycle, peaking at ovulation. In males, continuous secretion of FSH and testosterone stimulates and maintains spermatogenesis (formation of mature, functional sperm). Plasma levels fluctuate widely in females; to obtain a true baseline level, daily testing may be necessary (for 3 to 5 days), or multiple samples may be drawn on the same day.

What it all means

Reference values vary greatly, depending on the patient's age, stage of sexual development, and—for a female—phase of her menstrual cycle. These approximate values are for menstruating females:

- *follicular phase:* 5 to 20 mIU/ml (SI, 5 to 20 International Units/L)
- *ovulatory phase:* 15 to 30 mIU/ml (SI, 15 to 30 International Units/L)
- *luteal phase:* 5 to 15 mIU/ml (SI, 5 to 15 International Units/L).

Approximate values for adult males are 5 to 20 mIU/ml (SI, 5 to 20 International Units/L); for menopausal females, 50 to 100 mIU/ml (SI, 50 to 100 International Units/L).

The lowdown on levels

Decreased FSH levels may cause male or female infertility. Low FSH levels may indicate secondary hypogonadotropic states, which can result from anorexia nervosa, panhypopituitarism, or hypothalamic lesions.

High FSH levels in females may indicate ovarian failure associated with Turner's syndrome (primary hypogonadism) or Stein-Leventhal syndrome (polycystic ovary syndrome). Elevated levels may occur in patients with precocious puberty (idiopathic or with central nervous system lesions) and in postmenopausal women. In males, abnormally high FSH levels may indicate destruction of the testes (from mumps, orchitis, or X-ray exposure), testicular failure, seminoma, or male climacteric. Congenital absence of the gonads and early-stage acromegaly may cause FSH levels to rise in both sexes. (See *FSH test interference*.)

What needs to be done

• Withhold medications, such as estrogens and progestogen, that may interfere with accurate determination of test results for 48 hours before the test. If these medications must be continued, note this on the laboratory request.
• Make sure the patient is relaxed and recumbent for 30 minutes before the test.
• Perform a venipuncture, preferably before 6 a.m. and 8 a.m., and collect a blood sample using a 7-ml clot-activator tube, or a tube volume in accordance with laboratory policy, and send the sample to the laboratory immediately.
• If the patient is female, indicate the phase of her menstrual cycle on the laboratory request. If she's menopausal, note this as well.

Stay on the ball

FSH test interference

• Ovarian steroid hormones, such as estrogen or progesterone, and related compounds, as well as phenothiazines (such as chlorpromazine), may possibly cause decrease of follicle-stimulating hormone (FSH).

Plasma luteinizing hormone

The plasma luteinizing hormone test (also called the *interstitial-cell-stimulating hormone test*) measures the amount of LH in the blood's serum. It's usually ordered for anovulation and infertility studies. For an accurate diagnosis, results must be evaluated in light of findings obtained from related hormone tests (FSH, estrogen, and testosterone levels, for example).

LH testing can detect ovulation, help assess infertility, and help monitor ovulation induction therapy.

Cycling by

In females, cyclic LH secretion (with FSH) causes ovulation and transforms the ovarian follicle into the corpus luteum which, in turn, secretes progesterone. (See *LH secretion cycle*, page 102.)

In males, continuous LH secretion stimulates the release of testosterone, which stimulates and maintains spermatogenesis (with FSH).

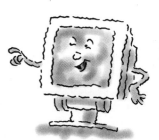

Now I get it!

LH secretion cycle

The menstrual cycle has three distinct phases: menstrual phase (days 1 to 5); proliferative, or follicular, phase (days 6 to 13); and, after ovulation on day 14, secretory, or luteal, phase (days 15 to 28). In a normal cycle, the menstrual phase is characterized by endometrial sloughing, corpus luteum degeneration, and new follicle growth. Estrogen and progesterone levels are low, triggering increased secretion of follicle-stimulating hormone (FSH) and luteinizing hormone (LH).

During the follicular phase, the follicle stimulated by FSH reaches full size and increases its estrogen secretion. Simultaneously, FSH decreases while LH increases slowly but steadily.

During the late follicular phase, LH rises sharply and FSH rises slightly. On about the 14th day, within hours of this abrupt LH surge, plasma estrogen levels drop and ovulation occurs. After ovulation, levels of both LH and FSH fall rapidly.

During the final, or luteal, phase, the follicle reorganizes as the corpus luteum and secretes progesterone and estrogen. Within 7 or 8 days after ovulation, if fertilization hasn't occurred, the corpus luteum regresses and progesterone and estrogen levels decrease. The endometrium sloughs, and the menstrual cycle begins again.

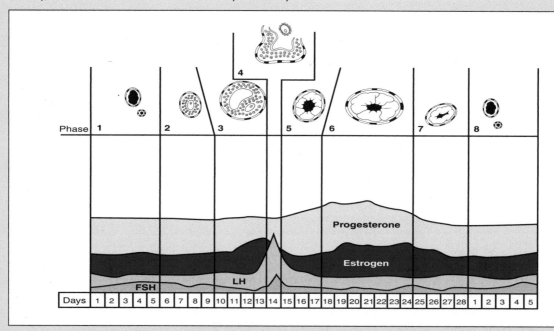

1. Menstrual phase (degeneration of corpus luteum)
2. Early follicular phase (development of follicle)
3. Late follicular phase (development of follicle)
4. Ovulation at midcycle (rupture of follicle)
5. Early luteal phase (development of corpus luteum)
6. Midluteal phase (development of corpus luteum)
7. Late luteal phase (development of corpus luteum)
8. Menstrual phase (degeneration of corpus luteum)

What it all means

Normal values vary widely:
- *adult women:* vary depending on the phase of the patient's menstrual cycle; follicular phase—5 to 15 mIU/ml (SI, 5 to 15 International Units/L); ovulatory phase—30 to 60 mIU/ml (SI, 30 to 60 International Units/L); luteal phase—5 to 15 mIU/ml (SI, 5 to 15 International Units/L)
- *postmenopausal women:* 50 to 100 mIU/ml (SI, 50 to 100 International Units/L)
- *adult men:* 5 to 20 mIU/ml (SI, 5 to 20 International Units/L)
- *children:* 4 to 20 mIU/ml (SI, 4 to 20 International Units/L).

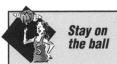

Stay on the ball

Plasma LH test interference

- Steroids, anticonvulsants, hormonal contraceptives, and digoxin may decrease levels.

Trouble for the ovaries

In females, absence of a midcycle peak in LH secretion may indicate anovulation. Decreased or low-normal levels may indicate hypogonadism, a finding commonly associated with amenorrhea. High LH levels may indicate congenital absence of ovaries or ovarian failure, which is associated with Stein-Leventhal syndrome (polycystic ovary syndrome), Turner's syndrome (ovarian dysgenesis), menopause, or early-stage acromegaly. Infertility can result from either primary or secondary gonadal dysfunction.

Dysfunction and failure

In males, low values may indicate secondary gonadal dysfunction (of hypothalamic or pituitary origin); high values may indicate testicular failure (primary hypogonadism) or destruction or congenital absence of testes. (See *Plasma LH test interference.*)

What needs to be done

- Withhold drugs, such as steroids (including estrogens or progesterone), that may interfere with plasma LH levels for 48 hours before the test. If these medications must be continued, note this on the laboratory request.
- Perform a venipuncture, collect the sample in a 7-ml clot-activator tube or a tube volume in accordance with laboratory policy, and send it to the laboratory immediately.
- If the patient is a female, indicate the phase of her menstrual cycle on the laboratory request. If the patient is menopausal, note this on the laboratory request.

Thyroid-stimulating hormone

Thyroid-stimulating hormone (TSH) is a protein secreted by the anterior pituitary. It stimulates an increase in the size, number, and secretory activity of thyroid cells; heightens "iodine pump activity," commonly raising the ratio of intracellular to extracellular iodine; and stimulates the release of triiodothyronine (T_3) and thyroxine (T_4). These hormones affect total body metabolism and are essential for normal growth and development.

Gettin' hip to hypothyroidism

This test, also known as the *serum thyrotropin test*, measures serum TSH levels by immunoassay. It can detect primary hypothyroidism and can determine whether it results from thyroid gland failure or from pituitary or hypothalamic dysfunction. Normal serum TSH levels rule out primary hypothyroidism. This test may not distinguish between low-normal and subnormal levels, especially in secondary hypothyroidism.

The thyrotropin-releasing hormone (TRH) challenge test evaluates thyroid function and can be performed after a baseline TSH reading has been obtained.

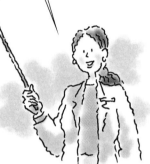

TSH levels can diagnose primary hypothyroidism and distinguish it from secondary hypothyroidism. They also help monitor therapy for hypothyroidism.

What it all means

Normal values for adults and children range from undetectable to 15 µIU/ml (SI, 15 mU/L). TSH levels that exceed 20 µIU/ml (SI, 20 mU/L) suggest primary hypothyroidism or, possibly, an endemic goiter (associated with dietary iodine deficiency). TSH levels may be slightly elevated in patients with normal thyroid function who have thyroid cancer.

Low TSH

Low or undetectable TSH levels may be normal but may occasionally indicate secondary hypothyroidism. Low TSH levels may also result from hyperthyroidism (Graves' disease) or thyroiditis. Testing with TRH is necessary to confirm the diagnosis.

What needs to be done

• Keep the patient relaxed and recumbent for 30 minutes before the test.
• As ordered, withhold steroids, thyroid hormones, aspirin, and other drugs that may influence test results. If these medications must be continued, note this on the laboratory request.
• Between 6 a.m. and 8 a.m., perform a venipuncture, collect the sample in a 5-ml clot-activator tube or a tube volume in accordance with laboratory policy, and send it to the laboratory immediately.

Neonatal thyroid-stimulating hormone

The neonatal TSH test, also known as the *neonatal thyrotropin test*, confirms congenital hypothyroidism after an initial screening test detects low T_4 levels.

The birth surge

TSH levels normally surge after birth and trigger a rise in thyroid hormone, which is essential for neurologic development. In primary congenital hypothyroidism, the thyroid gland doesn't respond to TSH stimulation, which results in lower thyroid hormone levels and higher TSH levels. Early detection and treatment of congenital hypothyroidism are critical to prevent mental retardation and cretinism.

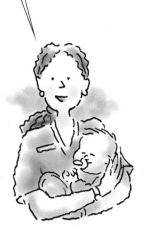

The neonatal TSH test can help diagnose congenital hypothyroidism. Early diagnosis and treatment can prevent permanent brain damage.

What it all means

At age 1 to 2 days, TSH levels are normally 25 to 30 µIU/ml (SI, 25 to 30 mU/L). At age 3 days and older, levels are normally less than 25 µIU/ml (SI, 25 mU/L).

The lowdown on levels

Neonatal TSH levels must be interpreted in light of T_4 concentrations. Elevated TSH that's accompanied by decreased T_4 indicates primary congenital hypothyroidism. Depressed TSH and depressed T_4 may be present in secondary congenital hypothyroidism. When TSH is normal and is accompanied by depressed T_4, it may indicate hypothyroidism caused by a congenital defect or it may indicate transient congenital hypothyroidism caused by prematurity or prenatal hypoxia. A complete thyroid workup must be done to confirm the cause of hypothyroidism before treatment can begin. (See *Neonatal TSH test interference*.)

What needs to be done

This test can be performed using samples collected from serum or from filter paper. (See *Collecting a filter paper sample*, page 106.)

For a serum sample, perform a venipuncture and collect the sample in a 3-ml clot-activator tube or a tube volume in accordance with laboratory policy. Label the sample, and send it to the laboratory immediately.

Stay on the ball

Neonatal TSH test interference

• Corticosteroids, triiodothyronine, and thyroxine lower thyroid-stimulating hormone (TSH) levels.

• Lithium carbonate, potassium iodide, excessive topical resorcinol, and TSH injection raise TSH levels.

Collecting a filter paper sample

To collect a specimen for neonatal thyroid-stimulating hormone testing using the filter paper method, gather the following equipment:
- alcohol or povidone-iodine swabs
- sterile lancet
- specially marked filter paper
- sterile 2″ × 2″ gauze pads
- adhesive bandage
- labels
- gloves.
  Then follow these easy steps:
- Assemble the necessary equipment, wash your hands thoroughly, and put on gloves.
- Wipe the infant's heel with an alcohol or povidone-iodine swab; then dry it thoroughly with a gauze pad.
- Perform a heelstick and squeeze the infant's heel gently, filling the circles on the filter paper with blood. Make sure the blood saturates the paper.
- Gently apply pressure with a gauze pad to ensure hemostasis at the puncture site.
- Allow the filter paper to dry, label it appropriately, and send it to the laboratory.

Thyroid and parathyroid hormones

Thyroxine

T_4 is an amine secreted by the thyroid gland in response to TSH from the pituitary and, indirectly, to TRH from the hypothalamus. The rate of secretion is normally regulated by a complex system of negative and positive feedback involving three glands: the thyroid, the anterior pituitary, and the hypothalamus. The suspected precursor, or prohormone, of T_3 is T_4, which is converted to T_3 mainly in the liver and kidneys.

The T_4 that binds

Only a fraction of T_4 (about 0.3%) circulates freely in the blood; the rest binds strongly to plasma proteins, primarily to thyroxine-binding globulin (TBG). This minute fraction of free-circulating T_4 is responsible for the clinical effects of thyroid hormone. TBG binds so tenaciously that T_4 survives in the plasma for a relatively long time, with a half-life of about 6 days. This test measures the total circulating T_4 level when TBG is normal.

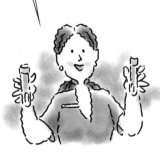

The T_4 test helps evaluate thyroid function and monitor thyroid replacement therapy.

What it all means

Normal total T_4 levels range from 5 to 13.5 mcg/dl (SI, 60 to 165 nmol/L). Normal T_4 levels don't guarantee normal thyroid functioning; for example, normal readings occur in T_3 thyrotoxicosis.

Results and further testing

Abnormally elevated levels of T_4 are consistent with primary and secondary hyperthyroidism, including excessive T_4 (levothyroxine) replacement therapy.

Subnormal levels of T_4 suggest primary or secondary hypothyroidism or T_4 suppression by normal, elevated, or replacement levels of T_3. Overt signs of hyperthyroidism require further testing, and in doubtful cases of hypothyroidism, the TSH or TRH test may be indicated. (See *T_4 test interference.*)

What needs to be done

• As ordered, withhold any medications that may interfere with test results. If these medications must be continued, note this on the laboratory request. (If this test is being performed to monitor thyroid therapy, the patient continues to receive daily thyroid supplements.)
• Perform a venipuncture, collect the sample in a 7-ml clot-activator tube or in a tube volume in accordance with laboratory policy, and send the sample to the laboratory immediately.

Stay on the ball

T_4 test interference

• Estrogens, progestins, levothyroxine, and methadone increase thyroxine (T_4) levels.
• Free fatty acids, heparin, iodides, liothyronine sodium, lithium, phenylbutazone, phenytoin, propylthiouracil, salicylates (high doses), steroids, sulfonamides, and sulfonylureas decrease T_4.
• Clofibrate can increase or decrease T_4.

Triiodothyronine

This highly specific immunoassay measures total serum content of T_3 to investigate clinical indications of thyroid dysfunction. T_3, the more potent thyroid hormone, is derived primarily from T_4. At least 50%, and as much as 90%, of T_3 is thought to be derived from T_4. The remaining 10% or more is secreted directly by the thyroid gland.

This test aids in the diagnosis of T_3 toxicosis, helps diagnose hypothyroidism or hyperthyroidism, and helps monitor the course of thyroid replacement therapy.

T_3 versus T_4

Like T_4 secretion, T_3 secretion occurs in response to TSH released by the pituitary and, secondarily, to TRH from the hypothalamus.

Although T_3 is present in the bloodstream in minute quantities and is metabolically active for only a short time, its impact on body metabolism dominates that of T_4. T_3 binds less firmly to TBG and therefore persists in the bloodstream for a short time—half of

The triiodothyronine test helps diagnose hypothyroidism and hyperthyroidism when TBG is normal.

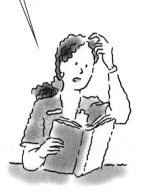

it disappears in about 1 day—whereas half of T_4 disappears in 6 days.

What it all means

Normally, serum T_3 levels range from 80 to 200 ng/dl (SI, 1.2 to 3 nmol/l).

Serum T_3 and T_4 levels usually rise and fall in tandem. However, in T_3 toxicosis, only T_3 levels rise while total and free T_4 levels remain normal. T_3 toxicosis occurs in patients with Graves' disease, toxic adenoma, or toxic nodular goiter. T_3 levels also surpass T_4 levels in patients receiving thyroid replacement containing more T_3 than T_4. In iodine-deficient areas, the thyroid may produce larger amounts of the more cellularly active T_3 than of T_4 in an effort to maintain the euthyroid state.

The lowdown on levels

Generally, T_3 levels appear to be a more accurate diagnostic indicator of hyperthyroidism than do T_4 levels. Although hyperthyroidism increases both T_3 and T_4 levels in about 90% of patients, it causes a disproportionate increase in T_3. In some patients with hypothyroidism, T_3 levels may fall within the normal range and may not be sufficient for diagnosis.

In pregnant patients, it's normal to see a rise in serum T_3 levels. Low T_3 levels may appear in euthyroid patients with systemic illness, during severe acute illness, or after trauma or major surgery; in such patients, however, TSH levels are within normal limits. Low serum T_3 levels are also sometimes found in euthyroid patients with malnutrition. (See *T_3 test interference*.)

What needs to be done

• As ordered, withhold medications that may influence thyroid function, such as steroids, propranolol, and cholestyramine. If such medications must be continued, record this information on the laboratory request.
• Perform a venipuncture, collect the sample in a 7-ml clot-activator tube or in a tube volume in accordance with laboratory policy, and send it to the laboratory immediately.
• If a patient must receive thyroid preparations such as T_3, note the time of drug administration on the laboratory request.

Thyroxine-binding globulin

The TBG test measures the serum level of TBG, the predominant protein carrier for circulating T_4 and T_3. TBG values may be identified by saturating the sample for TBG determination with radioac-

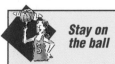

Stay on the ball

T_3 test interference

• Clofibrate, ethionamide, free fatty acids, heparin, iodides, lithium, methimazole, phenylbutazone, phenytoin, propranolol, propylthiouracil, reserpine, salicylates (high doses), steroids, and sulfonamides decrease triiodothyronine (T_3) levels.
• Clofibrate, estrogen, liothyronine sodium, methadone, and progestins increase T_3 levels.

tive T_4, then subjecting this sample to electrophoresis and quantitating the amount of TBG by the amount of radioactive T_4 bound or by radioimmunoassay.

The free Ts

Any condition that affects TBG levels and subsequent binding capacity also affects the amount of free T_4 (FT_4) and free T_3 (FT_3) in circulation. This can be clinically significant because only T_4 and FT_3 are metabolically active. If there's an underlying TBG abnormality, the tests for total T_3 and T_4 are rendered inaccurate; however, this doesn't alter results for FT_3 and FT_4.

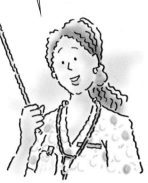

The TBG test helps evaluate abnormal thyrometabolic states that don't correlate with thyroid hormone values.

What it all means

Normal values for serum TBG by immunoassay range from 16 to 32 mcg/dl (SI, 120 to 180 mg/ml).

When TBGs are up...

Elevated TBG levels may indicate hypothyroidism and congenital excess, some forms of hepatic disease, or acute intermittent porphyria.

...and when they're down

Suppressed levels may indicate hyperthyroidism or congenital deficiency and can occur in active acromegaly, nephrotic syndrome, and malnutrition with hypoproteinemia, acute illness, or surgical stress.

Patients with TBG abnormalities require additional testing, such as the serum FT_3 and serum FT_4 tests, to evaluate thyroid function more precisely. (See *TBG test interference.*)

What needs to be done

• As ordered, withhold medications that may interfere with accurate testing, such as estrogens, anabolic steroids, phenytoin, salicylates, and thyroid preparations. If these medications must be continued, note this on the laboratory request.
• Perform a venipuncture, collect the sample in a 7-ml clot-activator tube or a tube volume in accordance with laboratory policy, and send it to the laboratory immediately.

Triiodothyronine uptake

The T_3 uptake test measures FT_4 levels. It does this indirectly by demonstrating the availability of serum protein-binding sites for T_4. The results of T_3 uptake are frequently combined with a T_4 radioimmunoassay or T_4 (D) (competitive protein-binding) test to

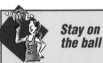

Stay on the ball

TBG test interference

• Estrogens and phenothiazines (perphenazine) elevate thyroxine-binding globulin (TBG) levels.
• Androgens, prednisone, phenytoin, and high doses of salicylates depress TBG levels.

determine the FT_4 index, a mathematical calculation that's thought to reflect FT_4 by correcting for thyroxine-TBG abnormalities.

The T_3 uptake test has become less popular recently because rapid tests for T_3, T_4, and TSH are readily available.

What it all means

Normal T_3 uptake values are 25% to 35%. In primary thyroid disease, T_4 uptake and T_3 uptake vary in the same direction: A high T_3 uptake percentage in the presence of elevated T_4 levels indicates hyperthyroidism. A low uptake percentage, together with low T_4 levels, indicates hypothyroidism.

Reading the variance

TBG abnormality is suggested when the variance in T_4 and T_3 uptake is conflicting. For example, a high T_3 uptake percentage and a low or normal FT_4 level suggests decreased TBG levels. Such decreased levels may result from protein loss (as in nephrotic syndrome), decreased production (due to androgen excess or genetic or idiopathic causes), or competition for T_4 binding sites by certain drugs (salicylates, phenylbutazone, and phenytoin).

Conversely, a low T_3 uptake percentage and a high or normal FT_4 level suggests increased TBG levels. Such increased levels may be caused by supplemental estrogen or estrogen produced by the body (pregnancy), or they may result from unknown causes. Thus, in primary disorders of TBG level, measured T_4 and free sites change in the same direction. (See *T_3 uptake test interference*.)

What needs to be done

• Withhold medications, such as estrogens, androgens, phenytoin, salicylates, and thyroid preparations that may interfere with test results. If they must be continued, note this on the laboratory request.

• Perform a venipuncture, collect the sample in a 7-ml clot-activator tube or a tube volume in accordance with laboratory policy, and send it to the laboratory immediately.

Free thyroxine and free triiodothyronine

These tests measure serum levels of FT_4 and FT_3, the minute portions of T_4 and T_3 not bound to TBG and other serum proteins.

Boundless hormones

As the active components of T_4 and T_3, these unbound hormones enter target cells and are responsible for the thyroid's effects on

---

Stay on the ball

T_3 uptake test interference

• Antithyroid agents, clofibrate, estrogen, hormonal contraceptives, and thiazide diuretics may decrease triiodothyronine (T_3) uptake.

The T_3 uptake test helps diagnose hypothyroidism, hyperthyroidism, and primary disorders of TBG levels.

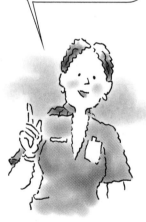

cellular metabolism. Because levels of circulating FT_4 and FT_3 are regulated by a feedback mechanism that compensates for changes in binding protein concentrations by adjusting total hormone levels, measurement of free hormone levels is the best indicator of thyroid function. Of the two tests, FT_3 is the better indicator. This test may be useful in the 5% of patients in whom the standard T_3 or T_4 tests fail to produce diagnostic results.

What it all means

Normal range for FT_4 is 0.9 to 2.3 ng/dl (SI, 10 to 30 nmol/L); for FT_3, 0.2 to 0.6 ng/dl (SI, 0.003 to 0.009 nmol/L). Values vary depending on the laboratory.

The lowdown on levels

Elevated FT_4 and FT_3 levels typically indicate hyperthyroidism. T_3 toxicosis, a distinct form of hyperthyroidism, yields high FT_3 levels, with normal or low FT_4 values. Low FT_4 levels usually indicate hypothyroidism, except in patients receiving replacement therapy with T_3. Patients receiving thyroid hormone replacement therapy may have varying levels of FT_4 and FT_3, depending on the preparation used and the time of sample collection. (See *FT_4 and FT_3 test interference.*)

What needs to be done

• Perform a venipuncture, collect the sample in a 7-ml clot-activator tube or a tube volume in accordance with laboratory policy, and send it to the laboratory immediately.

Plasma calcitonin

Plasma calcitonin, a radioimmunoassay, measures plasma levels of calcitonin (also known as *thyrocalcitonin*), a hormone secreted by specialized C cells of the thyroid gland in response to rising plasma calcium levels. Although the exact role of calcitonin in normal human physiology hasn't been determined, calcitonin is known to inhibit bone resorption by osteoclasts and osteocytes and to increase calcium excretion by the kidneys. Therefore, calcitonin acts as an antagonist to parathyroid hormone (PTH) and lowers serum calcium levels.

This test is usually indicated in suspected medullary carcinoma of the thyroid, which causes hypersecretion of calcitonin without associated hypocalcemia. Uncertain results require further testing with I.V. pentagastrin or calcium to rule out this disease.

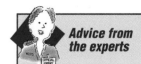

Advice from the experts

FT_4 and FT_3 test interference

Depending on the dosage, thyroid medication may increase levels. However, these medications shouldn't be withheld.

The plasma calcitonin test aids in the diagnosis of thyroid medullary carcinoma.

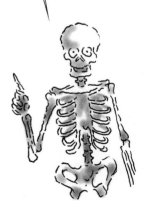

What it all means

Normal basal plasma calcitonin levels are:
- *males:* 40 pg/ml (SI, 40 ng/L)
- *females:* 20 pg/ml (SI, 20 ng/L).
    Values after testing with 4-hour calcium infusion are:
- *males:* 190 pg/ml (SI, 190 ng/L)
- *females:* 130 pg/ml (SI, 130 ng/L).
    Values after testing with pentagastrin infusion are:
- *males:* 110 pg/ml (SI, 110 ng/L)
- *females:* 30 pg/ml (SI, 30 ng/L).

Calcitonin and carcinoma

Elevated plasma calcitonin levels in the absence of hypocalcemia usually indicate thyroid cancer. Occasionally, increased calcitonin levels may be associated with ectopic calcitonin production resulting from oat cell cancer of the lung or from breast cancer.

What needs to be done

- Tell the patient to fast overnight.
- Perform a venipuncture, collect the sample in a 7-ml heparinized tube or a tube volume in accordance with laboratory policy, and send it to the laboratory immediately.

Parathyroid hormone

PTH, also known as *parathormone*, is secreted by the parathyroid glands and regulates plasma concentration of calcium and phosphorus.

Two tests are better than one

Currently, two tests are available to detect intact PTH and the N- and C-terminal fragments. Both tests can be used to confirm a diagnosis of hyperparathyroidism or hypoparathyroidism. The C-terminal PTH assay is more useful for diagnosing such chronic disturbances in PTH metabolism as secondary and tertiary hyperparathyroidism; it's also better for differentiating ectopic from primary hyperparathyroidism. The assay for intact PTH and the N-terminal fragment (both measured concomitantly) more accurately reflects acute changes in PTH metabolism and thus is useful in monitoring a patient's response to PTH therapy.

Measuring serum calcium, phosphorus, and creatinine levels with serum PTH is useful in identifying states of pathologic parathyroid function.

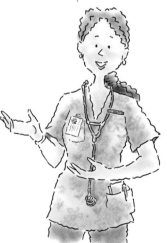

The PTH test helps diagnose parathyroid disorders.

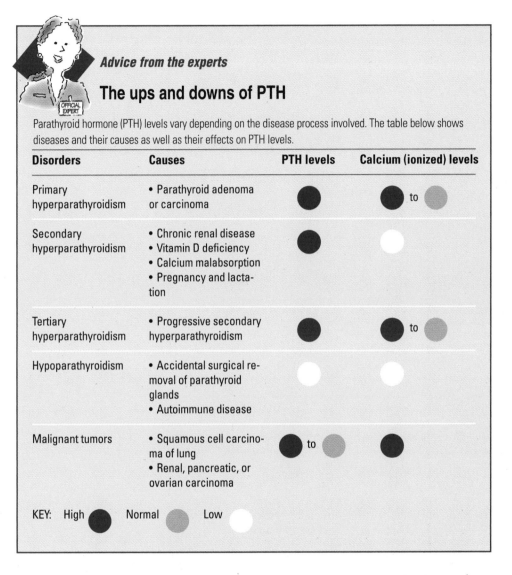

Advice from the experts

The ups and downs of PTH

Parathyroid hormone (PTH) levels vary depending on the disease process involved. The table below shows diseases and their causes as well as their effects on PTH levels.

Disorders	Causes	PTH levels	Calcium (ionized) levels
Primary hyperparathyroidism	• Parathyroid adenoma or carcinoma	High	High to Normal
Secondary hyperparathyroidism	• Chronic renal disease • Vitamin D deficiency • Calcium malabsorption • Pregnancy and lactation	High	Low
Tertiary hyperparathyroidism	• Progressive secondary hyperparathyroidism	High	High to Normal
Hypoparathyroidism	• Accidental surgical removal of parathyroid glands • Autoimmune disease	Low	Low
Malignant tumors	• Squamous cell carcinoma of lung • Renal, pancreatic, or ovarian carcinoma	High to Normal	High

KEY: High ●   Normal ●   Low ○

Suppression or stimulation tests may confirm the diagnosis.

What it all means

Normal serum PTH levels vary depending on the laboratory and must be interpreted in relation to serum calcium levels. The following values are normal:

- *intact PTH:* 10 to 50 pg/ml (SI, 1.1 to 5.3 pmol/L)
- *N-terminal fraction:* 8 to 24 pg/ml (SI, 0.8 to 2.5 pmol/L)
- *C-terminal fraction:* 0 to 340 pg/ml (SI, 0 to 35.8 pmol/L).

Measured together with serum calcium levels, abnormally elevated PTH values may indicate primary, secondary, or tertiary hyperparathyroidism. Abnormally low PTH levels may result from hypoparathyroidism and from certain malignant diseases. (See *The ups and downs of PTH*, page 113.)

What needs to be done

• Tell the patient that he must fast for at least 8 hours before the test.
• Perform a venipuncture, draw 3 ml of blood into two separate 7-ml clot-activator tubes or a tube volume in accordance with laboratory policy, and send them to the laboratory immediately so the serum can be separated and frozen for assay.

Adrenal and renal hormones

Serum aldosterone

The serum aldosterone test measures serum aldosterone levels. Aldosterone, secreted by the adrenal cortex, regulates ion transport across cell membranes in the renal tubules to promote reabsorption of sodium and chloride in exchange for potassium and hydrogen ions.

Consequently, aldosterone helps maintain blood pressure and blood volume and helps regulate fluid and electrolyte balance.

The serum aldosterone test identifies aldosteronism and, when supported by plasma renin levels, distinguishes between the primary and secondary forms of this disorder. Thus, it's helpful in identifying adrenal adenoma and adrenal hyperplasia, which are causes of primary aldosteronism. Secondary aldosteronism is commonly associated with salt depletion, potassium excess, heart failure with ascites, and other conditions that increase activity of the renin-angiotensin system.

What it all means

The following are normal serum aldosterone levels, which vary with the time of day and posture. Upright posture is accompanied by higher aldosterone levels, as indicated by these normal values:
• *upright individuals:* 7 to 30 ng/dl (SI, 190 to 832 pmol/L)

The serum aldosterone test aids in the diagnosis of fluid and electrolyte imbalances.

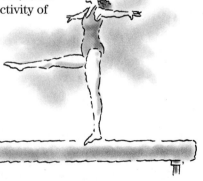

• *supine individuals:* 3 to 16 ng/dl (SI, 80 to 440 pmol/L).

Are we talkin' primary or secondary?

Excessive aldosterone secretion may indicate a primary or secondary disease. Primary aldosteronism (also known as *Conn's syndrome*) may result from adrenocortical adenoma or carcinoma or from bilateral adrenal hyperplasia. Secondary aldosteronism can result from renovascular hypertension, heart failure, cirrhosis of the liver, nephrotic syndrome, cyclic edema with no known cause, or the third trimester of pregnancy.

Depressed serum aldosterone levels may indicate primary hypoaldosteronism, salt-losing syndrome, toxemia of pregnancy, or Addison's disease. (See *Serum aldosterone test interference.*)

What needs to be done

• As ordered, withhold all drugs that alter fluid, sodium, and potassium balance, especially diuretics, antihypertensives, corticosteroids, progesterone agents, and estrogens, for at least 2 weeks or, preferably, 30 days before the test.
• Also withhold all renin inhibitors, such as propranolol, for 1 week before the test. If these medications must be continued, note this on the laboratory request.
• Warn the patient that licorice produces an aldosterone-like effect and should be avoided for at least 2 weeks before the test.
• Tell the patient he needs to maintain a low-carbohydrate, normal-sodium diet for at least 2 weeks or, preferably, 30 days before the test.
• Before the patient rises from sleep, perform a venipuncture, collect the sample in a 7-ml clot-activator tube or a tube volume in accordance with laboratory policy, and send it to the laboratory immediately.
• To evaluate the effect of postural change, draw another sample in a 7-ml clot-activator collection tube, or a tube volume in accordance with laboratory policy, 4 hours later, with the patient in a standing position after he has been up and moving around.
• Alternatively, use a 24-hour urine collection.
• Record on the laboratory request whether the patient was in a supine position or stood during the venipuncture. If the patient is a premenopausal female, specify the phase of her menstrual cycle because aldosterone levels may fluctuate during the menstrual cycle.

Stay on the ball

Serum aldosterone test interference

• Certain antihypertensives (such as methyldopa) that promote sodium and water retention cause possible decrease.
• Diuretics cause possible increase.
• Some corticosteroids (such as fludrocortisone) that mimic mineralocorticoid activity cause possible decrease.

Plasma cortisol

Cortisol helps metabolize nutrients, mediate physiologic stress, and regulate the immune system. Cortisol secretion normally follows a diurnal (daily) pattern: Levels rise during the early morning hours and peak around 8 a.m., and then decline to very low levels in the evening and during the early phase of sleep. (See *Viewing the cortisol secretion cycle.*)

Cortisol production is influenced by physical or emotional stress, which activates corticotropin. Thus, intense heat or cold, infection, trauma, exercise, obesity, and debilitating disease influence cortisol secretion.

The plasma cortisol test is usually ordered for patients with signs of adrenal dysfunction, but dynamic tests, suppression tests for hyperfunction, and stimulation tests for hypofunction are generally required to confirm the diagnosis.

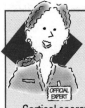

Advice from the experts

Viewing the cortisol secretion cycle

Cortisol secretion rises in the early morning, peaking after the patient awakens. Levels decline sharply in the evening and during the early phase of sleep. They rise again during the night and peak by the next morning.

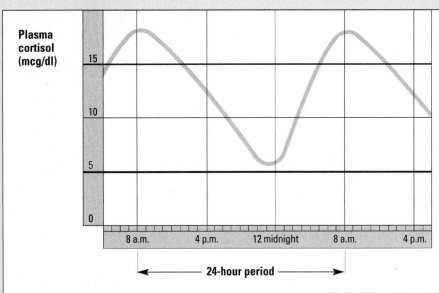

What it all means

Normally, plasma cortisol levels range from 9 to 35 mcg/dl (SI, 250 to 690 nmol/L) in the morning and from 3 to 12 mcg/dl (SI, 80 to 330 nmol/L) in the afternoon; the afternoon level is usually half the morning level.

Doin' the diurnal dance

Increased plasma cortisol levels may indicate adrenocortical hyperfunction in Cushing's disease or Cushing's syndrome. In patients with Cushing's syndrome, little or no difference in values is found between morning samples and afternoon samples. Diurnal variations may also be absent in otherwise healthy people who are under considerable emotional or physical stress.

Decreased cortisol levels may indicate primary adrenal hypofunction (Addison's disease). Tuberculosis, fungal invasion, and hemorrhage can cause adrenocortical destruction. Low cortisol levels resulting from secondary adrenal insufficiency may occur in conditions of impaired corticotropin secretion, such as hypophysectomy, postpartum pituitary necrosis, craniopharyngioma, or chromophobe adenoma. (See *Plasma cortisol test interference.*)

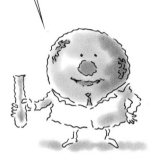

Measuring plasma cortisol levels can help diagnose Cushing's disease, Cushing's syndrome, and Addison's disease.

What needs to be done

• As ordered, withhold all medications that may interfere with plasma cortisol levels, such as estrogens, androgens, and phenytoin, for 48 hours before the test.
• If the patient is receiving replacement therapy and is dependent on exogenous steroids for survival, note this—as well as any other medications that must be continued—on the laboratory request.
• Tell the patient to maintain a normal-sodium diet for 3 days before the test and to fast and limit physical activity for 10 to 12 hours before the test.
• Make sure the patient is relaxed and recumbent for at least 30 minutes before the test.
• Perform a venipuncture, collect the sample in a 7-ml heparinized tube, or a tube volume in accordance with laboratory policy, at approximately 8 a.m. Label it appropriately, and send it to the laboratory immediately. For diurnal variation testing, draw another sample at approximately 4 p.m. Collect it in a heparinized tube, label it appropriately, and send it to the laboratory immediately.
• Record the collection time on the laboratory request.

Stay on the ball

Plasma cortisol test interference

• Levels are falsely elevated by hormonal contraceptives or pregnancy. Obesity, stress, or severe hepatic or renal disease may cause a possible increase in cortisol level.
• Androgens and phenytoin may decrease levels.

Plasma catecholamines

The plasma catecholamine test is clinically significant in patients with hypertension and signs of adrenal medullary tumor and in patients with neural tumors that affect endocrine function. In patients with elevated plasma catecholamine levels, supportive confirmation by urinalysis that shows such catecholamine degradation products as metanephrine are needed.

Fight or flight

Major catecholamines include the hormones epinephrine and norepinephrine. When secreted into the bloodstream, adrenal medullary catecholamines prepare the body for the fight-or-flight reaction: They increase heart rate and contractility, constrict blood vessels, redistribute circulating blood toward the skeletal and coronary muscles, mobilize carbohydrate and lipid reserves, and sharpen alertness. (See *Fight-or-flight reaction: The protective response.*)

Sweating it out

The effects of the fight-or-flight reaction resemble those produced by direct stimulation of the sympathetic nervous system, but they're intensified and prolonged. Excessive catecholamine secretion by tumors causes hypertension, weight loss, episodic sweating, headache, palpitations, and anxiety.

Plasma levels commonly fluctuate in response to temperature, stress, postural change, diet, smoking, anoxia, volume depletion, renal failure, obesity, and use of certain drugs.

> Plasma catecholamine levels help rule out pheochromocytoma in patients with hypertension. They also help identify neural tumors and diagnose autonomic nervous system dysfunction.

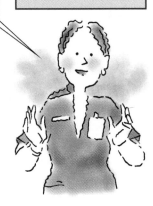

What it all means

The range of catecholamine levels is:
• *supine:* epinephrine, undetectable to 110 pg/ml (SI, undetectable to 600 pmol/L); norepinephrine, 70 to 750 pg/ml (SI, 413 to 4,432 pmol/L)
• *standing:* epinephrine, undetectable to 140 pg/ml (SI, undetectable to 764 pmol/L); norepinephrine, 200 to 1,700 pg/ml (SI, 1,182 to 10,047 pmol/L).

High catecholamine levels may indicate pheochromocytoma, neuroblastoma, ganglioneuroblastoma, or ganglioneuroma. (See *Clonidine suppression test.*)

Elevations are possible with—but don't directly confirm—thyroid disorders, hypoglycemia, or cardiac disease. Electroconvulsive therapy or shock resulting from hemorrhage, endotoxins, or anaphylaxis also raises catecholamine levels.

Clonidine suppression test

This test uses clonidine to help differentiate pheochromocytoma and essential hypertension. To perform the test, place the patient in the supine position. Collect a blood sample to obtain baseline catecholamine levels, and then administer 0.3 mg of oral clonidine. Collect a blood sample after 3 hours to measure catecholamine levels again and allow for comparison of findings.

Interpreting results
Patients with pheochromocytoma show no decrease in catecholamine levels after clonidine administration. In contrast, those with essential hypertension have normal catecholamine levels.

Fight-or-flight reaction: The protective response

The fight-or-flight reaction enables the body to confront a threat appropriately and resolve the situation. This innate stress reaction, which is automatic and immediate, helps us survive in dangerous situations. The events that take place during the fight-or-flight reaction are shown in the illustrations below.

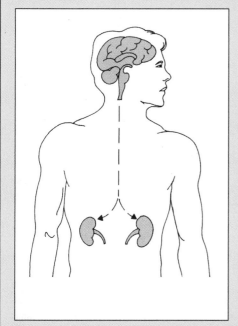

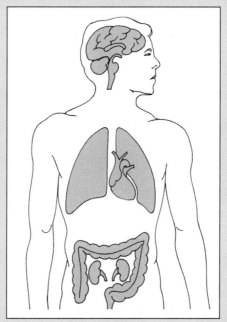

Stress triggers nerve impulse transmission by way of the sympathetic nervous system to the adrenal medulla. The medulla releases epinephrine and norepinephrine.

The fight-or-flight reaction increases respiratory rate, cardiac output, blood pressure, and pulse rate; boosts blood supply to major organs; and decreases blood supply to the skin and intestines.

What's the cause?

Fractional analysis helps identify the cause of elevated catecholamine levels. For example, adrenal medullary tumors secrete epinephrine, whereas ganglioneuromas, ganglioblastomas, and neuroblastomas secrete norepinephrine.

In the patient with normal or low baseline catecholamine levels, failure to show an increase in the sample taken after standing suggests autonomic nervous system dysfunction. (See *Plasma catecholamine test interference*.)

Stay on the ball

Plasma catecholamine test interference

• Epinephrine, levodopa, amphetamines, phenothiazines, sympathomimetics, decongestants, and tricyclic antidepressants raise plasma catecholamine levels; reserpine lowers them.

What needs to be done

- If the patient is hospitalized, withhold medications that affect catecholamine levels, such as amphetamines, phenothiazines, sympathomimetics, and tricyclic antidepressants, as ordered.
- Insert an indwelling venous catheter (saline lock) 24 hours before the test as ordered. This may be needed because the stress of the venipuncture itself may significantly raise catecholamine levels.
- Make sure the patient is relaxed and recumbent for 45 to 60 minutes before the test.
- If necessary, provide blankets to keep the patient warm because low temperatures stimulate catecholamine secretion.
- Tell the patient that the test requires one or two blood samples.
- Tell the patient to strictly follow these pretest instructions: He must refrain from using self-prescribed medications, especially cold or allergy remedies that may contain sympathomimetics, for 2 weeks; he must exclude amine-rich foods and beverages, such as bananas, avocados, cheese, coffee, tea, cocoa, beer, and Chianti wine, from his diet for 48 hours; he must maintain vitamin C intake; he must abstain from smoking for 24 hours; and he must fast for 10 to 12 hours before the test.
- Perform a venipuncture between 6 a.m. and 8 a.m. Collect the sample in a 10-ml chilled tube containing EDTA, or a tube volume in accordance with laboratory policy.
- If a second sample is requested, have the patient stand for 10 minutes, and draw the sample into another tube exactly like the first. If a saline lock is used, you may need to discard the first 1 or 2 ml of blood.
- After collecting each sample, roll the tube slowly between your palms to distribute the EDTA without agitating the blood.
- Pack the tube in crushed ice to minimize deactivation of catecholamines, and send it to the laboratory immediately. Indicate on the laboratory request whether the patient was supine or standing and the time the sample was drawn.

Erythropoietin

This test of renal hormone production measures erythropoietin. It's used to evaluate anemia, polycythemia, and kidney tumors. It's also used to evaluate abuse of commercially prepared erythropoietin by athletes who use the drug to enhance their performance.

What it all means

- The normal range by radioimmunoassay is 5 to 36 mU/ml (SI, 5 to 36 International Units/L).

Erythropoietin testing can detect abuse of the substance and helps diagnose anemia, polycythemia, and kidney tumors. The Tour de France and other athletic organizations have banned erythropoietin use.

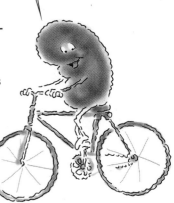

• Low levels of erythropoietin appear in anemic patients with inadequate or absent hormone production and may occur in severe renal disease. Congenital absence of erythropoietin can also occur.

• Elevated levels occur in anemias as a compensatory mechanism in the reestablishment of homeostasis. Inappropriate elevations (when the hematocrit, or HCT, is normal to high) are seen in polycythemia and erythropoietin-secreting tumors.

What needs to be done

• Keep the patient relaxed and recumbent for 30 minutes before the test.

• Explain to the patient that this test determines whether hormonal secretion is causing changes in his red blood cells.

• Tell the patient that he must fast for 8 to 10 hours before the test.

• During and after the test:
  – Perform a venipuncture, collect the sample in a 5-ml clot-activator tube or a tube volume in accordance with laboratory policy, and send it to the laboratory immediately.
  – If requested, an HCT test may be performed at the same time by collecting an additional sample in a 2-ml tube with EDTA added, or a tube volume in accordance with laboratory policy.

Pancreatic and gastric hormones

Serum insulin

The serum insulin radioimmunoassay is a quantitative analysis of serum insulin levels, which are usually measured concomitantly with glucose levels because glucose is the primary stimulus for insulin release from pancreatic islet cells. The test helps evaluate patients suspected of having hyperinsulinemia resulting from pancreatic tumor or hyperplasia.

Efficient insulin

Insulin regulates the metabolism and transport or mobilization of carbohydrates, amino acids, proteins, and lipids. Stimulated by increased plasma levels of glucose, insulin secretion reaches peak levels after meals, when metabolism and food storage are greatest.

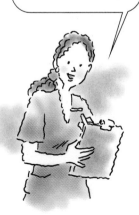

Measuring serum insulin can help diagnose hypoglycemia, glucocorticoid deficiency, severe hepatic disease, diabetes mellitus, and insulin resistance.

Stay on the ball

Serum insulin test interference

- Corticotropin, corticosteroids, thyroid hormones, and epinephrine may raise levels.
- Use of insulin by type 2 diabetes patients may lower levels.

What it all means

Serum insulin levels normally range from 0 to 35 µU/ml (SI, 144 to 243 pmol/L).

Conjunction junction

Insulin levels are interpreted in conjunction with glucose concentration: A normal insulin level may be inappropriate for the glucose results. High insulin and low glucose levels after a significant fast suggest an islet cell tumor. Prolonged fasting or stimulation testing may be required to confirm the diagnosis. In type 1 diabetes, insulin levels are elevated; in type 2 diabetes, they're low. (See *Serum insulin test interference*.)

What needs to be done

- As ordered, withhold corticotropin, corticosteroids (including hormonal contraceptives), thyroid supplements, epinephrine, and other medications that may interfere with test results. If they must be continued, note this on the laboratory request.
- Make sure the patient is relaxed and recumbent for 30 minutes before the test.
- Tell the patient that he must fast for 10 to 12 hours before the test and that a repeat test may be required.
- Tell the patient that, frequently, a simultaneous glucose tolerance test in which he must drink a glucose solution may be required.
- Perform a venipuncture, and collect one sample for insulin testing in a 7-ml tube with EDTA added, or a tube volume in accordance with laboratory policy; then collect a sample for glucose testing in a tube with sodium fluoride and potassium oxalate added, if requested.
- Pack the sample for insulin testing in ice, and immediately send it, along with the glucose sample, to the laboratory.
- In the patient with an islet cell tumor, fasting for this test may precipitate dangerously severe hypoglycemia. Keep glucose I.V. (50%) available to combat this reaction.

Guide to color-top collection tubes

The tube color used to collect a blood sample varies according to the purpose of the test. Listed here are tube colors, draw volumes, and additives for blood samples. Always check with your facility before following these guidelines because some requirements vary.

Purpose	Tube color	Draw volume	Additive
For collection of serum	Red	2 to 20 ml	None
For coagulation studies on plasma	Blue	1.8 to 5 ml	Buffered sodium citrate
For collection of plasma	Green	2 to 10 ml	Heparin
For collection of whole blood	Lavender	3 to 10 ml	EDTA
For collection of serum	Tiger	2.5 to 13 ml	Polymer gel and clot activator
For glucose determinations on serum or plasma	White	3 to 10 ml	Anticoagulant and glycolytic inhibitor
For preservation of red blood cells and whole blood studies	Yellow	10 to 12 ml	Acid citrate dextrose solution

Venipuncture

Venipuncture is performed to obtain venous blood samples for testing. The most commonly used venipuncture sites are on the forearm, followed by those on the hand. Blood values remain constant regardless of site as long as venous blood (not arterial blood) is sampled.

Forearm veins

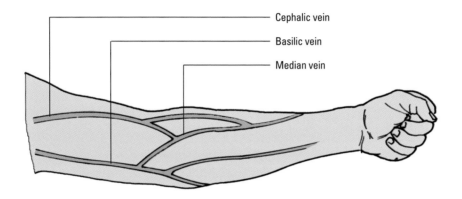

Cephalic vein

Basilic vein

Median vein

Hand veins

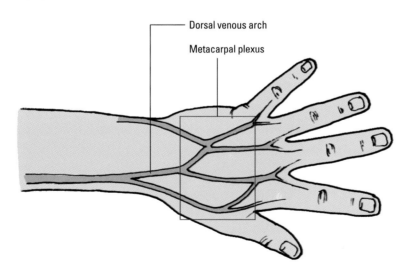

Dorsal venous arch

Metacarpal plexus

Collecting a venous sample

Follow these instructions to collect a venous sample.
- Gather the necessary equipment.
- Wash your hands and put on gloves.
- Identify the patient.
- Prepare the equipment.
- Select the site.
- Tie a tourniquet 3" (7.6 cm) proximal to the area you choose, pull the ends tightly in the opposite direction, and tuck one end under the other.

- Clean the site with an antimicrobial agent.
- Perform the venipuncture with the bevel of the needle facing up, entering the vein at a 30-degree angle.

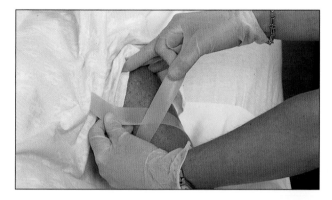

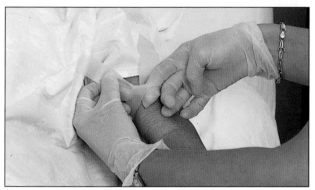

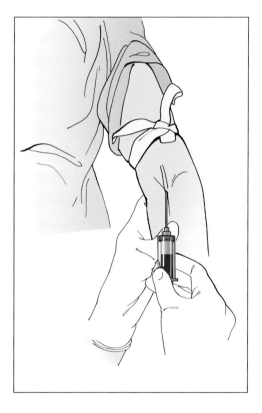

Arterial puncture technique

• The angle of needle penetration in arterial blood gas sampling depends on which artery is being used.

• For the radial artery, which is most commonly used, the needle should enter bevel-up at a 30- to 45-degree angle over the radial artery (as shown).

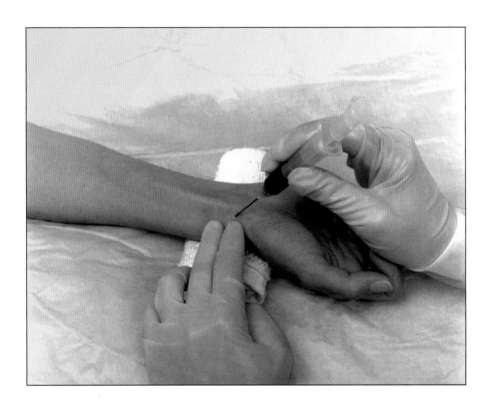

Plasma glucagon

Glucagon, a polypeptide hormone, is secreted by alpha cells of the islets of Langerhans in the pancreas. It acts primarily on the liver to promote glucose production and control glucose. This test is a quantitative analysis of plasma glucagon by radioimmunoassay.

What it all means

Glucagon levels are normally less than 60 pg/ml (SI, less than 60 ng/L).

The lowdown on levels

Elevated fasting glucagon levels (900 to 7,800 pg/ml [SI, 900 to 7,800 ng/L]) can occur in glucagonoma, diabetes mellitus, acute pancreatitis, and pheochromocytoma.

Abnormally low glucagon levels are associated with idiopathic glucagon deficiency and hypoglycemia due to chronic pancreatitis. (See *Plasma glucagon test interference*.)

What needs to be done

• As ordered, withhold insulin, catecholamines, and other drugs that could influence the test results. If they must be continued, note this on the laboratory slip.
• Have the patient lie down and relax for 30 minutes before the test.
• Tell the patient that he must fast for 10 to 12 hours before the test.
• Perform a venipuncture, and collect the sample in a chilled, 10-ml tube with EDTA added, or a tube volume in accordance with laboratory policy.
• Place the sample on ice, and send it to the laboratory immediately.

Measuring glucagon levels helps diagnose glucagonoma, hypoglycemia, and idiopathic glucagon deficiency.

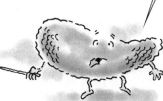

Gastrin

Gastrin is a polypeptide hormone produced and stored primarily in the antrum of the stomach and, to a lesser degree, in the islets of Langerhans. Gastrin's main function is to promote food digestion by triggering gastric acid secretion. Gastrin's secondary functions are to stimulate the release of pancreatic enzymes and the gastric enzyme pepsin, increase gastric and intestinal motility, and stimulate bile flow from the liver.

Abnormal gastrin secretion can result from tumors (gastrinomas) and from pathologic disorders affecting the stomach, pan-

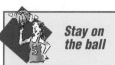

Gastrin stimulation tests: The whys and hows

Because some patients with duodenal or gastric ulcers have normal fasting gastrin levels, provocative testing is necessary to identify them; a protein-rich test meal serves this purpose. With duodenal gastric ulcers, gastrin levels increase markedly after such a meal.

Other indications

Provocative testing also distinguishes duodenal or gastric ulcers from Zollinger-Ellison syndrome, both of which may cause similar baseline gastrin levels. One test involves I.V. infusion of calcium gluconate (5 mg/kg of body weight over 3 hours). After the infusion, 10 ml of venous blood is drawn and sent to the laboratory. In Zollinger-Ellison syndrome, gastrin levels double, rising to about 500 pg/ml (SI, 500 ng/L); in duodenal or gastric ulcers, levels rise only moderately or don't change at all.

A third indication for provocative testing is an abnormally—but not strikingly—high fasting serum gastrin level, as in Zollinger-Ellison syndrome and pernicious anemia. To distinguish between the two, hydrochloric acid may be infused into the stomach through a nasogastric tube. Such infusion causes a sharp drop in gastrin levels in patients with pernicious anemia but not in those with Zollinger-Ellison syndrome.

Gastrin test interference

- Gastrin secretion is increased by amino acids (especially glycine), calcium carbonate, acetylcholine, calcium chloride, and ethanol; it's decreased by anticholinergics (atropine), hydrochloric acid, and secretin (a strongly basic polypeptide).
- Insulin-induced hypoglycemia increases gastrin secretion.

creas and, less commonly, esophagus and small bowel. (See *Gastrin stimulation tests: The whys and hows*.)

Unclear ulcers

Gastrin analysis is useful in patients with suspected gastrinomas (Zollinger-Ellison syndrome). If the situation is doubtful, provocative testing may be necessary.

What it all means

- Normal serum gastrin levels are 50 to 150 pg/ml (SI, 50 to 150 ng/L).
- Strikingly high serum gastrin levels (over 1,000 pg/ml [SI, 1,000 ng/L]) confirm Zollinger-Ellison syndrome.

Gastrin levels and pH

Gastrin levels may be high in various conditions, but the finding of very low gastric juice pH in conjunction with a very high serum gastrin level indicates autonomous hormone secretion not governed by a negative feedback mechanism. Increased serum levels of gastrin may occur in a few patients with duodenal ulceration (less than 1%), in patients with achlorhydria (with or without pernicious anemia), or in patients with extensive stomach carcinoma (because of hyposecretion of gastric juices and hydrochloric acid). (See *Gastrin test interference*.)

Analyzing gastrin levels helps confirm gastrinoma or the gastrin-secreting tumor in Zollinger-Ellison syndrome. It can also help distinguish between gastric and duodenal ulcers.

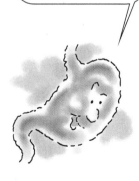

What needs to be done

• As ordered, withhold all medications that may interfere with test results, especially anticholinergics—such as atropine and belladonna—and insulin. If these medications must be continued, note this on the laboratory request.

• Because stress can increase gastrin levels, make sure the patient is relaxed and recumbent for at least 30 minutes before the test.

• Tell the patient that he must abstain from alcohol for at least 24 hours and fast for 12 hours before the test (water is permitted).

• Perform a venipuncture, and collect the sample in a 5-ml clot-activator tube or a tube volume in accordance with laboratory policy.

• To prevent destruction of serum gastrin by proteolytic enzymes, send the sample to the laboratory immediately to have the serum separated and frozen.

C-peptide

C-peptide is a biologically inactive chain formed during the proteolytic conversion of proinsulin to insulin in the pancreatic beta cells. As insulin enters the bloodstream, the C-peptide chain splits off from the hormone. The C-peptide test helps to:

• determine the cause of hypoglycemia

• indirectly measure insulin secretion in the presence of circulating insulin antibodies

• detect residual tissue after total pancreatectomy for carcinoma

• determine beta-cell function in the patient with diabetes mellitus.

What it all means

Normally, serum C-peptide levels generally parallel those of insulin. Normal fasting values range between 0.78 and 1.89 ng/ml (SI, 0.26 to 0.63 mmol). Elevated levels may indicate endogenous hyperinsulinism (insulinemia), oral hypoglycemic drug ingestion, pancreas or B-cell transplantation, renal failure, or type 2 diabetes mellitus. Decreased levels may indicate factitious hypoglycemia (surreptitious insulin administration), radical pancreatectomy, or type 1 diabetes. (See *C-peptide test interference.*)

What needs to be done

• Instruct the patient to fast for 8 to 12 hours before testing; he doesn't have to restrict water.

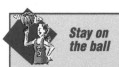
Stay on the ball

C-peptide test interference

• Hormonal contraceptives, prednisone, and rifampin may increase C-peptide levels.

• Atenolol and calcitonin may decrease levels.

• Failure to fast prior to the test alters results.

- If the patient is to receive radioisotope testing, it should take place after blood is drawn for C-peptide levels.
- Blood glucose levels are usually drawn at the same time as C-peptide levels.
- If the patient receives a C-peptide stimulation test, give I.V. glucagon after a baseline blood sample is drawn.
- Withhold medications that may interfere with test results. If the patient must continue them, note this on the laboratory request.
- Perform a venipuncture, and collect a 1-ml sample in a chilled clot-activator tube or a tube volume in accordance with laboratory policy. The blood is separated and frozen to be tested later.
- Collect a sample for testing glucose level in a tube with sodium fluoride and potassium oxalate, if ordered.
- Pack the sample in ice, and send it immediately, along with the glucose sample, to the laboratory.
- Instruct the patient that he may resume his usual activities, diet, and medications discontinued before the test.

Gonadal hormones

Estrogens

Estrogens and progesterone are secreted by the ovaries. They're responsible for the development of secondary female sexual characteristics and for normal menstruation.

Estrogen through the years

Usually undetectable in children, these hormones are secreted by ovarian follicular cells during the first half of the menstrual cycle and by the corpus luteum during the luteal phase and during pregnancy. In menopause, estrogen secretion drops to a constant, low level. Three estrogens are present in the blood in measurable amounts: estrone, estradiol (which is the most potent), and estriol.

Radioimmunoassay measures serum levels of estradiol and estriol, which are used to evaluate abnormal ovarian function. (See *Predicting premature labor.*)

Tests of hypothalamic-pituitary function may be required to confirm the diagnosis.

What it all means

Normal serum estradiol levels for women vary widely during the menstrual cycle, ranging from 26 to 149 pg/ml (SI, 90 to 550

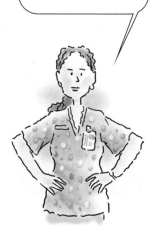

Estrogen tests help determine fetal well-being, infertility, precocious or delayed puberty, and menstrual disorders.

Predicting premature labor

A simple salivary test can help determine whether a pregnant woman is at risk for premature labor. The test, known as *SalEst,* measures salivary levels of estriol, an estrogen that increases 1,000-fold during pregnancy. For at-risk women, the SalEst test is 98% accurate in ruling out premature labor and delivery.

Positive means premature

The test is performed on women between weeks 22 and 36 of gestation using their saliva and the SalEst test kit. Estriol has been found to increase 2 to 3 weeks before spontaneous onset of labor and delivery. A positive test confirms that the patient is at risk for premature labor.

Stay on the ball

Estrogen test interference

• Pregnancy and pretest use of estrogens, such as hormonal contraceptives, may increase estrogen levels.
• Clomiphene, an estrogen antagonist, may cause a possible decrease.
• Steroids and pituitary-based hormones, such as dexamethasone, may alter test results.

pmol/L). The range for postmenopausal women is 0 to 34 pg/ml (SI, 0 to 125 pmol/L). Serum estradiol levels in men range from 12 to 34 pg/ml (SI, 40 to 125 pmol/L). In children under age 6, the normal level of serum estradiol is 3 to 10 pg/ml (SI, 10 to 36 pmol/L).

Estriol is secreted in large amounts by the placenta during pregnancy. Levels range from 2 ng/ml (SI, 7 nmol/L) by 30 weeks' gestation to 30 ng/ml (SI, 105 nmol/L) by week 40.

Estrogen effects

Decreased estrogen levels may indicate primary hypogonadism, or ovarian failure, such as in Turner's syndrome or ovarian agenesis; secondary hypogonadism, such as in hypopituitarism; or menopause.

Abnormally high estrogen levels may occur with estrogen-producing tumors, in precocious puberty, and in severe hepatic disease, such as cirrhosis, that prevents clearance of plasma estrogens. High levels may also result from congenital adrenal hyperplasia (increased conversion of androgens to estrogen). (See *Estrogen test interference.*)

What needs to be done

• Withhold all steroid and pituitary-based hormones. If they must be continued, note this on the laboratory slip.
• Perform a venipuncture, and collect the sample in a 10-ml clot-activator tube or a tube volume in accordance with laboratory policy.
• If the patient is premenopausal, indicate the phase of her menstrual cycle on the laboratory slip.
• Send the sample to the laboratory immediately.

Plasma progesterone

Progesterone, an ovarian steroid hormone secreted by the corpus luteum, helps prepare the endometrium for implantation of the fertilized ovum. Progesterone levels peak during the midluteal phase of the menstrual cycle, and they may prolong the surge of LH after ovulation. If implantation doesn't occur, progesterone (and estrogen) levels drop sharply and menstruation begins about 2 days later.

> Plasma progesterone levels can help assess placental function during pregnancy, confirm ovulation, and help assess corpus luteum function.

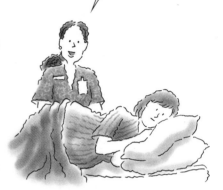

Progesterone and pregnancy

During pregnancy, the placenta releases about 10 times the normal monthly amount of progesterone to maintain the pregnancy. Increased secretion begins toward the end of the first trimester and continues until delivery.

The plasma progesterone test measures plasma progesterone levels. It provides reliable information about corpus luteum function in fertility studies or placental function in pregnancy. Serial determinations are recommended. Although plasma levels provide accurate information, progesterone can also be monitored by measuring urine pregnanediol, a catabolite of progesterone.

What it all means

Normal values during menstruation are:
- *follicular phase:* less than 150 ng/dl (SI, less than 5 nmol/L)
- *luteal phase:* 300 to 1,200 ng/dl (SI, 10 to 40 nmol/L).
  Normal values during pregnancy are:
- *first trimester:* 1,500 to 5,000 ng/dl (SI, 50 to 160 nmol/L)
- *second and third trimesters:* 8,000 to 20,000 ng/dl (SI, 250 to 650 nmol/L).
  Normal values for menopausal women are 10 to 22 ng/dl (SI, 0 to 2 nmol/L).

The lowdown on levels

Elevated progesterone levels may indicate ovulation, luteinizing tumors, ovarian cysts that produce progesterone, or adrenocortical hyperplasias and tumors that produce progesterone along with other steroidal hormones.

Low progesterone levels are associated with amenorrhea, which can have several causes (such as panhypopituitarism or gonadal dysfunction), toxemia of pregnancy, threatened abortion, and fetal death. (See *Plasma progesterone test interference*.)

Stay on the ball

Plasma progesterone test interference

- Progesterone or estrogen therapy may alter test results.

What needs to be done

- Tell the patient that this test may be repeated at specific times coinciding with phases of her menstrual cycle or at each prenatal visit.
- Perform a venipuncture, and collect the sample in a 7-ml heparinized tube or a tube volume in accordance with laboratory policy.
- Completely fill the collection tube; then invert it gently at least 10 times to adequately mix the sample and the anticoagulant.
- Indicate the date of the patient's last menstrual period and the phase of her cycle on the laboratory request. If the patient is pregnant, indicate the month of gestation.
- Send the sample to the laboratory immediately.

Testosterone

As the principal androgen secreted by the interstitial cells of the testes (Leydig cells), testosterone induces puberty in the male and maintains male secondary sex characteristics.

Time for testosterone

Testosterone production begins increasing at the onset of puberty and continues to rise during adulthood. Production begins to taper off at about age 40, eventually dropping to about one-fifth the peak level by age 80. In females, the adrenal glands and the ovaries secrete small amounts of testosterone.

Testing testosterone

This test measures plasma or serum testosterone levels. When results are combined with measurements of plasma gonadotropin (FSH and LH) levels, it reliably aids evaluation of gonadal dysfunction in males and females.

What it all means

Normal levels of testosterone are (laboratory values vary slightly):
- *men:* 300 to 1,200 ng/dl (SI, 10.4 to 41.6 nmol/L)
- *women:* 20 to 80 ng/dl (SI, 0.7 to 2.8 nmol/L)
- *prepubertal children:* values lower than adult levels.

Testosterone highs

Elevated testosterone levels in prepubertal males may indicate true sexual precocity (development occurs earlier than expected) caused by excessive gonadotropin secretion, or they may indicate pseudoprecocious puberty caused by male hormone pro-

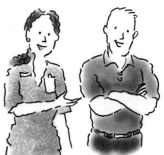

Testosterone levels help evaluate male infertility or other sexual dysfunction and also diagnose hypogonadism.

duction by a testicular tumor. They can also indicate congenital adrenal hyperplasia (excessive proliferation of normal cells), which results in precocious puberty in males (from ages 2 to 3) and pseudohermaphroditism and milder development of secondary sexual characteristics of females. Increased levels can occur with a benign or malignant adrenal tumor, hyperthyroidism, or beginning puberty. In females with ovarian tumors or polycystic ovarian syndrome, testosterone levels may rise, leading to hirsutism (excessive hair growth in unusual places).

Testosterone lows

Depressed testosterone levels can indicate primary hypogonadism (as in Klinefelter's syndrome) or secondary hypogonadism (hypogonadotropic eunuchoidism) from hypothalamic-pituitary dysfunction. Depressed testosterone levels can also follow orchiectomy, testicular or prostatic cancer, delayed male puberty, estrogen therapy, or cirrhosis. (See *Testosterone test interference.*)

What needs to be done

• Perform a venipuncture, and collect the sample in a 7-ml clot-activator tube or a tube volume in accordance with laboratory policy. Use a heparinized tube if plasma is to be collected.
• Indicate the patient's age, sex, and history of hormone therapy on the laboratory request.
• The sample is stable and requires no refrigeration or preservative for up to 1 week. Frozen samples are stable for at least 6 months.

Placental hormone

Human chorionic gonadotropin

Human chorionic gonadotropin (hCG) is a hormone produced by the trophoblastic cells of the placenta. When conception occurs, the hCG assay may detect this hormone in the blood as early as 9 days after ovulation. This interval coincides with implantation of the fertilized ovum into the uterine wall.

hCG comes early

Although the precise function of this hormone is still unclear, hCG, along with progesterone, appears to maintain the corpus luteum during early pregnancy. Production of hCG increases

Stay on the ball

Testosterone test interference

• Exposure to exogenous sources of estrogens or androgens may alter results.
• Estrogens decrease free testosterone levels by increasing sex hormone–binding globulin, which binds testosterone.
• Androgens cause possible increase of testosterone levels.

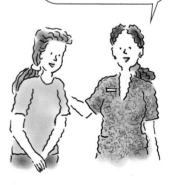

Testing hCG can detect pregnancy early and can also be used to monitor ovulation and conception, determine adequate hormone production in high-risk pregnancy, and help diagnose certain tumors.

steadily during the first trimester, peaking around the 10th week of gestation.

This serum immunoassay is more sensitive (and costly) than the routine pregnancy test using a urine specimen.

What it all means

Normal values for hCG are less than 4 mIU/L (SI, less than 4 International Units/L). During pregnancy, hCG levels are quite variable and depend partially on the number of days since the last normal menstrual period.

The lowdown on levels

Elevated hCG levels indicate pregnancy; significantly higher concentrations are present in a multiple pregnancy. Increased levels may also suggest hydatidiform mole, trophoblastic neoplasm of the placenta, or nontrophoblastic carcinomas that secrete hCG (including gastric, pancreatic, and ovarian adenocarcinomas). Because levels are high in both conditions, hCG levels can't differentiate between pregnancy and tumor recurrence.

Low hCG levels can occur in ectopic pregnancy or pregnancy of fewer than 9 days. (See *Interference with hCG tests.*)

What needs to be done

• Perform a venipuncture, and collect the sample in a 7-ml clot-activator tube or a tube volume in accordance with laboratory policy.

• Send the sample to the laboratory immediately.

Stay on the ball

Interference with hCG tests

• Epostane and mifepristone may decrease human chorionic gonadotropin (hCG) levels.

• Use of phenothiazines may produce false-positive or false-negative results.

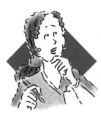

Quick quiz

1. Which test assesses corpus luteum function?

   A.   Plasma progesterone

   B.   Estrogen

   C.   Placental hormone

   D.   Testosterone

Answer: A. The plasma progesterone test assesses corpus luteum function as part of infertility studies.

2. Which drug can cause false hCG results?
A. Estrogens
B. Insulin
C. Phenothiazines
D. Diuretics

Answer: C. Phenothiazines can reduce hCG secretion.

3. Which pretest precaution must the patient follow when preparing for a plasma catecholamine test?
A. Limit vitamin C intake.
B. Stay in a cool environment.
C. Avoid amine-rich foods.
D. Be sure to eat breakfast.

Answer: C. The patient must exclude amine-rich foods and beverages from the diet for 48 hours before a catecholamine test.

4. Which test helps diagnose anemia and polycythemia?
A. Catecholamines
B. Erythropoietin
C. Plasma cortisol
D. Triiodothyronine

Answer: B. An erythropoietin test can help diagnose anemia and polycythemia.

5. A serum gastrin level above 1,000 pg/ml (SI, greater than 1,000 ng/L) confirms which disorder?
A. Pancreatic cancer
B. Ganglioblastoma
C. Addison's disease
D. Zollinger-Ellison syndrome

Answer: D. A serum gastrin level above 1,000 pg/ml (SI, 1,000 ng/L) confirms Zollinger-Ellison syndrome.

Scoring

☆☆☆ If you answered all five questions correctly, wow! You're the Hercules of hormones!

☆☆ If you answered three or four questions correctly, excellent! You're cruisin' with cortisol!

☆ If you answered fewer than three questions correctly, hang in there! You'll be doing the hormone hoedown before you know it!

Immunologic tests

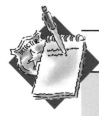

Just the facts

In this chapter, you'll learn:

♦ about immunologic tests and how they're performed

♦ the patient care associated with immunologic tests

♦ factors that can interfere with these tests

♦ what immunologic test results may indicate.

A look at immunologic tests

Before he undergoes immunologic testing, make sure that your patient understands the test to be performed. Use a clear, simple explanation. Inform him that the test requires a venipuncture that will cause some brief discomfort and that he'll feel brief pressure from the tourniquet. After you draw the blood samples, handle the samples gently to prevent hemolysis, which can alter test results. Be sure to label the samples clearly. Monitor the venipuncture site for bleeding. If a hematoma develops, apply warm soaks. If the hematoma is large, monitor circulation in the extremity distal to the venipuncture site.

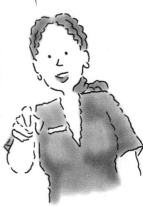

Easy does it! Be gentle with samples.

Immunohematology

ABO blood typing

ABO blood typing classifies blood according to the presence of major antigens A and B on red blood cell (RBC) surfaces and according to the serum antibodies anti-A and anti-B. ABO blood typing is required before transfusions to prevent a lethal reaction—

even if the patient is carrying an ABO blood group identification card.

There are four blood types in the ABO system: A, B, AB, and O.

Antigens

An antigen is a substance that can stimulate the formation of an antibody. RBCs carry antigens, which can initiate an immune response. Each blood group in the ABO system is named for antigens—A, B, both of these, or neither—that are carried on a person's RBCs. An antigen may induce formation of a corresponding antibody if given to a person who doesn't normally carry the antigen.

Antibodies

An antibody is an immunoglobulin molecule synthesized in response to a specific antigen. The ABO system includes two naturally occurring antibodies: anti-A and anti-B. One or both, or neither, of these antibodies may be found in plasma. The interaction of corresponding antigens and antibodies of the ABO system can cause agglutination (clumping together).

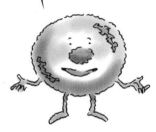

ABO testing determines whether blood is type A, B, AB, or O, indicating whether a blood donor and recipient are compatible for transfusion.

O, you're everybody's type

Because group O lacks both A and B antigens, it can be transfused in limited amounts in an emergency to any patient—regardless of the recipient's blood type—with little risk of adverse reaction. (See *ABO blood types.*)

What it all means

Testing reveals blood type as type A, type B, type AB, or type O. (See *ABO blood typing interference.*)

What needs to be done

• Check the patient history for recent administration of blood, dextran, or I.V. contrast media.
• Perform a venipuncture, and collect the sample in a 10-ml tube without additives, or a tube volume in accordance with laboratory policy, as ordered.
• Label the sample with the patient's name, the hospital or blood bank number, the date, and the initials of the person who drew the sample.
• Send the sample to the laboratory immediately with a properly completed laboratory request.

Now I get it!

ABO blood types

Precise typing of donor blood and recipient blood helps avoid transfusing incompatible blood, which can be fatal. This illustration shows the recipient's blood type and the compatible donor type.

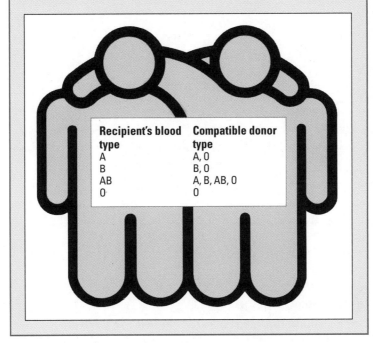

Recipient's blood type	Compatible donor type
A	A, O
B	B, O
AB	A, B, AB, O
O	O

Stay on the ball

ABO blood typing interference

• Recent administration of dextran or I.V. contrast media causes cellular aggregation that resembles agglutination.
• New antibodies may interfere with compatibility testing if the patient has received blood or has been pregnant in the past 3 months.

Rh typing establishes blood type according to the Rhesus system and helps determine donor-recipient blood compatibility.

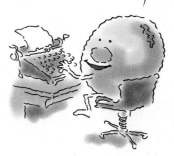

Rh typing

The Rhesus (Rh) system classifies blood by the presence or absence of the $Rh_0(D)$ antigen on the surface of RBCs. In this test, a patient's RBCs are mixed with serum containing anti-$Rh_0(D)$ antibodies and are observed for clumping. If clumping occurs, the $Rh_0(D)$ antigen is present and the patient's blood is typed Rh-positive; if clumping doesn't occur, the antigen is absent and the patient's blood is typed Rh-negative.

What it all means

Classified as *Rh-positive*, *Rh-negative*, or *Rh(D^u)-positive*, donor blood may be transfused only if it's compatible with the

The ABCs of Rh$_0$(D) typing

Classified as *Rh$_0$(D)-positive*, *Rh$_0$(D)-negative*, or *Rh(D^u)-positive*, donor blood may be transfused only if it's compatible with the recipient's blood, as shown below.

Rh$_0$(D) recipient types	Compatible Rh$_0$(D) donor types	Incompatible Rh$_0$(D) donor types
Rh$_0$(D)-positive	Rh$_0$(D)-positive or Rh$_0$(D)-negative	None
Rh$_0$(D)-negative	Rh$_0$(D)-negative	Rh$_0$(D)-positive
Rh(D^u)-positive	Rh(D^u)-positive, Rh$_0$(D)-negative, or Rh$_0$(D)-positive (the least desirable choice because it may cause a mild hemolytic reaction)	None

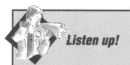

Listen up!

An ounce of prevention

If an Rh-negative woman delivers an Rh-positive baby or aborts a fetus whose Rh-type is unknown, she should receive an injection of Rh$_0$(D) immune globulin within 72 hours to prevent future hemolytic disease of the neonate.

recipient's blood. (See *The ABCs of Rh$_0$(D) typing* and *An ounce of prevention*.)

What needs to be done

• Perform a venipuncture, and collect the sample in a 7-ml tube with EDTA added, or a tube volume in accordance with laboratory policy, as ordered.
• Label the sample with the patient's name, the hospital or blood bank number, the date, and the initials of the person who drew the sample.
• Send the sample to the laboratory immediately.
• If a transfusion is ordered, a transfusion request form must accompany the sample to the laboratory. (See *Rh typing interference*.)

Fetal-maternal erythrocyte distribution

Some transfer of RBCs from fetal to maternal circulation occurs during most spontaneous or elective abortions and most normal deliveries. Fetal-maternal erythrocyte distribution measures the

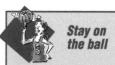

Stay on the ball

Rh typing interference

• Methyldopa, cephalosporins, and levodopa may cause a false-positive result for the D^u antigen.

number of fetal RBCs in maternal circulation to allow calculation of the $Rh_o(D)$ immune globulin dosage needed for protection against maternal immunization to the $Rh_o(D)$ antigen, which can develop.

What it all means

Maternal whole blood should contain no fetal RBCs.

Elevated levels

An elevated fetal RBC volume in maternal circulation necessitates administration of more than one dose of $Rh_o(D)$ immune globulin. The number of vials needed is determined by dividing the calculated fetomaternal hemorrhage by 30 (a single vial of $Rh_o[D]$ immune globulin will provide protection against a 30-ml fetomaternal hemorrhage).

Don't delay

Administration of $Rh_o(D)$ immune globulin to an unsensitized Rh-negative mother as soon as possible (no later than 72 hours) after the birth of an Rh-positive infant or after a spontaneous or elective abortion prevents complications in subsequent pregnancies. Most practitioners now administer $Rh_o(D)$ immune globulin preventively at 28 weeks' gestation to women who are Rh-negative but have no detectable Rh antibodies.

Who needs the screen?

These patients should be screened for Rh isoimmunization or irregular antibodies: all Rh-negative mothers during their first prenatal visit and at 28 weeks' gestation, and all Rh-positive mothers with a history of transfusion, a jaundiced infant, stillbirth, cesarean delivery, or induced or spontaneous abortion.

What needs to be done

• Explain to the patient that this blood test determines blood group and helps determine how many doses of $Rh_o(D)$ immune globulin she'll require to prevent immunization as a result of this pregnancy.
• Check the patient history for recent administration of dextran or I.V. contrast media that may alter results.
• Perform a venipuncture, and collect the sample in a 7-ml tube with EDTA added, or a tube volume in accordance with laboratory policy, as ordered.
• Label the sample with the patient's name, the hospital or blood bank number, the date, and the initials of the person who drew the sample.

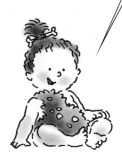

Testing for fetal-maternal erythrocyte distribution measures blood transfer and helps determine the amount of $Rh_o(D)$ immune globulin needed to prevent maternal immunization to the $Rh_o(D)$ antigen.

• Send the sample to the laboratory immediately with a properly completed laboratory request.

Crossmatching

Crossmatching establishes the compatibility or incompatibility of a donor's and a recipient's blood. It's the best antibody detection test available for avoiding lethal transfusion reactions.

Major matching

After the donor's and the recipient's ABO blood type and Rh factor type are determined, major crossmatching tests for compatibility between the donor's RBCs and the recipient's serum. They're compatible if the recipient's serum has no antibodies that would destroy transfused cells and possibly cause an acute hemolytic reaction.

Minor matching

Minor crossmatching tests for compatibility between the donor's serum and the recipient's RBCs. This crossmatch is less important, however, because the donor's antibodies are greatly diluted in the recipient's plasma. Because the antibody-screening test is routinely performed on all blood donors, minor crossmatching is commonly omitted.

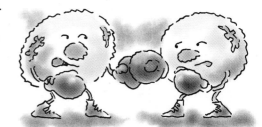

Crossmatching, which prevents deadly transfusion reactions, is the final check for compatibility between donor and recipient blood.

What it all means

Absence of clumping indicates compatibility between the donor's blood and the recipient's blood, which means that the transfusion of donor blood can proceed.

Positive = no match

A positive crossmatch indicates incompatibility between the donor's blood and the recipient's blood, which means the donor's blood can't be transfused to the recipient. The sign of a positive crossmatch is clumping after the donor's RBCs and the recipient's serum are correctly mixed and incubated. Clumping indicates an undesirable antigen-antibody reaction. The donor's blood must be withheld and the crossmatch continued to determine why the blood is incompatible and to identify the antibody.

Negative = probable compatibility

A negative crossmatch—the absence of clumping—indicates probable compatibility between the donor's blood and the recipient's blood, which means the transfusion of the donor's blood can proceed. It doesn't guarantee a safe transfusion, but it's the best method available to prevent an acute hemolytic reaction. (See *Crossmatching test interference*.)

What needs to be done

• Check the patient history for recent administration of blood, dextran, or I.V. contrast media.
• Perform a venipuncture, and collect the sample in a 10-ml tube or a tube volume in accordance with laboratory policy, without additives or with EDTA added. ABO typing, Rh typing, and crossmatching are all done together.
• Label the sample with the patient's name, the hospital or blood bank number, the date, and the initials of the person who drew the sample.
• Indicate on the laboratory request form the amount and type of blood component needed.
• Send the sample to the laboratory immediately. Crossmatching must be performed on the sample within 72 hours.
• If more than 72 hours has elapsed since a previous transfusion, previously crossmatched donor blood must be crossmatched again with a new recipient serum sample to detect newly acquired incompatibilities before the transfusion.

Stay on the ball

Crossmatching test interference

• Previous administration of dextran or I.V. contrast media causes clumping. A previous blood transfusion may produce antibodies to donor blood.

Direct antiglobulin

Also known as the *direct Coombs' test*, the direct antiglobulin test detects antibodies on the surfaces of RBCs. These antibodies coat RBCs when they become sensitized to an antigen such as Rh factor.

One step direct

In this test, antiglobulin (Coombs') serum added to saline-washed RBCs results in clumping if antibodies or complement is present. This test is "direct" because it requires only one step: the addition of Coombs' serum to washed cells.

What it all means

A negative test in which neither antibodies nor complement appears on the RBCs is normal.

Crossed and coated

A positive test on umbilical cord blood indicates that maternal antibodies have crossed the placenta and have coated fetal RBCs, causing hemolytic disease of the newborn (HDN).

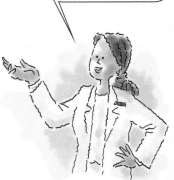

The direct antiglobulin test can do a lot! It helps diagnose hemolytic disease of the newborn and congenital anemias. It can also be used to investigate hemolytic transfusion reactions.

I beg to differ

In other patients, a positive test result may indicate hemolytic anemia and may help differentiate between autoimmune and secondary hemolytic anemia, which can be drug-induced or associated with an underlying disease such as lymphoma. A positive test result can also indicate sepsis.

Borderline

A borderline or slightly positive test result may suggest a transfusion reaction in which the patient's antibodies react with transfused RBCs containing the corresponding antigen. (See *Direct antiglobulin test interference*.)

What needs to be done

- If the patient is a neonate, explain to the parents that this blood test helps diagnose HDN.
- If the patient is suspected of having hemolytic anemia, explain that this test determines whether the anemia is caused by an immune system abnormality, from the use of certain drugs, or from some unknown cause.
- As ordered, withhold medications that may induce autoimmune hemolytic anemia.
- For an adult, perform a venipuncture and collect the sample in two 5-ml tubes with EDTA added, or a tube volume in accordance with laboratory policy.
- For a neonate, draw 5 ml of cord blood into a tube with EDTA or no additives, or a tube volume in accordance with laboratory policy, as ordered, after the cord is clamped and cut.
- The test must be performed within 24 hours; send the sample to the laboratory immediately.
- Label the sample with the patient's full name, the facility or blood bank number, the date, and the initials of the person who drew the sample.

Stay on the ball

Direct antiglobulin test interference

Positive results may occur with use of quinidine, methyldopa, cephalosporins, sulfonamides, chlorpromazine, diphenylhydantoin, ethosuximide, hydralazine, levodopa, mefenamic acid, melphalan, penicillin, procainamide, rifampin, streptomycin, tetracyclines, or isoniazid.

Antibody screening

The antibody screening test, also known as the *indirect Coombs' test* and the *indirect antiglobulin test*, detects unexpected circulating antibodies in the patient's serum. After incubating the serum with group O RBCs, which are unaffected by anti-A or anti-B antibodies, an antiglobulin (Coombs') serum is added. Clumping occurs if the patient's serum contains an antibody to one or more antigens on the RBCs.

> By detecting unexpected antibodies in circulation, the antibody screening test prevents conflicts between the blood of donors and recipients.

Checkin' ID

The antibody screening test detects 95% to 99% of the circulating antibodies. Then the antibody identification test determines the specific identity of the antibodies. (See *What the antibody identification test shows*.)

What it all means

A negative test result is normal—that is, clumping doesn't occur, indicating that the patient's serum contains no circulating antibodies (other than anti-A and anti-B).

Positively unexpected

A positive result indicates the presence of unexpected circulating antibodies to RBC antigens, which demonstrates donor and recipient incompatibility.

Now I get it!

What the antibody identification test shows

The antibody identification test identifies unexpected circulating antibodies detected by the antibody screening test (indirect Coombs' test). In this test, group O red blood cells (RBCs)—at least three with and three without a specific antigen—are combined with serum containing unknown antibodies and are observed for clumping. If the serum contains the corresponding antibody to the RBC antigen, a positive reaction occurs with RBCs that have the antigen but not with those that lack the antigen. For example, serum that reacts with Rh-positive cells but not Rh-negative cells probably contains the anti-Rh_0(D) antibody.

At least three RBCs containing the antigen and three without it are used in each test to reduce error. Serum that contains rare or multiple antibodies requires more complicated procedures.

Antibody presence

A positive result in a pregnant patient with Rh-negative blood may indicate the presence of antibodies to the Rh factor from a previous transfusion with incompatible blood or from a previous pregnancy with an Rh-positive fetus.

Pregnancy may necessitate repetition

A positive result indicates that the fetus may develop HDN. As a result, repeated testing throughout the patient's pregnancy is necessary to evaluate progressive development of circulating antibody levels. (See *Antibody screening interference.*)

What needs to be done

• Check the patient history for recent administration of blood, dextran, or I.V. contrast media, and note any such administration on the laboratory request.
• Perform a venipuncture, and collect a blood sample in two 10-ml tubes or a tube volume in accordance with laboratory policy. If the antibody screen is positive, antibody identification is performed on the blood.
• Label the sample appropriately, noting the patient's diagnosis, pregnancy status, history of transfusions, and current drug therapy. Send the sample to the laboratory immediately. The antibody screening must be done within 72 hours after the sample is drawn.

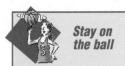

Stay on the ball

Antibody screening interference

• Previous administration of blood, dextran, or I.V. contrast media causes clumping.

Leukoagglutinins

The leukoagglutinin test detects leukoagglutinins (also known as *white cell antibodies* or *human leukocyte antigen [HLA] antibodies*), which are antibodies that react with white blood cells (WBCs) and may cause a transfusion reaction. These antibodies usually develop after exposure to foreign WBCs through transfusions, pregnancies, or allografts.

What it all means

A negative test result is normal—that is, clumping doesn't occur, indicating that the patient's serum contains no antibodies. There are no known factors that interfere with the leukoagglutinin test.

Heated reaction

A positive result in a blood recipient indicates the presence of agglutinins, identifying his transfusion reaction as a febrile nonhemolytic reaction to these antibodies. Recipients who test positive for HLA antibodies may need HLA-matched platelets to con-

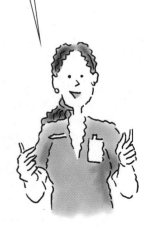

Testing for leukoagglutinins can differentiate between hemolytic and febrile nonhemolytic transfusion reactions.

trol bleeding episodes caused by thrombocytopenia. (See *Precautions before the next transfusion.*)

What needs to be done

• Check the patient history for recent administration of blood, dextran, or I.V. contrast media, and note any such administration on the laboratory request.
• Perform a venipuncture, and collect the sample in a 10-ml clot-activator tube or a tube volume in accordance with laboratory policy. The laboratory needs 3 to 4 ml of serum for testing.
• Label the sample with the patient's name, the hospital or blood bank number, the date, and the initials of the person who drew the sample. Be sure to include on the laboratory request the patient's suspected diagnosis and any history of blood transfusions, pregnancies, and drug therapy.

General cellular function

T- and B-lymphocyte assays

Lymphocytes—key cells in the immune system—have the capacity to recognize antigens through special receptors found on their surfaces. The two primary kinds of lymphocytes, T cells and B cells, originate in the bone marrow. T cells mature under the influence of the thymus gland; B cells evolve without thymic influence.

No difference

T- and B-lymphocyte assays recover approximately 80% of the lymphocytes but don't differentiate between T and B cells. The percentage of T and B cells is determined by attaching a label or marker and using different identification techniques. Null cells are usually determined by subtracting the sum of T and B cells from total lymphocytes.

What it all means

T-cell and B-cell values may differ from one laboratory to another, depending on test technique. Generally, T cells constitute 68% to 75% of total lymphocytes; B cells, 10% to 20%; and null cells, 5% to 20%.

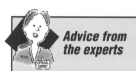

Advice from the experts

Precautions before the next transfusion

If a patient who received a transfusion has a positive leukoagglutinin test, he should receive acetaminophen 1 to 2 hours before the next transfusion. To prevent further reactions, he should also receive specially prepared leukocyte-poor blood or a leukocyte removal blood filter should be used during administration.

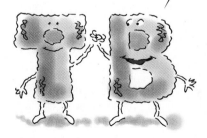

T- and B-lymphocyte assays can help diagnose immunodeficiency diseases and monitor immunotherapy.

Suggestive material

An abnormal T-cell or B-cell count suggests but doesn't confirm specific diseases. The B-cell count is elevated in chronic lymphocytic leukemia, multiple myeloma, Waldenström's macroglobulinemia, and DiGeorge syndrome (a congenital T-cell deficiency). The B-cell count decreases in acute lymphocytic leukemia and in certain congenital or acquired immunoglobulin deficiency diseases. In other immunoglobulin deficiency diseases, especially if only one immunoglobulin class is deficient, the B-cell count remains normal.

T cells on the rise

The T-cell count rises occasionally in infectious mononucleosis; it rises more commonly in multiple myeloma and acute lymphocytic leukemia. T cells decrease in congenital T-cell deficiency diseases, such as DiGeorge, Nezelof, and Wiskott-Aldrich syndromes, and in chronic lymphocytic leukemia, Waldenström's macroglobulinemia, and acquired immunodeficiency syndrome (AIDS). (See *T- and B-lymphocyte assay interference*.)

What needs to be done

• Perform a venipuncture, and collect the sample in a 7-ml heparinized tube or a tube volume in accordance with laboratory policy.
• Fill the collection tube completely, and invert it gently several times.
• Transport the sample to the laboratory immediately; keep it at room temperature.
• If antilymphocyte antibodies are suspected, notify the laboratory.

Stay on the ball

T- and B-lymphocyte assay interference

• Changes in health status, stress, surgery, chemotherapy, steroid or immunosuppressive therapy, and radiography can rapidly change T- and B-cell counts.
• Immunoglobulins that sometimes occur in autoimmune disease can alter test results.

Lymphocyte transformation

Transformation tests evaluate the ability of lymphocytes to change into actively multiplying cells without injection of antigens into the patient's skin. These in vitro tests eliminate the risk of adverse effects but can still accurately assess the ability of lymphocytes to reproduce and to recognize and respond to antigens.

Long division

The mitogen assay evaluates the cell division response of T lymphocytes and B lymphocytes to a foreign antigen. The antigen assay uses specific substances—such as purified protein derivative, Candida, mumps, tetanus toxoid, and streptokinase—to stimulate lymphocyte transformation. The mixed lymphocyte culture (MLC)

Lymphocyte transformation testing helps assess immunodeficiency states, provides histocompatibility typing of tissue transplant recipients and donors, and determines exposure to certain pathogens.

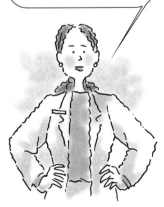

Neutrophil function tests

Neutrophil function tests may reveal the inability of neutrophils to kill a target bacteria or to migrate to the bacterial site (chemotaxis). The killing ability can be evaluated by the nitroblue tetrazolium (NBT) test, which relies on neutrophil generation of bactericidal enzymes and toxins during killing. This action increases oxygen consumption and glucose metabolism, which reduces colorless NBT to blue formazan. The reduced dye is then extracted with pyridine and measured photometrically; the level of reduction indicates phagocytic activity.

Neutrophil-killing activity can also be evaluated by noting the neutrophil's chemiluminescence (its ability to emit light). After a neutrophil phagocytizes a microorganism, oxygen-containing substances form within phagocytic vacuoles. As the cell is stimulated, it emits light in proportion to the amount of oxygen-containing substances that are formed, thereby providing an indirect measurement of phagocytosis.

Chemotaxis can be assessed in vitro by placing bacteria in the lower half of a two-part chamber and phagocytic neutrophils in the upper half. After incubation, migrating cells are counted microscopically and compared with standard values.

---

assay helps match transplant recipients and donors and tests immunocompetence. The neutrophils' ability to engulf and destroy bacteria and foreign particles can also be determined. (See *Neutrophil function tests.*)

What it all means

Results depend on the mitogens used. Reference ranges accompany test results. In general, a positive test is normal; a negative test indicates deficiency.

An impression of depression

In the mitogen and antigen assays, a low stimulation index or unresponsiveness indicates a depressed or defective immune system. Serial testing can monitor the effectiveness of therapy in a patient with an immunodeficiency disease.

Are we compatible?

• In the MLC test, the stimulation index is a measure of compatibility. A high index indicates poor compatibility; conversely, a low stimulation index indicates good compatibility.
• A high stimulation index in response to the relevant pathogen can also demonstrate exposure to malaria, hepatitis, mycoplasmal

pneumonia, periodontal disease, and certain viral infections in patients who no longer have detectable serum antibodies. (See *Lymphocyte transformation test interference.*)

What needs to be done

• If a radioisotope scan is scheduled, make sure the serum sample for this test is drawn first.
• Perform a venipuncture. For an adult, collect the sample in a 7-ml heparinized tube or in a tube volume in accordance with laboratory policy; for a child, use a 5-ml heparinized tube or a tube volume in accordance with laboratory policy.
• Fill the collection tube completely, and invert it gently several times to mix the sample and anticoagulant adequately. Send the sample to the laboratory immediately.

General humoral function

Immunoglobulins G, A, and M

Immunoglobulins—proteins that can function as specific antibodies in response to antigen stimulation—account for humoral immunity. Deviations from normal immunoglobulin percentages occur in many immune disorders, including cancer, hepatic disorders, rheumatoid arthritis, and systemic lupus erythematosus (SLE).

Immunoelectrophoresis identifies immunoglobulin (Ig) G, IgA, and IgM in a serum sample; levels are measured by radial immunodiffusion or nephelometry. Some laboratories detect imunoglobulin by indirect immunofluorescence and radioimmunoassay.

What it all means

Serum Ig levels for adults range as follows:
• *IgG:* 800 to 1,800 mg/dl (SI, 8 to 18 g/L)
• *IgA:* 100 to 400 mg/dl (SI, 1 to 4 g/L)
• *IgM:* 55 to 150 mg/dl (SI, 0.55 to 1.5 g/L).

The lowdown on levels

IgG, IgA, and IgM levels change in various disorders. (See *Serum immunoglobulin levels in various disorders.*) In congenital and acquired hypogammaglobulinemias (decreased levels of gamma globulin in the blood), myelomas, and macroglobulinemia, the find-

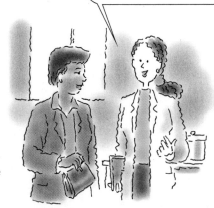

Measuring immunoglobulins helps diagnose multiple myeloma and Waldenström's macroglobulinemia as well as cirrhosis and hepatitis. It can also monitor the effectiveness of chemotherapy or radiation therapy.

Serum immunoglobulin levels in various disorders

Disorder	IgG	IgA	IgM
Immunoglobulin disorders			
Lymphoid aplasia	D	D	D
Agammaglobulinemia	D	D	D
Type I dysgammaglobulinemia (selective immunoglobulin [Ig] G and IgA deficiency)	D	D	N or I
Type II dysgammaglobulinemia (absent IgA and IgM)	N	D	D
IgA globulinemia	N	D	N
Ataxia-telangiectasia	N	D	N
Multiple myeloma, macroglobulinemia, lymphomas			
Heavy chain disease (Franklin's disease)	D	D	D
IgG myeloma	I	D	D
IgA myeloma	D	I	D
Macroglobulinemia	D	D	I
Acute lymphocytic leukemia	N	D	N
Chronic lymphocytic leukemia	D	D	D
Acute myelocytic leukemia	N	N	N
Chronic myelocytic leukemia	N	D	N
Hodgkin's disease	N	N	N

Key: N = normal; I = increased; D = decreased

(continued)

ings confirm the diagnosis. (See *IgG, IgA, and IgM test interference*, page 149.)

Serum immunoglobulin levels in various disorders *(continued)*

Disorder	IgG	IgA	IgM
Hepatic disorders			
Hepatitis	I	I	I
Laënnec's cirrhosis	I	I	N
Biliary cirrhosis	N	N	I
Hepatoma	N	N	D
Other disorders			
Rheumatoid arthritis	I	I	I
Systemic lupus erythematosus	I	I	I
Nephrotic syndrome	D	D	N
Trypanosomiasis	N	N	I
Pulmonary tuberculosis	I	N	N

Key: N = normal; I = increased; D = decreased

What needs to be done

• Tell the patient to restrict food and fluids, except for water, for 12 to 14 hours before the test.
• Perform a venipuncture, and collect the sample in a 7-ml clot-activator tube or a tube volume in accordance with laboratory policy.
• Send the sample to the laboratory immediately to prevent deterioration of immunoglobulins.

Immune complex assays

When immune complexes are produced faster than they can be cleared by the lymph system, immune complex disease, such as postinfectious syndromes, serum sickness, drug sensitivity, rheumatoid arthritis, and SLE, may occur. Immune complexes can develop when a certain ratio of antigen reacts with antibodies of isotopes immunoglobulin (Ig) G 1, 2, 3, or IgM in tissues. These

Stay on the ball

IgG, IgA, and IgM test interference

- Aminophenazone, anticonvulsants, asparaginase, hydralazine, hydantoin derivatives, hormonal contraceptives, and phenylbutazone may raise levels.
- Methotrexate and severe hypersensitivity to bacillus Calmette-Guérin vaccine may lower levels.
- Dextrans, phenytoin, and high methylprednisolone doses lower IgG and IgA levels; dextrans and methylprednisolone lower IgM levels.
- Methadone raises IgA levels.
- Alcohol or opioid drug abuse may affect results.

complexes can fix the first component of complement (C1) and activate the complement cascade. Subsequent complement-mediated activity leads to inflammation and local tissue necrosis. In the blood, soluble circulating immune complexes may also activate complement and eventually cause damage, usually in the renal glomeruli, the aorta, and other large blood vessels.

Diplomatic immunity

Histologic examination of tissue obtained by biopsy and the use of fluorescence or staining with antibodies specific for immunologic types generally detect immune complexes. However, because tissue biopsies can't provide information about titers of complexes still in circulation, serum assays, which detect circulating immune complexes indirectly, may be required. Because of the inherent variability of these complexes, several serum test methods may be appropriate, using C1, rheumatoid factor, or cellular substrates such as Raji cells as reagents.

What it all means

Normally, immune complexes aren't detectable in serum.

Complex presence

Immune complexes may be present in serum in many autoimmune diseases, such as SLE and rheumatoid arthritis. However, for a definitive diagnosis, the presence of these complexes must be con-

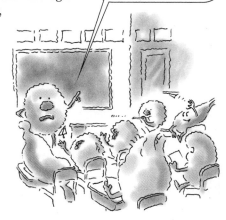

Immune complex assays detect immune complexes in serum. They help monitor response to therapy and assess disease severity.

sidered with other test results. For example, in SLE, immune complexes are associated with high titers of antinuclear antibodies (ANA) and circulating antinative deoxyribonucleic acid (DNA) antibodies. (See *Immune complex assay interference*.)

What needs to be done

• If the patient is scheduled for a C1q (a component of C1) assay, check his history for recent heparin therapy. Report such therapy to the laboratory because it may affect test results.
• Perform a venipuncture, and collect the sample in a 7-ml clot-activator tube or a tube volume in accordance with laboratory policy.
• Send the sample to the laboratory immediately to prevent deterioration of immune complexes.

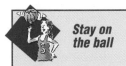

Stay on the ball

Immune complex assay interference

Cryoglobulins in the serum can alter results.

Complement assays

Complement is a collective term for a system of at least 20 serum proteins designed to destroy foreign cells and to help remove foreign materials. The system may be triggered by contact with antigen-antibody complexes or by clotting factor XIIa. A cascade of events follows, resulting in the formation of a complex that ruptures cell membranes.

Complement components are numerically designated as C1 through C9, with C1 having three subcomponents: C1q, C1r, and C1s. These components constitute 3% to 4% of total serum globulins and play a key role in antibody-mediated immune reactions.

Complements can function as a defense by promoting the removal of infectious agents or as a threat by triggering destructive reactions in host tissues. Complement deficiency can increase susceptibility to infection and predispose a patient to other diseases. Complement assays are indicated in patients with known or suspected immune-mediated disease or repeatedly abnormal response to infection.

Various laboratory methods are used to evaluate and measure total complement and its components; hemolytic assay, laser nephelometry, and radial immunodiffusion are the most common.

Not all of the story

Although complement assays provide valuable information about a patient's immune system, the results must be considered in light of serum immunoglobulin and autoantibody tests for a definitive diagnosis of immune-mediated disease or abnormal response to infection.

> Complement assays help detect immune-mediated disease or genetic complement deficiency. They also help monitor the effectiveness of therapy.

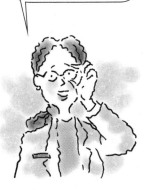

What it all means

Normal values for complement range as follows:
- *total complement:* 25 to 110 units/ml (SI, 0.25 to 1.1 g/L)
- *C3:* 70 to 150 mg/dl (SI, 0.7 to 1.5 g/L)
- *C4:* 15 to 45 mg/dl (SI, 0.15 to 0.45 g/L).

Short on complement

Complement abnormalities may be genetic or acquired; acquired abnormalities are most common. Depressed total complement levels (which are clinically more significant than elevations) may result from excessive formation of antigen-antibody complexes, insufficient synthesis of complement, inhibitor formation, or increased complement catabolism; decreased levels are characteristic in such conditions as SLE, acute poststreptococcal glomerulonephritis, and acute serum sickness. Low levels may also occur in some patients with advanced cirrhosis of the liver, multiple myeloma, hypogammaglobulinemia, and rapidly rejecting allografts.

Too complementary

Elevated total complement may occur in obstructive jaundice, thyroiditis, acute rheumatic fever, rheumatoid arthritis, acute myocardial infarction, ulcerative colitis, and diabetes.

C1 esterase inhibitor deficiency is characteristic in hereditary angioedema, the most common genetic abnormality associated with complement. C3 deficiency is characteristic in recurrent pyogenic infection, and C4 deficiency is characteristic in SLE and rheumatoid arthritis; its level is increased in autoimmune hemolytic anemia. (See *Complement assay interference.*)

What needs to be done

- Perform a venipuncture, and collect the sample in a 7-ml tube without additives, or a tube volume in accordance with laboratory policy.
- Send the sample to the laboratory immediately because complement is heat labile and deteriorates rapidly.

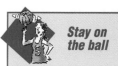

Stay on the ball

Complement assay interference

Recent heparin therapy can alter test results.

Radioallergosorbent test

The radioallergosorbent test (RAST) measures IgE antibodies in serum by radioimmunoassay and identifies specific allergens that cause rashes, asthma, hay fever, drug reactions, or other atopic complaints. RAST is easier to perform and more specific than skin testing; it's also less painful for and less dangerous to the patient.

However, careful selection of specific allergens, based on the patient's clinical history, is crucial for effective testing.

Skin testing is preferred

Although skin testing is still the preferred means of diagnosing IgE-mediated hypersensitivities, RAST may be more useful when a skin disorder makes accurate reading of skin tests difficult, when a patient requires continual antihistamine therapy, or when skin tests are negative but the patient's clinical history supports IgE-mediated hypersensitivity.

What it all means

RAST results are interpreted in relation to a control or reference serum, which differs among laboratories.

Overly sensitive

Elevated serum IgE levels suggest hypersensitivity to the specific allergen or allergens used. (See *RAST test interference*.)

What needs to be done

• If the patient is scheduled for a radioactive scan, make sure the sample is collected before the scan.
• Perform a venipuncture, and collect the sample in a 7-ml clot-activator tube or a tube volume in accordance with laboratory policy. Generally, 1 ml of serum is sufficient for five allergen assays. Be sure to note on the laboratory request the specific allergens tested.

Human leukocyte antigen

The HLA test identifies a group of antigens that's present on the surfaces of all nucleated cells but that's most easily detected on lymphocytes.

Antiserum breakup

Three types of HLA (HLA-A, HLA-B, and HLA-C) are measured with a lymphocyte microcytotoxicity assay. A lymphocyte sample is mixed with known antisera to these antigens and complement. Lymphocytes react with a specific antiserum, which causes the cells to break up and allow a dye to enter; they may then be detected by phase microscopy.

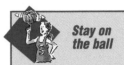

Stay on the ball

RAST test interference

A radioactive scan within 1 week before sample collection may alter test results.

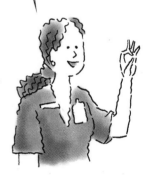

The radioallergosorbent test helps identify allergens to which the patient has immediate, or IgE-mediated, hypersensitivity.

Mixed reaction

A fourth type of HLA, HLA-D, is measured by a mixed leukocyte reaction. Leukocytes from the recipient and the donor are combined in culture to determine HLA-D compatibility.

> The HLA test helps provide histocompatibility typing of tissue recipients and donors and can aid genetic counseling and paternity testing.

What it all means

In HLA-A, HLA-B, and HLA-C testing, lymphocytes that react with the test antiserum break up and are detected by phase microscopy. In HLA-D testing, leukocyte incompatibility is marked by blast formation, DNA synthesis, and reproduction.

Incompatible HLA-A, HLA-B, HLA-C, or HLA-D groups may cause unsuccessful tissue transplantation.

Strong association

Many diseases have a strong association with certain types of HLA. For example, HLA-DR5 is associated with Hashimoto's thyroiditis. HLA-B8 and HLA-Dw3 are associated with Graves' disease, whereas HLA-B8 alone is associated with chronic autoimmune hepatitis, celiac disease, and myasthenia gravis. HLA-Dw3 alone is associated with Addison's disease, Sjögren's syndrome, dermatitis herpetiformis, and SLE.

Fatherly ID

In paternity testing, an alleged father who presents a phenotype (two haplotypes: one from the father and one from the mother) with no haplotype or antigen pair identical to one of the child's is excluded as the father. An alleged father with one haplotype identical to one of the child's may be the father; the probability varies with the incidence of the haplotype in the population. (See *HLA test interference.*)

What needs to be done

• Check the patient history for recent blood transfusions, and report them to the doctor, who may want to postpone HLA testing.
• Perform a venipuncture, and collect the sample in a tube with anticoagulant acid citrate dextrose solution added, or a tube volume in accordance with laboratory policy.

Stay on the ball

HLA test interference

Human leukocyte antigen (HLA) from blood transfused before sample collection may alter test results.

Autoantibodies

Antinuclear antibodies

In such conditions as SLE, scleroderma, and certain infections, the body's immune system may perceive portions of its own cell nuclei as foreign and may produce ANA. Specific types of ANA include antibodies to DNA, nucleoprotein, histones, nuclear ribonucleoprotein, and other nuclear constituents.

Guilty by association

Although ANA are harmless on their own because they don't penetrate living cells, they sometimes form antigen-antibody complexes that cause damage, as in SLE. Because of multi-organ involvement, test results aren't diagnostic and can only partially confirm clinical evidence. (See *ANA incidence in various disorders.*)

What it all means

Using Hep-2 cells, the test for ANA is negative at a titer of 1:40 or below. If mouse kidney substrate is being used, the test is negative at a titer of less than 1:20. Results are reported as positive, with pattern and serum titer noted, or negative.

Sensitive but nonspecific

Although this test is a sensitive indicator of ANA, it isn't specific for SLE. Low titers may occur in patients with viral diseases, chronic hepatic disease, collagen vascular disease, or autoimmune diseases as well as in some healthy adults; incidence increases with age. The higher the titer, the more specific the test is for SLE, for which the titer commonly exceeds 1:256. (See *ANA test interference.*)

> ANA testing helps to screen SLE and can monitor the effectiveness of treatment.

What needs to be done

• If appropriate, inform the patient that the test will be repeated to monitor response to therapy.
• Check the patient history for drugs that may affect test results. Note such drug use on the laboratory request.
• Perform a venipuncture, and collect the sample in a 7-ml tube with no additives, or a tube volume in accordance with laboratory policy.
• Keep a clean, dry bandage over the site for at least 24 hours.

ANA test interference

Certain drugs—most commonly isoniazid, hydralazine, and procainamide—can produce a syndrome resembling systemic lupus erythematosus.

A long list
Other drugs with this effect include chlorpromazine, clofibrate, phenytoin, griseofulvin, ethosuximide, gold salts, methyldopa, hormonal contraceptives, penicillin, phenylbutazone, methysergide, streptomycin, sulfonamides, tetracyclines, mephenytoin, quinidine, primidone, reserpine, and trimethadione.

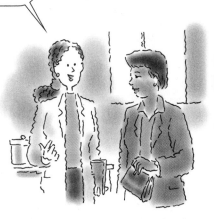

ANA incidence in various disorders

This chart shows the percentage of patients with certain disorders whose serum contains antinuclear antibodies (ANA). About 40% of elderly people and 5% of the general population also have positive ANA findings.

Disorder	Positive ANA
Systemic lupus erythematosus (SLE)	95% to 100%
Lupoid hepatitis	95% to 100%
Felty's syndrome	95% to 100%
Progressive systemic sclerosis (scleroderma)	75% to 80%
Drug-associated SLE-like syndrome (hydralazine, procainamide, isoniazid)	Approximately 50%
Sjögren's syndrome	40% to 75%
Rheumatoid arthritis	25% to 60%
Healthy family member of SLE patient	Approximately 25%
Chronic discoid lupus erythematosus	15% to 50%
Juvenile arthritis	15% to 30%
Polyarteritis nodosa	15% to 25%
Miscellaneous diseases	10% to 50%
Dermatomyositis, polymyositis	10% to 30%
Rheumatic fever	Approximately 5%

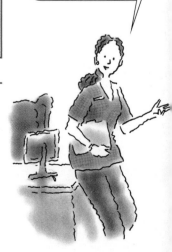

Measuring antithyroid antibodies helps confirm Hashimoto's thyroiditis, Graves' disease, and other thyroid disorders.

Antithyroid antibodies

In such autoimmune disorders as Hashimoto's thyroiditis and Graves' disease (hyperthyroidism), thyroglobulin—the major colloidal storage compound—is released into blood. Antithyroglobulin antibodies are produced to attack this foreign substance; the ensuing autoimmune response damages the thyroid gland.

What it all means

The normal titer is less than 1:100 for both antithyroglobulin and antimicrosomal antibodies. Low levels of these antibodies are normal in 10% of the general population and in 20% or more of people age 70 and older. There are no known factors that interfere with the antithyroid antibody test.

Suggestive titers

The presence of antithyroglobulin or antimicrosomal antibodies in serum can indicate subclinical autoimmune thyroid disease, Graves' disease, or idiopathic myxedema. High titers (1:400 or more) strongly suggest Hashimoto's thyroiditis.

These antibodies may also occur in patients with other autoimmune disorders, such as SLE, rheumatoid arthritis, or autoimmune hemolytic anemia.

What needs to be done

• Perform a venipuncture, and collect the sample in a 7-ml tube with no additives, or a tube volume in accordance with laboratory policy.

Thyroid-stimulating immunoglobulin

Thyroid-stimulating immunoglobulin (TSI), formerly called *long-acting thyroid stimulator*, appears in the blood of most patients with Graves' disease. This autoantibody reacts with the cell-surface receptors that usually combine with thyroid-stimulating hormone. TSI stimulates the thyroid gland to produce and excrete excessive amounts of thyroid hormones.

What it all means

TSI doesn't normally appear in serum. However, it may be present in 5% of people without hyperthyroidism or exophthalmos.

TSI on the rise

Increased TSI levels are associated with exophthalmos, Graves' disease (thyrotoxicosis), and recurrence of hyperthyroidism. (See *TSI test interference*.)

What needs to be done

• Perform a venipuncture, and collect the sample in a 5-ml clot-activator tube or a tube volume in accordance with laboratory policy.

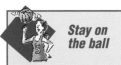

Stay on the ball

TSI test interference

Administration of radioactive iodine within 48 hours before the test may affect the accuracy of results.

• Note on the laboratory request whether the patient had a radioactive iodine scan within 48 hours before the test.

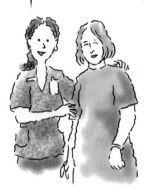

> Testing for RF is the best way to confirm that you have rheumatoid arthritis.

Rheumatoid factor

The rheumatoid factor (RF) test is the most useful immunologic test for confirming rheumatoid arthritis (RA). In this disease, "renegade" IgG antibodies, produced by lymphocytes in the synovial joints, react with other IgG or IgM molecules to produce immune complexes, complement activation, and tissue destruction. How IgG molecules become antigenic is still unknown, but they may be altered by aggregating with viruses or other antigens. These immune complexes can migrate from the synovial fluid to other areas of the body, causing vasculitis, subcutaneous nodules, or lymphadenopathy. The IgG or IgM molecules that react with altered IgG are called *rheumatoid factors*.

What it all means

• Normal RF titer is less than 1:20; normal rheumatoid screening test is nonreactive.
• Non-RA and RA populations aren't clearly separated with regard to the presence of RF: Approximately 25% of patients with RA have a nonreactive titer; 8% of non-RA patients are reactive at greater than 39 International Units/ml, and only 3% of non-RA patients are reactive at greater than 80 International Units/ml.
• Patients with various non-RA diseases characterized by chronic inflammation—such as SLE, scleroderma, polymyositis, tuberculosis, infectious mononucleosis, syphilis, viral hepatic disease, and influenza—may test positive for RF. (See *RF test interference*.)

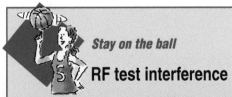

Stay on the ball

RF test interference

• Serum with high immunoglobulin (Ig) G levels may cause false-negative results through competition with IgG on the surface of latex particles or sheep red blood cells used as substrate.

What needs to be done

• Perform a venipuncture, and collect the sample in a 7-ml clot-activator tube or a tube volume in accordance with laboratory policy.

• Because a patient with RA may be immunocompromised from the disease or from corticosteroid therapy, keep the venipuncture site covered with a clean, dry bandage for 24 hours. Check regularly for signs of infection.

Cold agglutinins

Cold agglutinins are antibodies (usually of the IgM type) that cause RBCs to aggregate at low temperatures. Transient elevations of these antibodies develop during certain infectious diseases, notably primary atypical pneumonia. Small amounts may also occur in healthy people. The test for cold agglutinins reliably detects such pneumonia within 1 to 2 weeks after onset.

What it all means

Results are reported as positive or negative. Positive results are titered. Normal titers are less than 1:16.

Riding high with infection

High titers may occur as primary phenomena or secondary to infections or lymphoreticular malignancy (cancer involving the phagocytic cells in the lymph system). Levels may be elevated in infectious mononucleosis, cytomegalovirus (CMV) infection, hemolytic anemia, multiple myeloma, scleroderma, malaria, cirrhosis, congenital syphilis, peripheral vascular disease, pulmonary embolism, trypanosomiasis, tonsillitis, staphylococcemia, scarlatina, influenza and, occasionally, pregnancy.

Chronically high with pneumonia

Chronically elevated titers are most commonly associated with pneumonia and lymphoreticular malignancy; an acute transient elevation commonly accompanies many viral infections.

Positive, peak, then disappear

In primary atypical pneumonia, cold agglutinins appear in serum in one-half to two-thirds of all patients during the 1st week of acute infection. Titers usually become positive at 7 days, peak above 1:32 in 4 weeks, and disappear rapidly after 6 weeks. When sequential titers verify this pattern and clinical evidence of pneumonia exists, the diagnosis is confirmed.

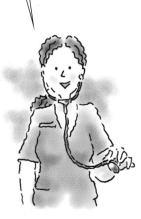

Testing for cold agglutinins helps confirm pneumonia and viral infection.

Sounding the alarm on lymphoma

Extremely high titers (1:2,000 or higher) can occur with idiopathic cold agglutinin disease that precedes development of lymphoma. Patients with extremely high titers are susceptible to intravascular agglutination, which causes significant clinical problems. (See *Cold agglutinins test interference.*)

What needs to be done

• If appropriate, inform the patient that the test will be repeated to monitor his response to therapy.
• If the patient is receiving antimicrobial drugs, note this on the laboratory request because these drugs may interfere with the development of cold agglutinins.
• Perform a venipuncture, and collect the sample in a 7-ml tube without additives that has been prewarmed to 98.6° F (37° C), or a tube volume in accordance with laboratory policy.
• Send the sample to the laboratory immediately.
• Don't refrigerate the sample; cold agglutinins will coat the RBCs, leaving none in the serum.

Stay on the ball

Cold agglutinins test interference

Antimicrobials can interfere with cold agglutinins, producing a false-negative test result.

Acetylcholine receptor antibodies

The acetylcholine receptor (AChR) antibodies test is the most useful test for confirming myasthenia gravis, a disorder of neuromuscular transmission. In normal muscle contraction, acetylcholine (ACh) is released from the terminal end of the nerve and binds to AChR sites on the muscle motor end plate. In myasthenia gravis, antibodies block and destroy AChR sites, causing muscle weakness that can be either generalized or localized to the ocular muscles.

Two test methods—a binding assay and a blocking assay—are available to determine the relative concentration of AChR antibodies in serum. Determination of AChR antibodies by either method also helps monitor immunosuppressive therapy for myasthenia gravis, although antibody levels don't usually parallel the severity of the disease.

Presence of AchR antibodies confirms myasthenia gravis. Further testing can monitor myasthenia gravis therapy.

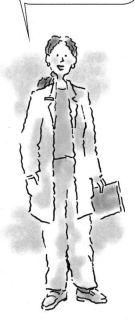

What it all means

Normal serum is negative for AChR-binding antibodies and is negative for AChR-blocking antibodies.

Confirming results

Positive AChR antibodies in symptomatic adults confirm the diagnosis of myasthenia gravis. Patients with only ocular symptoms

Stay on the ball

AchR antibody test interference

• Patients undergoing thymectomy, thoracic duct drainage, immuno-suppressive therapy, or plasmapheresis may show reduced AChR antibody levels.
• Patients with amyotrophic lateral sclerosis may show false-positive results.

tend to have lower antibody titers than those with generalized symptoms. (See *AchR antibody test interference.*)

What needs to be done

• Check the patient history for immunosuppressive drugs that may affect test results, and note their use on the laboratory request.
• Perform a venipuncture, and collect the sample in a 7-ml tube without additives, or a tube volume in accordance with laboratory policy.
• Check the venipuncture site for infection, and promptly report any change; patients with autoimmune disease have compromised immune systems. Keep a clean, dry bandage over the site for at least 24 hours.
• Keep the sample at room temperature, and send it to the laboratory immediately.

Anti-insulin antibodies

Some diabetic patients form antibodies to the insulin they take. These antibodies bind with some of the insulin, making less insulin available for glucose metabolism and necessitating increased insulin dosages. This phenomenon is known as *insulin resistance.*

Detective work

Performed on the blood of a diabetic patient receiving insulin, the anti-insulin antibody test detects insulin antibodies. Insulin antibodies are immunoglobulins and are called *anti-insulin Ab*. The most common type of anti-insulin Ab is IgG, but anti-insulin Ab is also found in the other four classes of Ig—A, D, E, and M. IgM may

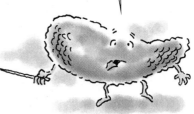

Testing for anti-insulin antibodies confirms insulin resistance.

cause insulin resistance, and IgE has been associated with allergic reactions.

What it all means

Less than 3% of the patient's serum should bind with labeled human and pork insulin.

Abnormal response, or resistance?

Elevated levels may occur in insulin allergy or resistance and in factitious hypoglycemia. (See *Anti-insulin antibody test interference.*)

What needs to be done

• If the patient has recently had a radioactive test, note this on the laboratory request.
• Perform a venipuncture, and collect the sample in a 7-ml tube with no additives, or a tube volume in accordance with laboratory policy.

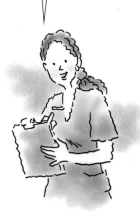

Stay on the ball

Anti-insulin antibody test interference

Radioactive test within 1 week before the test may alter results.

Anti-double-stranded DNA antibodies

About two-thirds of patients with active SLE have measurable levels of autoantibodies to double-stranded, or native, DNA (known as *anti-ds-DNA*). These antibodies are rarely detected in patients with other connective tissue diseases.

In autoimmune diseases such as SLE, native DNA is thought to be the antigen that forms a complex with antibody and complement, causing local tissue damage where these complexes are deposited. Serum anti-ds-DNA levels are directly related to the extent of renal or vascular damage caused by the disease.

The anti-ds-DNA antibody test measures and differentiates these antibody levels in a blood sample. If anti-ds-DNA antibodies are present, they combine with native DNA and form complexes that are too large to pass through a membrane filter. The test counts these oversized complexes.

Testing for anti-ds-DNA antibodies helps confirm SLE and monitor its therapy.

What it all means

An anti-ds-DNA antibody level less than 25 International Units/ml (SI, less than 25 kIU/L) is considered negative for SLE.

The lowdown on levels

Elevated anti-ds-DNA antibody levels may indicate SLE. Values of 25 to 30 International Units/ml (SI, 25 to 30 kIU/L) are considered borderline positive. Values of 31 to 200 International Units/ml (SI,

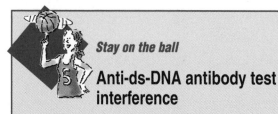

Stay on the ball

Anti-ds-DNA antibody test interference

Radioactive scan within 1 week before collection of a sample may alter results.

31 to 200 kIU/L) are positive, and those greater than 200 International Units/ml (SI, greater than 200 kIU/L) are strongly positive.

Depressed anti-ds-DNA antibody levels may follow immunosuppressive therapy, demonstrating effective treatment of SLE. (See *Anti-ds-DNA antibody test interference.*)

What needs to be done

• If the patient has recently had a radioactive test, note this on the laboratory request.
• Perform a venipuncture, and collect the sample in a 7-ml tube with no additives, or a tube volume in accordance with laboratory policy. Some laboratories may specify a tube with either EDTA or sodium fluoride and potassium oxalate added.

Viruses

Rubella antibodies

Although rubella (German measles) is generally a mild viral infection in children and young adults, it can produce severe infection in a fetus, resulting in spontaneous abortion, stillbirth, or congenital rubella syndrome. Because rubella infection normally induces IgG and IgM antibody production, measuring rubella antibodies can determine current infection and immunity resulting from past infection. (See *When immunity status is unknown.*)

What it all means

Titer of 1:8 or less indicates little or no immunity against rubella; titer greater than 1:10 indicates adequate protection against rubella.

> Testing for rubella antibodies is pretty important to me. It can diagnose rubella infection and determine susceptibility in women of childbearing age and in children.

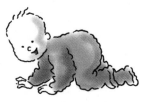

When immunity status is unknown

Rubella exposure risk may be evaluated using two serum samples, as follows:
• The first sample should be drawn in the acute phase of clinical symptoms. If clinical symptoms aren't apparent, the sample should be drawn as soon as possible after the suspected exposure.
• The second sample should be drawn 3 to 4 weeks later, during the convalescent phase.

The lowdown on levels

The presence of rubella-specific IgM antibodies indicates recent infection in an adult and congenital rubella in an infant.

What needs to be done

• Explain to the patient that if a current infection is suspected, a second blood sample will be needed in 2 to 3 weeks to identify a rise in the titer.
• Perform a venipuncture, and collect the sample in a 7-ml clot-activator tube or a tube volume in accordance with laboratory policy.

Hepatitis B surface antigen

Hepatitis B surface antigen (HBsAg) appears in the serum of patients with hepatitis B virus, formerly called *serum hepatitis* or *long-incubation hepatitis*. This antigen, also known as *hepatitis-associated antigen* and *Australia antigen*, can be detected during the extended incubation period and usually during the first 3 weeks of acute infection or if the patient is a carrier.

Grave complication

Because transmission of hepatitis is one of the gravest complications associated with blood transfusions, all donors must be screened for hepatitis B before their blood is stored. This screening, required by the Food and Drug Administration's Bureau of Biologics, has helped reduce the incidence of hepatitis. This test doesn't screen for hepatitis A (infectious hepatitis). (For information on related testing, see *Viral hepatitis test panel*, page 164.)

What it all means

Serum should be negative for HBsAg.

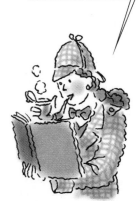

The HBsAg test screens blood donors as well as people at risk for contracting the disease.

Viral hepatitis test panel

The six types of viral hepatitis produce similar symptoms but differ in transmission mode, course of treatment, prognosis, and carrier status. When the clinical history is insufficient for differentiation, serologic tests can aid in a diagnosis. Testing helps to identify antibodies specific to the causative virus and establish the type of hepatitis:

- Type A: Detection of an antibody to hepatitis A confirms the diagnosis.
- Type B: The presence of hepatitis B surface antigens and hepatitis B antibodies confirms the diagnosis.
- Type C: Diagnosis depends on serologic testing for the specific antibody 1 or more months after the onset of acute illness; until then, diagnosis is established principally by obtaining negative test results for hepatitis A, B, and D.
- Type D: Detection of intrahepatic delta antigens or immunoglobulin (Ig) M antidelta antigens in acute disease (or IgM and IgG in chronic disease) establishes the diagnosis.
- Type E: Detection of hepatitis E antigens supports the diagnosis and possibly rules out hepatitis C.
- Type G: Detection of hepatitis G ribonucleic acid supports the diagnosis (serologic assays are being developed).

Additional findings from liver function studies that support the diagnosis include:
- serum aspartate aminotransferase and serum alanine aminotransferase levels increased in the prodromal stage of acute viral hepatitis
- serum alkaline phosphatase levels slightly increased
- serum bilirubin levels elevated, with levels possibly remaining elevated late in the disease, especially with severe disease
- prolonged prothrombin time (PT) (PT of more than 3 seconds longer than normal, indicating severe liver damage)
- white blood cell counts commonly revealing transient neutropenia and lymphopenia followed by lymphocytosis.

Retest if positive

The presence of HBsAg in a patient with hepatitis confirms hepatitis B. In chronic carriers and persons with chronic active hepatitis, HBsAg may be present in serum several months after the onset of acute infection. HBsAg may also appear in the serum of more than 5% of patients with certain diseases other than hepatitis, such as hemophilia, Hodgkin's disease, and leukemia. If the antigen is found in donor blood, the blood must be discarded because of the high risk of transmitting hepatitis. Blood samples that test positive should be retested because inaccurate results do occur. (See *HBsAg test interference.*)

What needs to be done

- Check the patient history for hepatitis B vaccine.

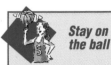

Stay on the ball

HBsAg test interference

Patients who have received the hepatitis B vaccine may test positive.

- If the patient is giving blood, explain the donation procedure to him.
- Perform a venipuncture, and collect the sample in a 10-ml clot-activator tube or a tube volume in accordance with laboratory policy.
- Because hepatitis B is easily transmitted, wash your hands carefully after the procedure. Remember to wear gloves when drawing blood and to dispose of the needle properly.

Hepatitis A antibodies

Hepatitis A antibodies are present in blood and feces only briefly before symptoms appear. This test identifies hepatitis A antibodies that appear in the serum or body fluid of patients with hepatitis A virus (HAV) and aids in the differential diagnosis of viral hepatitis.

What it all means

Normally, the serum is negative for hepatitis A antibodies. A single positive test result may indicate previous exposure to the virus, but because these antibodies persist so long in the bloodstream, only evidence of rising anti-HAV titers confirms HAV as the cause of current or very recent infection. (See *Hepatitis A antibody test interference.*)

What needs to be done

- Check the patient history for administration of hepatitis vaccine.
- Inform the patient that he need not restrict food or fluids before the test.
- Perform a venipuncture, and collect the sample in two 3- or 4.5-ml EDTA tubes or a tube volume in accordance with laboratory policy.
- Tell the patient that confirmed viral hepatitis is reported to public health authorities in most states.

Heterophil antibodies

Heterophil antibody tests detect and identify two IgM antibodies in human serum that react against foreign RBCs: Epstein-Barr virus (EBV) antibodies and Forssman antibodies.

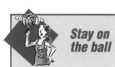

Stay on the ball

Hepatitis A antibody test interference

Previous administration of the hepatitis vaccine can result in a possible positive test result for hepatitis A antibodies.

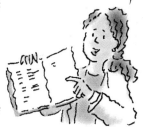

This test aids in the differential diagnosis of viral hepatitis.

What it all means

Normally, the titer is less than 1:56 but may be higher in elderly people. Some laboratories refer to a normal titer as "negative" or as having "no reaction."

Abnormal results

Although heterophil antibodies are present in the sera of about 80% of patients with infectious mononucleosis 1 month after on-set, a positive finding—a titer higher than 1:56—doesn't confirm this disorder; a high titer can also result from SLE, syphilis, cryo-globulinemia, or the presence of antibodies to nonsyphilitic trepo-nematosis, such as yaws, pinta, and bejel. A gradual increase in titer during week 3 or 4 followed by a gradual decrease during weeks 4 to 8 proves most conclusive for infectious mononucleo-sis.

Delayed reaction

A negative titer doesn't always rule out this disorder; occasionally, the titer becomes reactive 2 weeks later. Therefore, if symptoms persist, the test should be repeated in 2 weeks. Confirmation of in-fectious mononucleosis depends on heterophil agglutination tests and hematologic tests. (See *Explaining mononucleosis* and *Het-erophil antibody test interference.*)

What needs to be done

Perform a venipuncture, and collect the sample in a 7-ml clot-acti-vator tube or a tube volume in accordance with laboratory policy.

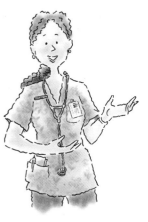

Heterophil antibody tests aid in the diagnosis of infectious mononucleosis.

Listen up!

Explaining mononucleosis

If your patient's heterophil antibody titer is positive and infectious mononucleosis is confirmed, explain the treatment plan.

If the titer is positive but infectious mononucleosis isn't confirmed, or if the titer is negative but symptoms persist, explain that additional testing will be necessary in a few days or weeks to confirm the diagno-sis and plan effective treatment.

Stay on the ball

Heterophil antibody test interference

• Opioid and phenytoin therapy can produce false-positive results.
• Patients with lym-phoma, hepatitis, or leukemia may have false-positive results.

Epstein-Barr virus antibodies

EBV, a member of the herpesvirus group, is the causative agent in infectious mononucleosis, Burkitt's lymphoma, and nasopharyngeal carcinoma. Although the virus doesn't reproduce in standard cell cultures, most EBV infections can be recognized by testing the patient's serum for antibodies (monospot test), which usually appear within the first 3 weeks of illness and then decline rapidly within a few weeks. (See *Monospot test for infectious mononucleosis*.)

Alternatively, EBV-specific antibodies, which develop into several antigens, can be measured with high sensitivity and specificity by indirect immunofluorescence tests. The test profile can help determine whether the patient was infected recently or in the remote past.

What it all means

Serum from patients who have never been infected with EBV will have no detectable antibodies to the virus measured by either the monospot or indirect immunofluorescence test. The monospot test is positive only during the acute phase of EBV infection; the indirect immunofluorescence test will detect and discriminate between acute and past infection.

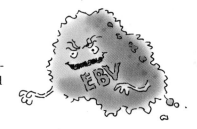

Just call me EBV. Testing for antibodies to me helps diagnose heterophil-negative infectious mononucleosis.

Now I get it!

Monospot test for infectious mononucleosis

The monospot test detects the infectious mononucleosis antibody. Heterophil antibodies, normally present in the blood, are produced in large amounts in patients with infectious mononucleosis. These antibodies quickly clump together with horse red blood cells (RBCs).

In a more common version of the monospot test, the patient's serum is added to horse RBCs on a slide. If clumping (agglutination) occurs, heterophil antibodies are present, confirming infectious mononucleosis.

What needs to be done

• Perform a venipuncture, and collect 5 ml of blood in a clot-activator tube or a tube volume in accordance with laboratory policy. Allow the blood to clot for at least 1 hour at room temperature.

Respiratory syncytial virus antibodies

Respiratory syncytial virus (RSV) is the major viral cause of severe lower respiratory tract disease in infants, but it may cause infections in persons of any age. RSV infections are most common and produce the most severe disease during the first 6 months of life.

IgG and IgM class antibodies can be easily measured using the indirect immunofluorescence test. Specific results for IgM are obtained only after separating this class of antibody from IgG. Prevalence of IgG antibodies to RSV is extremely high (greater than 95%), especially in adults.

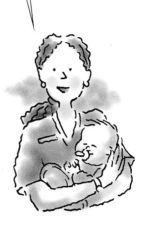

The RSV test diagnoses infections caused by RSV.

What it all means

Serum from patients who have never been infected with RSV will have no detectable antibodies to the virus (less than 1:5). In infants, serologic diagnosis of RSV infections is difficult because of the presence of maternal IgG antibodies; thus, the presence of IgM antibodies is most significant.

Ruling out RSV

RSV infection can be ruled out in patients whose serum samples have no detectable antibodies to the virus. The presence of IgM or a fourfold or greater increase in IgG antibodies indicates active RSV infection.

What needs to be done

• Perform a venipuncture, and collect 5 ml of blood in a clot-activator tube or a tube volume in accordance with laboratory policy. Allow the blood to clot for at least 1 hour at room temperature.
• Transfer the serum to a sterile tube or vial, and send it to the laboratory immediately. If transfer must be delayed, store the serum at 39.2° F (4° C) for 1 to 2 days or at –4° F (–20° C) for longer periods to avoid bacterial contamination.

Herpes simplex antibodies

Herpes simplex virus (HSV), a member of the herpesvirus group, causes severe signs and symptoms, including genital lesions, keratitis or conjunctivitis, generalized dermal lesions, and pneumonia. Severe involvement is associated with intrauterine or neonatal infections and encephalitis; such infections are most severe in immunosuppressed patients.

Two types

Of the two closely related types, type 1 usually causes infections above the waistline; type 2 primarily involves the external genitalia. Primary contact with this virus occurs in early childhood as acute stomatitis or, more commonly, as an inapparent infection. More than 50% of adults have antibodies to HSV.

Sensitive tests are used to demonstrate IgM class antibodies to HSV or to detect a fourfold or greater increase in IgG class antibodies between acute- and convalescent-phase serum.

What it all means

Serum from patients who have never been infected with HSV will have no detectable antibodies (less than 1:5). Patients with primary HSV infection develop IgM and IgG class antibodies. Reportedly, more than 50% of adults have IgG class antibodies to HSV because of prior infection. Reactivated infections caused by HSV can be recognized serologically only by an increase in IgG class antibodies between acute- and convalescent-phase serum.

Fourfold or greater = HSV

HSV infection can be ruled out in patients whose serum shows no detectable antibodies to the virus. The presence of IgM antibodies or a fourfold or greater increase in IgG antibodies indicates active HSV infection. A patient infected within the last 3 months may not have developed an antibody response and may have a false-negative test result.

What needs to be done

• Perform a venipuncture, and collect 5 ml of blood, or a tube volume in accordance with laboratory policy, in a tube (color of top to be designated by the laboratory). Allow the blood to clot for at least 1 hour at room temperature.

Human immunodeficiency virus antibodies

The human immunodeficiency virus (HIV) antibodies test detects antibodies to HIV in serum. HIV is the virus that causes AIDS. Transmission occurs by direct exposure of a person's blood to body fluids containing the virus. The virus may be transmitted from one person to another through exchange of contaminated

Testing for HIV

More and newer tests are available to help identify human immunodeficiency virus (HIV)–infected antibodies quicker and more conveniently, including a test to identify genetic changes that may alter the patient's course of treatment.

The Centers for Disease Control and Prevention and the American Medical Association recommend HIV testing for all patients between the ages of 13 and 64.

OraQuick rapid HIV-1 antibody test

For the many people each year who don't check back for test results, rapid HIV testing may be performed in any outpatient setting. The OraQuick rapid HIV-1 antibody test, approved by the Food and Drug Administration (FDA), allows results to be obtained in less than 20 minutes using 1 drop of blood. A color indicator similar to a home pregnancy test is used. If the test result is positive, another test must be done to confirm the results.

Nucleic acid test

The FDA has also approved a nucleic acid test to screen plasma donation for HIV and hepatitis C. This test has dramatically reduced the waiting time involved until blood and blood products may be used.

Gene-based test

Spikes of HIV virus in the bloodstream commonly mean that the individual being treated for HIV is growing resistant to his current drug treatment. The government has approved the first gene-based test to help determine whether an HIV-infected person's virus is mutating, thereby causing therapy to fail. This test can help the physician select more appropriate treatment.

---

blood and blood products, through sexual intercourse with an infected partner, through I.V. drug sharing, and from an infected mother to her child during pregnancy or breastfeeding.

Initial identification of HIV is usually done through the enzyme-linked immunosorbent assay (ELISA). Positive results are confirmed by Western blot test and immunofluorescence. Other available tests may be performed to detect antibodies. (See *Testing for HIV*.)

What it all means

Test results should be nonreactive. No known factors interfere with HIV antibodies.

Earlier exposure

This test detects previous exposure to HIV. A negative result doesn't necessarily mean that HIV antibodies aren't present. For example, the tests don't identify individuals who have been exposed to the virus but who haven't yet developed antibodies. A positive test for the HIV antibody can't determine whether the person harbors the actively replicating virus or when he'll present signs and symptoms of AIDS.

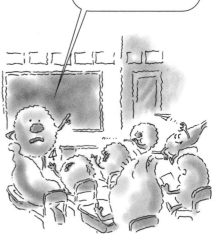

The HIV test can be used to screen patients and donated blood for HIV.

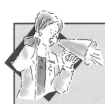

Many apparently healthy people have been exposed to HIV and have circulating antibodies. The test results for such people aren't considered false-positives. Likewise, patients in the later stages of AIDS may exhibit no detectable antibody in their sera because they can no longer mount an antibody response. (See *When test results are positive.*)

What needs to be done

• Perform a venipuncture, and collect the sample in a 10-ml barrier tube, or a tube volume in accordance with laboratory policy, which helps prevent contamination when pouring the serum.

Cytomegalovirus antibody screen

After primary infection, CMV remains latent in WBCs. The presence of CMV antibodies indicates past infection with this virus.

Screening tests for CMV antibodies are qualitative; they detect the presence of antibody at a single low dilution. In quantitative methods, several dilutions of the serum sample are tested to indicate acute infection with CMV.

> Presence of CMV antibodies indicates infection. The test screens organ donors and helps detect prior CMV immunocompromised patients.

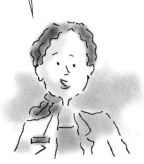

What it all means

Patients who have never been infected with CMV have no detectable antibodies to the virus. IgG and IgM are normally negative.

A serum sample collected early during the acute phase or late in the convalescent stage may not contain detectable IgG or IgM antibodies to CMV. Therefore, a negative result doesn't preclude recent infection. More than a single sample is needed to ensure accurate results.

Seronegative recipient needs seronegative donor

A serum sample that tests positive for antibodies at this single dilution indicates that the patient has been infected with CMV and that his WBCs contain latent virus capable of being reactivated in an immunocompromised host.

Immunosuppressed patients who lack antibodies to CMV should receive blood products or organ transplants from donors who are also seronegative. Patients with CMV antibodies don't require seronegative blood products.

What needs to be done

- Perform a venipuncture, and collect the sample in a 5-ml tube without additives, or a tube volume in accordance with laboratory policy.
- Allow the blood to clot for at least 1 hour at room temperature.

Bacteria and fungi

Fungal serology

Most fungal organisms enter the body as spores inhaled into the lungs or infiltrated through wounds in the skin or mucosa. If the body's defenses can't destroy the organisms initially, the fungi multiply to form lesions; blood and lymph vessels may then spread the mycosis (disease caused by a fungus) throughout the body.

Mycosis may be deep-seated or superficial. Deep-seated mycosis occurs primarily in the lungs; superficial mycosis occurs in the skin or the mucosal linings.

Culture club

Although cultures are usually performed to diagnose mycosis by identifying the causative organism, serologic tests occasionally provide the sole evidence of mycosis. These tests are used to detect blastomycosis, coccidioidomycosis, histoplasmosis, aspergillosis, sporotrichosis, and cryptococcosis. Fungal serologic tests use immunodiffusion, complement fixation, precipitin, latex agglutination, or agglutination methods to demonstrate the presence of mycotic antibodies.

What it all means

Depending on the test method, a negative finding or normal titer usually indicates the absence of mycosis. Elevated titers indicate that mycosis is present. (See *Fungal serology interference*.)

> Presence of antifungal antibodies indicates a fungal infection. Testing can monitor the effectiveness of mycosis therapy.

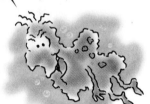

Stay on the ball

Fungal serology interference

- Recent skin testing with fungal antigens may elevate titers.
- Many mycoses depress the immune system, causing low titers or false-negative results.

What needs to be done

- If appropriate, explain to the patient that the test monitors his response to therapy and that it may be repeated during the course of his illness.
- Perform a venipuncture, and collect the sample in a 10-ml clot-activator tube or a tube volume in accordance with laboratory policy.

Bacterial meningitis antigen

The bacterial meningitis antigen test can detect specific antigens of *Streptococcus pneumoniae*, *Neisseria meningitidis*, and *Haemophilus influenzae* type b, the principal organisms that cause meningitis. This test can be performed on samples of serum, cerebrospinal fluid (CSF), urine, pleural fluid, or joint fluid; however, the preferred sample is CSF or urine.

> Testing for the bacterial meningitis antigen can identify the causative agent in meningitis.

What it all means

Normal results are negative for bacterial antigens.

A positive ID

Positive results identify the specific bacterial antigen: *S. pneumoniae*, *N. meningitidis*, *H. influenzae* type b, or group B streptococci. (See *Bacterial meningitis antigen test interference*, page 174.)

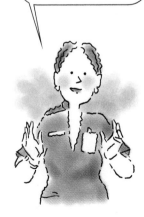

What needs to be done

- Explain the purpose of the test to the patient, and inform him that a urine or CSF specimen is required.

- If a CSF specimen is needed, describe how it will be obtained.
- Explain who'll perform the lumbar puncture and when and that transient discomfort may be felt from the needle puncture.
- Advise the patient that a headache is the most common adverse effect of lumbar puncture but that cooperation during the test minimizes this effect.
- Make sure the patient or a family member has signed a consent form (if a CSF specimen is being obtained).
- As required, collect a 10-ml urine specimen or a 1-ml CSF specimen in a sterile container.
- Promptly send the specimen to the laboratory on a refrigerated coolant.

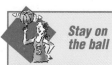

Stay on the ball

Bacterial meningitis antigen test interference

Previous antimicrobial therapy may alter test results.

Lyme disease serology

Lyme disease is a multisystem disorder characterized by dermatologic, neurologic, cardiac, and rheumatic manifestations in various stages. Studies point to a commonly tickborne spirochete, *Borrelia burgdorferi*, as the causative agent.

50% early versus 100% late

Serologic tests for Lyme disease measure antibody response to this spirochete and indicate current infection or past exposure. These tests can identify 50% of patients with early-stage Lyme disease; nearly 100% of patients with later complications of carditis, neuritis, or arthritis; and 100% of patients in remission.

What it all means

Normal serum values are nonreactive.

Suggestive but not definite

A positive Lyme serologic test strongly suggests the diagnosis but isn't definitive because other treponemal diseases and high RF titers can cause false-positive results.

Don't be misled

In addition, a negative result doesn't rule out Lyme disease because more than 15% of patients with Lyme disease fail to develop antibodies.

What needs to be done

- Perform a venipuncture, and collect the sample in a 7-ml clot-activator tube or a tube volume in accordance with laboratory policy.
- Send the specimen to the laboratory immediately.

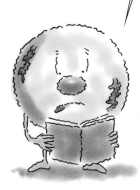

Lyme disease serology testing measures antibody response to the spirochete that causes Lyme disease.

Helicobacter pylori antibodies

Helicobacter pylori is a spiral, gram-negative bacterium associated with chronic gastritis and idiopathic chronic duodenal ulceration. Although a gastric specimen can be obtained by endoscopy and cultured for *H. pylori*, the *H. pylori* antibody blood test is a more useful noninvasive screening procedure and may be performed using the ELISA test.

Because you have GI symptoms, we're testing for H. pylori antibodies to diagnose an ulcer.

What it all means

Normally, no antibodies to *H. pylori* are revealed. Test results are reported as negative or positive. There are no known factors that interfere with *H. pylori* antibodies.

Bacterium antibodies

A positive *H. pylori* test result indicates that the patient has antibodies to the bacterium. The serologic results should be interpreted in light of the clinical findings. This test should be performed only on a patient with GI symptoms because of the large number of healthy people who have *H. pylori* antibodies.

What needs to be done

• Perform a venipuncture, and collect the sample in a 7-ml clot-activator tube or a tube volume in accordance with laboratory policy.
• Send the sample to the laboratory immediately.

Miscellaneous tests

Venereal Disease Research Laboratory test

The Venereal Disease Research Laboratory test, commonly known as the *VDRL test*, is widely used to screen for primary and secondary syphilis.

The VDRL test uses a serum sample but may also be performed on CSF to test for tertiary syphilis. However, the VDRL test of CSF is less sensitive than the fluorescent treponemal antibody absorption test. The rapid plasma reagin test can also be used to diagnose syphilis. (See *RPR test*, page 176.)

Now I get it!

RPR test

The rapid plasma reagin (RPR) test, a rapid serologic test, is an acceptable substitute for the Venereal Disease Research Laboratory (VDRL) test in diagnosing syphilis. Available as a kit, the RPR test uses a cardiolipin antigen to detect reagin, the antibody relatively specific for *Treponema pallidum,* the agent that causes syphilis.

In the RPR test, like the VDRL test, normal serum shows no flocculation.

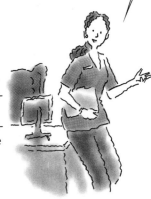

The VDRL test screens for primary and secondary syphilis and can monitor the patient's response to treatment.

What it all means

Absence of flocculation is reported as a nonreactive test.

Ifs, ands, or lesions

Definite flocculation is reported as a reactive test; slight flocculation is reported as a weakly reactive test. A reactive VDRL test occurs in about 50% of patients with primary syphilis and in nearly all patients with secondary syphilis. If syphilitic lesions exist, a reactive VDRL test is diagnostic. If no lesions are evident, a reactive VDRL test necessitates repeated testing. However, biologic false-positive reactions can be caused by conditions unrelated to syphilis, such as infectious mononucleosis, malaria, leprosy, hepatitis, SLE, rheumatoid arthritis, and such nonsyphilitic treponemal diseases as pinta or yaws.

On to the next stage

A reactive VDRL test using a CSF specimen indicates neurosyphilis, which can follow the primary and secondary stages in untreated persons. (See *What to tell the patient with suspected syphilis.*)

A nonreactive test doesn't rule out syphilis because *Treponemal pallidum* causes no detectable immunologic changes in the serum for 14 to 21 days after infection. However, dark-field microscopic examination of exudate from suspicious lesions can provide early diagnosis by identifying causative spirochetes. (See *VDRL test interference.*)

What needs to be done

• Tell the patient to abstain from alcohol for 24 hours before the test.

Stay on the ball

VDRL test interference

• Ingestion of alcohol within 24 hours before the test can affect test results.
• A faulty immune system can cause a false-negative result.

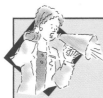

Listen up!

What to tell the patient with suspected syphilis

If your patient's VDRL test is nonreactive or borderline but syphilis hasn't been ruled out, instruct the patient to return for follow-up testing. Explain that borderline test results don't necessarily mean he's free from the disease.

If the test is reactive, explain the importance of proper treatment. Teach the patient about venereal disease and how it's spread, and stress the need for antibiotic therapy. Also, prepare him for mandatory inquiries from public health authorities. If the test is reactive but the patient shows no signs of syphilis, explain that many uninfected persons show false-positive reactions. Stress the need for further specific tests to rule out syphilis.

• Perform a venipuncture, and collect the sample in a 7-ml clot-activator tube or a tube volume in accordance with laboratory policy.

CA 15-3

CA 15-3 is a tumor marker used to monitor the response to treatment of invasive breast cancer and to watch for recurrence of the disease. A combination of markers may be used because of low sensitivity and specificity of the markers.

What it all means

Normal value for the tumor marker CA 15-3 (27, 29) is less than 30 units/ml. CA 15-3 greatly increases in metastatic breast cancer; it also increases in pancreas, lung, colorectal, ovarian, and liver cancers. It decreases with therapy; an increase after therapy suggests progressive disease.

What needs to be done

• Follow the specific directions from the laboratory or cancer center for the particular test ordered. This may involve fasting, and you may identify factors that may interfere with test results. Note interfering factors on the appropriate laboratory requests.

• Obtain a 10-ml venous blood sample, or a tube volume in accordance with laboratory policy, in the tube specified by the laboratory or cancer center, and transport the sample as directed.
• Provide emotional support to the patient.

CA 19-9

CA 19-9 carbohydrate antigen may be ordered in the patient with GI, pancreas, hepatobiliary, or liver cancer. A combination of markers may be used because of low sensitivity and specificity of the markers.

The main purposes of performing tumor markers are to assess the patient's response to therapy and to monitor and detect disease recurrence in stomach, pancreatic, colorectal, gallbladder, and liver cancer.

What it all means

Normal value for the tumor marker CA 19-9 is less than 70 units/ml.

Abnormal results

CA 19-9 increases in pancreatic, hepatobiliary, and lung cancers. It may be mildly increased in gastric and colorectal cancers. (See *CA 19-9 test interference.*)

What needs to be done

• Follow specific directions from the laboratory or cancer center for the particular test ordered. This may involve fasting, and you may identify factors that may interfere with test results. Note interfering factors on the appropriate laboratory requests.
• Obtain a 10-ml venous blood sample, or a tube volume in accordance with laboratory policy, in the tube specified by the laboratory or cancer center, and transport the sample as directed.
• Provide emotional support to the patient.

CA-50

The CA-50 may be ordered in the patient with GI or pancreatic cancer. A combination of markers may be used because of low sensitivity and specificity of the markers. Tumor markers are performed to assist tumor staging and identify possible metastasis, monitor and detect disease recurrence, and assess the patient's response to therapy.

Stay on the ball

CA19-9 test interference

• Radioactive scans or radiation 1 week before the test can alter test results

---

Tumor markers assist in tumor "staging," identifying possible metastasis, assessing the patient's response to therapy, and detecting disease recurrence.

What it all means

Normal value for the tumor marker CA-50 is less than 17 units/ml.

Abnormal results

CA-50 increases in GI and pancreatic cancers.

What needs to be done

• Follow specific directions from the laboratory or cancer center for the particular test ordered. This may involve fasting, and you may identify factors that may interfere with test results. Note interfering factors on the appropriate laboratory requests.
• Obtain a 10-ml venous blood sample, or a tube volume in accordance with laboratory policy, in the tube specified by the laboratory or cancer center, and transport the sample as directed.
• Provide emotional support to the patient.

CA-125

The CA-125 glycoprotein antigen and serum carbohydrate antigen is commonly associated with types of ovarian cancers. The test is performed to assist in the diagnosis of ovarian, endometrial, or cervical cancer and to monitor response to treatment of ovarian cancer.

What it all means

Normal value for the tumor marker CA-125 is less than 34 units/ml.

Abnormal results

CA-125 increases in epithelial ovary, fallopian tube, endometrial, endocervix, pancreas, and liver cancers. CA-125 increases less in colon, breast, lung, and GI cancers.

What needs to be done

• Follow specific directions from the laboratory or cancer center for the particular test ordered. This may involve fasting, and you may identify factors that may interfere with test results. Note interfering factors on the appropriate laboratory requests.
• Obtain a 10-ml venous blood sample, or a tube volume in accordance with laboratory policy, in the tube specified by the laboratory or cancer center, and transport the sample as directed.
• Provide emotional support to the patient.

Carcinoembryonic antigen

Carcinoembryonic antigen (CEA) is a protein normally found in embryonic endodermal epithelium and fetal tissue. CEA production usually stops before birth but may begin again later if a neoplasm develops.

Because CEA levels are raised by biliary obstruction, alcoholic hepatitis, chronic heavy smoking, and other conditions as well as by benign or malignant neoplasms, the CEA test can't be used as a general indicator of cancer. Measurement of CEA levels is useful for staging and monitoring treatment of certain cancers. Other tests are used to diagnose certain types of cancer. (See *Using CEA tests to monitor cancer treatment*.)

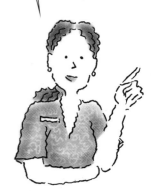

CEA testing is good way to monitor the effectiveness of cancer therapy. It can also help stage cancer and test for recurrence.

What it all means

Normal serum CEA values are less than 5 ng/ml (SI, 5 mg/L) in healthy nonsmokers. Approximately 5% of the population has above-normal CEA levels.

On the trail to success

If serum CEA levels are above normal before surgical resection, chemotherapy, or radiation therapy, a return to normal within 6 weeks after therapy suggests successful treatment. Persistent elevation of CEA levels, however, suggests residual or recurrent tumor.

Beware of heights

High CEA levels are characteristic in various malignant conditions, particularly in endodermally derived neoplasms of the GI organs and the lungs and in certain nonmalignant conditions, such as benign hepatic disease, hepatic cirrhosis, alcoholic pancreatitis, and inflammatory bowel disease. Elevated CEA levels may also result from nonendodermal cancers, such as breast cancer and ovarian cancer. (See *CEA test interference*.)

What needs to be done

- If appropriate, inform the patient that the test will be repeated to monitor the effectiveness of therapy.
- Perform a venipuncture, and collect the sample in a 7-ml tube without additives, or a tube volume in accordance with laboratory policy.
- Send the sample to the laboratory immediately.

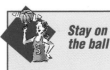

Stay on the ball

CEA test interference

- Cigarette smoking may elevate carcinoembryonic antigen (CEA) levels, altering test results.

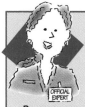

Advice from the experts

Using CEA tests to monitor cancer treatment

Because many patients in the early stages of colorectal cancer have normal or low levels of carcinoembryonic antigen (CEA), the CEA test doesn't screen successfully for early malignancy. However, it's a good tool for monitoring response to cancer therapy. After a patient's serum CEA level has decreased following surgery, chemotherapy, or other treatment, any increase suggests cancer recurrence or diminished effectiveness of treatment.

Both charts below show CEA levels in patients during and after colorectal cancer treatment. In the top chart, initial results show the usual dramatic drop in response to treatment; the subsequent rise in CEA indicates a diminishing response to chemotherapy. In the bottom chart, the progressive CEA rise signals cancer recurrence 8 months before clinical symptoms or radiologic evidence.

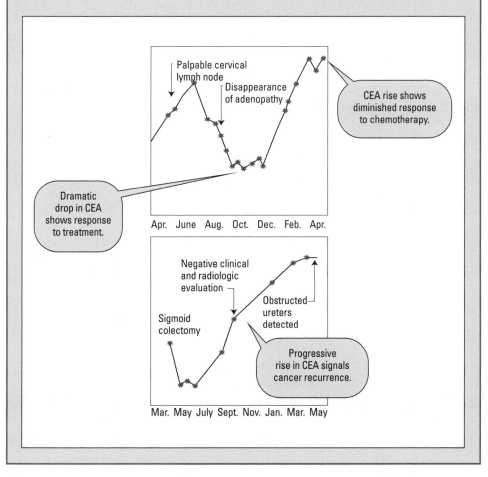

Alpha-fetoprotein

Alpha-fetoprotein (AFP) is a glycoprotein produced by fetal tissue and tumors that differentiate from midline embryonic structures. During fetal development, AFP levels in serum and amniotic fluid rise; because this protein crosses the placenta, it appears in maternal serum. Elevated AFP levels in the patient who isn't pregnant may occur in cancers or certain nonmalignant conditions such as ataxia-telangiectasia. In these conditions, AFP assays are more useful for monitoring the patient's response to therapy than for diagnosis.

What it all means

When testing by immunoassay, AFP values are less than 15 ng/ml (SI, 15 mg/L) in males and nonpregnant females. In pregnant females, AFP levels are less than 25 ng/ml (SI, less than 25 mg/L). At 15 to 18 weeks' gestation, values range from 10 to 150 ng/ml (SI, 10 to 150 mg/L).

Elevations in pregnant patients...

Elevated maternal serum AFP levels may suggest a neural tube defect or other neural tube anomalies. AFP levels rise sharply in approximately 90% of fetuses with anencephaly and in 50% of those with spina bifida. Definitive diagnosis requires ultrasonography and amniocentesis. High AFP levels may indicate intrauterine death or such anomalies as duodenal atresia, omphalocele, tetralogy of Fallot, or Turner's syndrome.

...and in nonpregnant patients

Elevated serum AFP levels in 70% of nonpregnant patients may indicate hepatocellular carcinoma (although low AFP levels don't rule it out) or germ cell tumor of gonadal, retroperitoneal, or mediastinal origin. Serum AFP level rises in patients with ataxia-telangiectasia; cancer of the pancreas, stomach, or biliary system; or nonseminiferous testicular tumors. Transient high elevations can occur in nonneoplastic hepatocellular disease, such as alcoholic cirrhosis and acute or chronic hepatitis. Elevation of AFP levels after remission suggests tumor recurrence.

Favorable response

In patients with hepatocellular carcinoma, a gradual decrease in serum AFP levels indicates a favorable response to therapy. In patients with germ cell tumors, serum AFP and human chorionic gonadotropin levels should be measured at the same time. (See *AFP test interference*.)

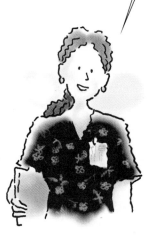

AFP levels can help determine the need for amniocentesis or high-resolution ultrasound in a pregnant woman. They can also monitor the effectiveness of therapy in some malignant diseases.

Stay on the ball

AFP test interference

Multiple pregnancy may cause false-positive results.

What needs to be done

• Advise the patient that she may need further testing.
• Perform a venipuncture, and collect the sample in a 7-ml clot-activator tube or a tube volume in accordance with laboratory policy.
• Record the patient's age, race, weight, and gestational period on the laboratory request.

TORCH test

The toxoplasmosis, rubella, cytomegalovirus, and herpes simplex antibodies (TORCH) test detects exposure to pathogens involved in congenital and neonatal infections. These pathogens are commonly associated with congenital or neonatal infections that aren't clinically apparent and may cause severe central nervous system impairment. This test confirms such infection serologically by detecting specific antibodies in infant blood.

What it all means

Test results should be negative for TORCH agents.

Exams in sequence

Toxoplasmosis is diagnosed by sequential examination that shows rising antibody titers, changing titers, and serologic conversion from negative to positive; a titer of 1:256 suggests recent toxoplasma infection. Approximately two-thirds of infected infants are asymptomatic at birth; one-third show signs of cerebral calcification and choroidoretinitis.

Hereditary factor

In infants younger than age 6 months, rubella infection is associated with a marked and persistent rise in complement-fixing antibody titer over time. Persistence of rubella antibody in an infant older than age 6 months strongly suggests congenital infection. Congenital rubella is associated with cardiac anomalies, neurosensory deafness, growth retardation, and encephalitic symptoms. Detection of herpes antibodies in CSF with signs of herpetic encephalitis and persistent HSV type 2 antibody levels confirms herpes simplex infection in a neonate without obvious herpetic lesions.

The TORCH test aids diagnosis of acute, congenital, and intrapartum infections.

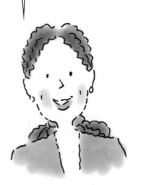

What needs to be done

• Obtain a 3-ml sample of venous or cord blood or a tube volume in accordance with laboratory policy.

• Send it to the laboratory promptly for serologic testing.

Tuberculin skin tests

Tuberculin skin tests are used to screen patients for previous infection by the tubercle bacillus. They're routinely performed in children, young adults, and people with radiographic findings that suggest this infection. In the purified protein derivative (PPD) tests, intradermal injection of the tuberculin antigen causes a delayed hypersensitivity reaction in patients with active or dormant tuberculosis (TB).

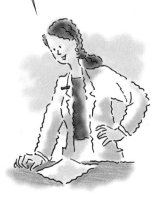

Tuberculin skin tests help determine whether a patient has been exposed to TB.

Accurate, or easy?

The Mantoux test uses a single-needle intradermal injection of PPD, which permits precise measurement of dosage. Multipuncture tests, such as the tine test, Mono-Vacc test, and Aplitest, involve intradermal injections using tines impregnated with Old tuberculin or PPD. Because multipuncture tests require less skill and are more rapidly administered than the Mantoux test, they're generally used for screening. However, a positive multipuncture test usually requires a Mantoux test for confirmation. (See *Performing tuberculin skin tests* and *Tuberculin skin test follow-up*.)

Performing tuberculin skin tests

Before you perform tuberculin skin testing, gather the following equipment: alcohol swabs, a vial of purified protein derivative (intermediate strength—5 tuberculin units per 0.1 ml), a 1-ml tuberculin syringe with a ½" (1.3-cm) or ³/₈" (1.6-cm) 25G or 26G needle for the Mantoux test, and a commercially available device (tine, Mono-Vacc, or Aplitest) for multipuncture tests. Be sure to have epinephrine (1:1,000) and a 3-ml syringe available to treat an anaphylactic or acute hypersensitivity reaction.

Next, have the patient sit with his arm extended and supported on a flat surface. Clean the volar surface of the upper forearm with alcohol, and let the area dry completely.

Test procedures
The procedure depends on which test you conduct:
• *Mantoux test*—Perform an intradermal injection.

• *Multipuncture tests*—Remove the protective cap on the injection device to expose the four tines. Hold the patient's forearm in one hand, stretching the forearm skin tightly. With your other hand, firmly depress the device into the skin (without twisting it). Hold the device in place for at least 1 second before removing it. If you have applied sufficient pressure, you'll see four puncture sites and a circular depression on the patient's skin.

After the test
Record where the test was given, the date and time, and when it's to be read. Tuberculin skin tests generally are read 48 to 72 hours after injection. However, the Mono-Vacc test can be read 48 to 96 hours after the test.

What it all means

For the Mantoux test, induration less than 5 mm in diameter or no induration indicates a negative reaction.

For the tine test and Aplitest, no induration or induration less than 2 mm in diameter indicates a negative reaction. No induration indicates a negative reaction for the Mono-Vacc test. (See *Reading tuberculin skin test results*.)

Equal opportunity test

A positive tuberculin reaction indicates previous infection by tubercle bacilli. It doesn't distinguish between an active and a dormant infection; nor does it provide a definitive diagnosis. If a positive reaction occurs, sputum smear and culture and chest X-rays are necessary to provide more information.

Borderline

In the Mantoux test, induration of 5 to 9 mm in diameter indicates a borderline reaction; larger induration, a positive reaction. Because patients with atypical mycobacteria other than tubercle bacilli may have borderline reactions, follow-up is necessary.

Vesicular presence

In the tine test or Aplitest, vesicles indicate a positive reaction; induration of 2 mm in diameter without vesicles requires confirmation by the Mantoux test. Any induration in the Mono-Vacc test indicates a positive reaction but requires confirmation by the Mantoux test. (See *Tuberculin skin test interference*, page 186.)

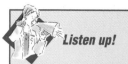

Listen up!

Tuberculin skin test follow-up

If you're performing a tuberculin test on an outpatient, instruct him to return at the specified time so test results can be read. Tell him that a positive reaction to a skin test appears as a red, hard, raised area at the injection site.

If it itches, don't scratch
Although the area may itch, instruct the patient not to scratch it. Stress that a positive reaction doesn't always indicate active tuberculosis.

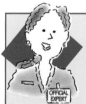

Advice from the experts

Reading tuberculin skin test results

Read the Mantoux, tine, and Aplitest skin tests 48 to 72 hours after injection. Read the Mono-Vacc test 48 to 96 hours afterward.

In a well-lighted room, flex the patient's forearm slightly. Observe the injection site for erythema and vesiculation; then gently rub your finger over the site to detect induration. If induration is present, measure the diameter in millimeters, preferably using a plastic ruler marked in concentric circles of specific diameter.

In multipuncture tests, you may find separate areas of induration around individual punctures or induration involving more than one puncture site. If so, measure the diameter of the largest single area of induration or coalesced induration.

What needs to be done

• Check the patient's history for active TB, the results of previous skin tests, and hypersensitivities. If the patient has had TB, don't perform a skin test; if he's had a positive reaction to previous skin tests, consult the doctor or follow your facility's policy.
• Tuberculin skin tests are contraindicated in patients with active TB, a current reaction to smallpox vaccinations, any type of rash, or a skin disorder.
• Don't perform a skin test in areas with excessive hair, acne, or insufficient subcutaneous tissue, such as over a tendon or bone.

Latex allergy testing

Latex is contained in many medical devices, such as gloves and catheters. Many people, including health care professionals, can experience an allergic reaction, which may be mild to severe in nature, when exposed to these products. Latex allergy testing measures IgE-mediated latex sensitivity. It doesn't measure irritation or delayed type reactions (Type IV) to latex.

What it all means

Latex allergy testing is done by the enzyme immunoassay (EIA) method, in which the color reaction is measured and is related directly to the amount of IgG specific for the test allergen in the sample. The normal value is negative for the latex allergen (less than 0.35 International Units/ml by EIA testing). A positive reaction for the latex allergen are values greater than 0.35 International Units/ml by EIA testing. A positive reaction is strongly associated with latex allergy.

What needs to be done

• Determine a history of exposure to latex allergens or of latex allergy reactions (swelling, itching, eczema, anaphylaxis). Test findings will be related to the clinical history of the patient.
• Tell the patient that there's no need to fast prior to testing.
• Collect a 7-ml blood serum sample in a red-topped tube or a tube volume in accordance with laboratory policy.
• Transport the specimen directly to the laboratory.

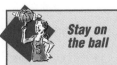

Stay on the ball

Tuberculin skin test interference

• Corticosteroids, other immunosuppressants, or live vaccine viruses (measles, mumps, rubella, or polio) given within the previous 4 to 6 weeks may suppress skin reactions.
• If less than 10 weeks has elapsed since tuberculosis infection, the skin reaction may be suppressed.

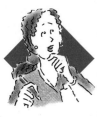

Quick quiz

1. Which blood type can be transfused in limited amounts in an emergency to any patient regardless of the recipient's blood type?
    A. Type O
    B. Type A
    C. Type B
    D. Type AB

Answer: A. Because type O blood lacks both A and B antigens, it can be transfused in limited amounts in an emergency to any recipient—with little risk of an adverse reaction.

2. Within which period must crossmatching be performed on a blood sample?
    A. 12 hours
    B. 24 hours
    C. 36 hours
    D. 72 hours

Answer: D. Crossmatching, which establishes the compatibility of donor and recipient blood, must be performed on a blood sample within 72 hours.

3. Infection by RSV can be ruled out when:
    A. serum samples have no detectable antibodies to the virus.
    B. IgM is present in the serum sample.
    C. IgG antibodies increase fourfold.
    D. serum samples are positive for antibodies.

Answer: A. In patients whose serum samples have no detectable antibodies to the virus, RSV can be ruled out.

4. The presence of HBsAg in a patient confirms:
    A. hepatitis A.
    B. hepatitis B.
    C. hepatitis G.
    D. hepatitis C.

Answer: B. The presence of HBsAg in a patient confirms hepatitis B. In chronic carriers and persons with chronic active hepatitis, HBsAg may be present several months after the onset of acute infection.

5. A Mantoux skin test should be read within which time range?
   A. 12 to 24 hours
   B. 24 to 36 hours
   C. 48 to 72 hours
   D. 72 to 96 hours

Answer: C. A Mantoux skin test should be read 48 to 72 hours after injection.

Scoring

☆☆☆ If you answered all five questions correctly, hooray! You're the Sultan of Serum Samples!

☆☆ If you answered three or four questions correctly, great! You're an immunologic icon!

☆ If you answered fewer than three questions correctly, don't worry! These assays will become easy in no time!

Urine tests

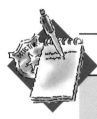

Just the facts

In this chapter, you'll learn:

♦ about urine tests

♦ what patient care is associated with these tests

♦ what factors can interfere with test results

♦ what urine test results may indicate.

A look at urine tests

Urine formation is one of the primary functions of the urinary system. When formed, normal urine consists of sodium, chloride, potassium, calcium, magnesium, sulfates, phosphates, bicarbonate, uric acid, ammonium ions, creatinine, and urobilinogen (a bilirubin derivative resulting from the action of intestinal bacteria). A few leukocytes and red blood cells (RBCs)—and in males, some spermatozoa—may enter urine as it passes from the kidney to the ureteral orifice.

The urine of a person receiving drugs normally excreted in urine contains drug substances as well. Because urine tests can reveal much about a patient's overall well-being, these tests are valuable tools for diagnosing many disorders. Before urine testing begins, explain the procedure to the patient.

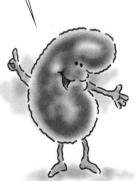

Urinalysis screens for renal or urinary tract disease and helps detect metabolic and systemic disease.

Urinalysis

Routine urinalysis serves many functions. It can be used to screen patients for kidney and urinary tract disease and can help detect metabolic or systemic disease.

During the course of a routine urinalysis, you'll:
• evaluate the urine's color, odor, and opacity
• determine the urine's specific gravity and pH
• detect and measure protein, glucose, and ketone bodies
• examine urine sediment for blood cells, casts, and crystals.

Normal findings in routine urinalysis

Element	Findings
Macroscopic	
Color	Straw-colored to dark yellow
Odor	Slightly aromatic
Appearance	Clear
Specific gravity	1.005 to 1.035
pH	4.5 to 8.0
Protein	None
Glucose	None
Ketones	None
Bilirubin	None
Urobilinogen	Normal
Hemoglobin	None
Red blood cells (RBCs)	None
Nitrite (bacteria)	None
White blood cells (WBCs)	None
Microscopic	
RBCs	0 to 2 per high-power field
WBCs	0 to 5 per high-power field
Epithelial cells	0 to 5 per high-power field
Casts	None, except 1 to 2 hyaline casts per low-power field
Crystals	Present
Bacteria	None
Yeast cells	None
Parasites	None

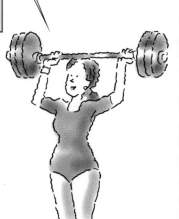

Specific gravity is a weighty issue! It measures the weight of a substance, such as urine, and compares it with the weight of an equal volume of another substance.

What it all means

Results of urine tests are based on the elements that make up urine. Even with normal findings, these elements have certain characteristics. (See *Normal findings in routine urinalysis*.)

Pondering the pathologic

Abnormal findings show an alteration in the normal characteristics of urine. These abnormal findings typically suggest a pathologic condition:

- *color change*—from diet, drugs, or disease
- *unusual odor*—due to ketone bodies, infection, or disease
- *turbidity* (cloudiness)—from kidney infection

• *low specific gravity* (less than 1.005)—from diabetes insipidus, acute tubular necrosis, or pyelonephritis
• *fixed specific gravity* (1.010 regardless of fluid intake)—from chronic glomerulonephritis with severe kidney damage
• *high specific gravity* (greater than 1.035)—from nephrotic syndrome, dehydration, acute glomerulonephritis, heart failure, liver failure, or shock
• *high pH* (alkaline urine)—from Fanconi syndrome, urinary tract infection, or metabolic or respiratory alkalosis
• *low pH* (acidic urine)—from renal tuberculosis, pyrexia, phenylketonuria, alkaptonuria, or acidosis
• *proteinuria* (excess serum proteins in urine)—from renal failure or, possibly, multiple myeloma
• *sugars in urine*—usually from diabetes mellitus but possibly from pheochromocytoma (brain tumor), Cushing syndrome, impaired tubular reabsorption, advanced kidney disease, increased intracranial pressure, or I.V. solutions containing glucose and total parenteral nutrition (TPN) containing 10% to 50% glucose
• *ketone bodies* (used as fuel by muscle and brain tissue)—from diabetes mellitus, starvation, pregnancy and lactation, or diarrhea or vomiting
• *bilirubin*—from liver disease or from fibrosis of the biliary canaliculi (as in cirrhosis)
• *increased urobilinogen levels*—liver damage, hemolytic disease, or severe infection (increased values)
• *decreased urobilinogen levels*—biliary obstruction, inflammatory disease, antimicrobial therapy, severe diarrhea, or renal insufficiency
• *blood cells*—infection, obstruction, inflammation, trauma, tumors, or other causes
• *excessive casts*—renal disease
• *calcium oxalate crystals*—hypercalcemia
• *cystine crystals*—inborn error of metabolism
• *bacteria, yeast cells, parasites*—genitourinary tract infection or contamination of external genitalia.

What needs to be done

• Tell the patient to avoid stress and strenuous exercise before the test.
• Check for drugs that influence urinalysis. (See *Drugs that influence routine urinalysis results,* pages 192 and 193.)
• Collect a random urine specimen of at least 15 ml, preferably a first-voided morning specimen.
• If the patient is being evaluated for renal colic, strain the specimen to catch calculi or calculus fragments.

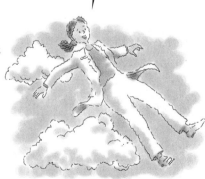

Turbidity refers to the cloudiness of a solution caused by particles or sediment.

(Text continues on page 194.)

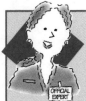

Advice from the experts

Drugs that influence routine urinalysis results

Drugs that change urine color
Chlorzoxazone (orange to purple-red)
Deferoxamine mesylate (red)
Fluorescein sodium I.V. (yellow-orange)
Furazolidone (brown)
Iron salts (black)
Levodopa (dark)
Methylene blue (blue-green)
Metronidazole (dark)
Nitrofurantoin (brown)
Oral anticoagulants, indandione derivatives (orange)
Phenazopyridine (orange, red, or orange-brown)
Phenothiazines (dark)
Quinacrine (deep yellow)
Riboflavin (yellow)
Rifabutin (red-orange)
Rifampin (red-orange)
Sulfasalazine (orange-yellow)

Drugs that cause urine odor
Antibiotics
Paraldehyde
Vitamins

Drugs that increase specific gravity
Albumin
Dextran
Glucose
Radiopaque contrast media

Drugs that decrease pH
Ammonium chloride
Ascorbic acid
Diazoxide
Metolazone

Drugs that increase pH
Amphotericin B
Carbonic anhydrase inhibitors
Mafenide
Potassium citrate
Sodium bicarbonate

Drugs that cause false-positive results for proteinuria
Acetazolamide (Combistix)
Aminosalicylic acid (sulfosalicylic acid or Extons method)
Methazolamide
Nafcillin (sulfosalicylic acid method)
Sodium bicarbonate
Tolbutamide (sulfosalicylic acid method)
Tolmetin (sulfosalicylic acid method)

Drugs that cause true proteinuria
Aminoglycosides
Amphotericin B
Bacitracin
Cephalosporins
Cisplatin
Gold preparations
Isotretinoin
Nonsteroidal anti-inflammatory drugs
Polymyxin B
Sulfonamides

Drugs that cause either true proteinuria or false-positive results
Penicillin in large doses (except with Ames reagent strips); however, some penicillins cause true proteinuria
Sulfonamides (sulfosalicylic acid method)

Drugs that influence routine urinalysis results (continued)

Drugs that cause false-positive results for glycosuria

Aminosalicylic acid (Benedict test)
Ascorbic acid (Clinistix, Diastix, Tes-Tape)
Ascorbic acid in large doses (Clinitest tablets)
Cephalosporins (Clinitest tablets)
Chloral hydrate (Benedict test)
Isoniazid (Benedict test)
Levodopa (Clinistix, Diastix, Tes-Tape)
Levodopa in large doses (Clinitest tablets)
Methyldopa (Tes-Tape)
Nalidixic acid (Benedict test or Clinitest tablets)
Nitrofurantoin (Benedict test)
Penicillin G in large doses (Benedict test)
Phenazopyridine (Clinistix, Diastix, Tes-Tape)
Probenecid (Benedict test, Clinitest tablets)
Salicylates in large doses (Clinitest tablets, Clinistix, Diastix, Tes-Tape)
Streptomycin (Benedict test)
Tetracycline (Clinistix, Diastix, Tes-Tape)
Tetracyclines, due to ascorbic acid buffer (Benedict test, Clinitest tablets)

Drugs that cause true glycosuria

Ammonium chloride
Asparaginase
Carbamazepine
Corticosteroids
Lithium carbonate
Nicotinic acid (large doses)
Phenothiazines (long-term)
Thiazide diuretics

Drugs that cause false-positive results for ketonuria

Levodopa (Ketostix, Labstix)
Phenazopyridine (Ketostix or Gerhardt's reagent strip shows atypical color)
Phenothiazines (Gerhardt's reagent strip shows atypical color)
Salicylates (Gerhardt's reagent strip shows reddish color)

Drugs that cause true ketonuria

Ether (anesthesia)
Insulin (excessive doses)
Isoniazid (intoxication)
Isopropyl alcohol (intoxication)

Drugs that increase white blood cell count

Allopurinol
Ampicillin
Aspirin (toxicity)
Kanamycin
Methicillin

Drugs that cause hematuria

Amphotericin B
Coumarin derivatives
Methicillin
Sulfonamides

Drugs that cause casts

Amphotericin B
Aspirin (toxicity)
Bacitracin
Ethacrynic acid
Furosemide
Gentamicin
Isoniazid
Kanamycin
Neomycin
Penicillin
Radiographic agents
Streptomycin
Sulfonamides

Drugs that cause crystals (if urine is acidic)

Acetazolamide
Aminosalicylic acid
Ascorbic acid
Nitrofurantoin
Theophylline
Thiazide diuretics

- Refrigerate the specimen if analysis will be delayed longer than 1 hour.

Urine osmolality

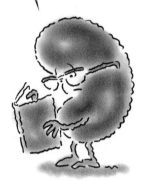

The urine osmolality test evaluates the concentration ability of the kidneys in acute and chronic renal failure.

Urine osmolality helps to evaluate renal tubular function and detect renal impairment. It evaluates the concentrating ability of the kidneys in acute and chronic renal failure by measuring the number of osmotically active ions or particles present per kilogram of water. Osmolality is high in concentrated urine and low in dilute urine. It's determined by the effect of solute particles on the freezing point of the fluid. Normal kidneys concentrate or dilute urine according to fluid intake. When intake is excessive, the kidneys excrete more water in the urine; when intake is limited, they excrete less. To make such variation possible, the distal segment of the tubule varies its permeability to water in response to antidiuretic hormone. Osmolality is a more sensitive indicator of renal function than are dilution techniques that measure specific gravity.

What it all means

The normal result for a random specimen is 50 to 1,400 mOsm/kg; in a 24-hour urine specimen, 300 to 900 mOsm/kg. The normal urine-to-sodium ratio is 1:1 to 3:1.

When capacity goes down

Decreased renal capacity to concentrate urine in response to fluid deprivation, or to dilute urine in response to fluid overload, may indicate tubular epithelial damage, decreased renal blood flow, loss of functional nephrons, or pituitary or cardiac dysfunction. Urine-to-sodium ratio is increased in prerenal azotemia and is decreased in acute tubular necrosis. (See *Urine osmolality test interference.*)

What needs to be done

- Withhold diuretics as ordered.
- To increase sensitivity, a high-protein diet may be ordered for 3 days before the test.
- Tell the patient that the test requires a urine specimen and collection of blood within 1 hour before or after the urine is collected.
- Teach the patient how to collect a 24-hour urine specimen, if required.

Stay on the ball

Urine osmolality test interference

• I.V. sodium or I.V. dextrose and water administration may interfere with test results.
• Use of furosemide, mannitol, metolazone, and vincristine may increase urine osmolality.
• Use of captopril, lithium, tolazamide, and verapamil may decrease urine osmolality.

• Collect a random urine specimen and draw a blood sample within 1 hour of urine collection using the tube volume and type indicated by the laboratory.
• If a 24-hour urine collection is necessary, record the total urine volume on the laboratory request. (Preservatives aren't required for a 24-hour container.)
• If the patient can't urinate into the specimen containers, give him a clean bedpan, urinal, or toilet specimen pan. Rinse the collection device after each use.
• If the patient is catheterized, empty the drainage bag before the test. Obtain the specimen from the catheter.
• Make sure the patient voids within 8 to 10 hours after the catheter has been removed.
• Send each specimen to the laboratory immediately after collection.

Enzymes

Urine amylase

Amylase is a starch-splitting enzyme produced primarily in the pancreas and salivary glands. It's usually secreted into the alimentary tract and then absorbed into the blood. Small amounts of amylase are also absorbed into the blood directly from the pancreas and salivary glands. After glomerular filtration, amylase is excreted in the urine.

What it all means

Urinary excretion of 1 to 17 amylase units/hour (SI, 0.017 to 0.29 μkat/hour) is generally considered normal.

Various conditions can cause elevated amylase levels, including acute pancreatitis; obstruction of the pancreatic duct, intestines, or salivary duct; carcinoma of the head of the pancreas; mumps; acute injury to the spleen; renal disease with impaired absorption; perforated peptic or duodenal ulcers; and gallbladder disease.

When amylase is lookin' low

Depressed amylase evels occur in association with chronic pancreatitis, cachexia, alcoholism, cancer of the liver, cirrhosis, hepatitis, and hepatic abscess.

What needs to be done

• If a female patient is menstruating, the test may have to be rescheduled.
• The test requires urine collection for 2, 6, 8, or 24 hours, and certain steps should be followed when collecting a specimen. (See *Teaching the patient to collect a timed urine specimen.*)
• These drugs may raise urine amylase levels and should be withheld for 24 hours before the test: morphine, meperidine, codeine, pentazocine, bethanechol, thiazide diuretics, indomethacin, and

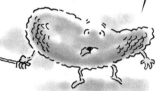

The urine amylase test helps diagnose acute pancreatitis and salivary gland disorders.

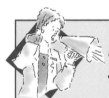

Listen up!

Teaching the patient to collect a timed urine specimen

Explain this process to the patient to make sure he properly collects a timed urine specimen.
• Provide a container for the patient to void into.
• Have the patient void and then discard this specimen.
• After this specimen is discarded, instruct him to pour every voided specimen into the collection bottle.
• If required, keep the specimen on ice or refrigerated (if collecting at home, keep the specimen in a brown paper bag separated from other refrigerator contents).
• Warn the patient not to void directly into the specimen container, especially if it contains a preservative.
• Ask the patient to void just before the collection period ends, if possible, and add it to the collection bottle.
• Seal the specimen bottle, attach a label, and send it to the laboratory.

ethyl alcohol. Fluoride may decrease levels. If any of the drugs must be continued, note this on the laboratory request.
• Collect a 2-, 6-, 8-, or 24-hour specimen.
• Cover and refrigerate the specimen during the collection period. If the patient is catheterized, keep the collection bag on ice.

Hormones

Urine aldosterone

Aldosterone promotes retention of sodium and excretion of potassium by the renal tubules, thereby helping regulate blood pressure and fluid and electrolyte balance.

The urine aldosterone test measures urine levels of aldosterone, the principal mineralocorticoid secreted by the zona glomerulosa of the adrenal cortex.

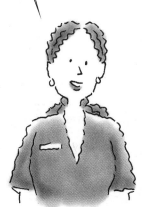

Urine aldosterone testing aids diagnosis of primary and secondary aldosteronisms.

What it all means

Normally, urine aldosterone levels range from 3 to 19 mcg/24 hours (SI, 8 to 51 nmol/24 day).

Primarily speaking...

Increased urine aldosterone levels suggest primary or secondary aldosteronism. The primary form usually arises from an aldosterone-secreting tumor of the adrenal cortex, but it may also result from adrenocortical hyperplasia (abnormal reproduction of normal cells). Patients with primary aldosteronism have increased aldosterone and decreased renin levels.

...and a secondary opinion

Secondary aldosteronism, the more common form, results from external stimulation of the adrenal cortex. The major systemic disorders that result in secondary aldosteronism are malignant hypertension, heart failure, cirrhosis of the liver, nephrotic syndrome, and idiopathic cyclic edema.

The lowdown on levels

Low urine aldosterone levels may result from Addison's disease, hypernatremia, overhydration, and toxemia of pregnancy. Aldosterone levels normally rise during pregnancy but rapidly decline following delivery. (See *Urine aldosterone test interference,* page 198.)

Stay on the ball

Urine aldosterone test interference

Licorice produces an aldosterone-like effect and should be avoided for 2 weeks before testing.

What needs to be done

• Check the patient's history for drugs that may affect aldosterone levels. Withhold renin inhibitors as ordered for 1 week before the test. If renin inhibitors must be continued, note it on the laboratory request.

• The patient should maintain a low-carbohydrate, normal sodium diet (135 mEq/day or 3 g/day) before the test, avoid sodium-rich foods, and avoid strenuous physical exercise and stressful situations during the collection period.

• The test requires collection of a 24-hour urine specimen.

• Collect a 24-hour specimen in a bottle containing a preservative, such as boric acid, to keep the specimen at a pH between 4.0 and 4.5.

• Refrigerate the specimen or place it on ice during the collection period.

Urine catecholamines

The urine catecholamine test measures urine levels of the major catecholamines—dopamine, epinephrine, and norepinephrine. Dopamine is secreted by the central nervous system (CNS); epinephrine, by the adrenal medulla; and norepinephrine, by both.

Catecholamines help regulate metabolism and prepare the body for the fight-or-flight response to stress. Certain tumors can also secrete catecholamines. One of the most common of these is a pheochromocytoma, which causes intermittent or persistent hypertension.

Conditions for collection

A 24-hour urine specimen is preferred for this test because catecholamine secretion fluctuates diurnally and in response to pain, heat, cold, emotional stress, physical exercise, hypoglycemia, injury, hemorrhage, asphyxia, and drugs.

What it all means

Normally, urine epinephrine values range from 0 to 20 mcg/24 hours (SI, 0 to 109 nmol/24 hours); norepinephrine, from 15 to 80 mcg/24 hours (SI, 89 to 473 nmol/24 hours); and dopamine from 65 to 100 mcg/24 hours (SI, 425 to 2610 nmol/24 hours).

Abnormal findings

In a patient with undiagnosed hypertension, elevated urine catecholamine levels following a hypertensive episode usually indicate a pheochromocytoma.

Elevated catecholamine levels without marked hypertension may be caused by a neuroblastoma or a ganglioneuroma. Myasthenia gravis and progressive muscular dystrophy commonly cause urine catecholamine levels to rise above normal, but this test is rarely performed to diagnose these disorders. Elevated catecholamine levels may also be seen in severe systemic situations (burns, peritonitis, shock, and septicemia), cor pulmonale, manic depressive disorders, or depressive neurosis.

Consistently low-normal catecholamine levels may indicate dysautonomia (a rare autonomic nervous system disease with mental retardation), which is marked by orthostatic hypotension. (See *Urine catecholamine test interference.*)

What needs to be done

• Check the patient's drug history for drugs that may affect catecholamine levels.
• Inform the patient that he should avoid chocolate, coffee, and bananas for 7 hours before the test. Stressful situations and exces-

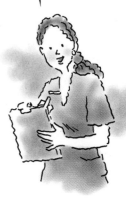

Measuring urine catecholamine levels aids pheochromocytoma diagnosis in patients with unexplained hypertension. It also aids diagnosis of neuroblastoma, ganglioneuroma, and dysautonomia.

Stay on the ball

Urine catecholamine test interference

• Caffeine, insulin, nitroglycerin, aminophylline, sympathomimetics, methyldopa, tricyclic antidepressants, chloral hydrate, quinidine, quinine, tetracycline, B-complex vitamins, isoproterenol, levodopa, and monoamine oxidase inhibitors may raise levels.
• Clonidine, guanethidine, reserpine, and iodine-containing contrast media may lower levels.
• Phenothiazines, erythromycin, and methenamine compounds may raise or lower levels.

sive physical activity should be avoided during the collection period.
• The test may require a 24-hour specimen or a random specimen.
• If this is a 24-hour urine specimen, collect it in a bottle containing a preservative to keep the specimen acidified to a pH of 3.0 or less; if it's a random specimen, collect it immediately after a hypertensive episode.
• Refrigerate a 24-hour specimen or place it on ice during the collection period.
• Instruct the patient that he may resume his usual activities, diet, and drugs as ordered.

Total urine estrogens

The total urine estrogens test is a quantitative analysis of total urine levels of estradiol, estrone, and estriol—the major estrogens present in significant amounts in urine.

What it all means

Total estrogen levels range as follows:
• *menstruating females:* 15 to 80 mcg/24 hours (SI, 55 to 294 nmol/day)
• *pregnant females:* first trimester: 0 to 800 mcg/24 hours (SI, 0 to 2,900 nmol/day); second trimester: 800 to 5,000 mcg/24 hours (SI, 2,900 to 18,350 nmol/day); third trimester: 5,000 to 50,000 mcg/24 hours (SI, 18,350 to 183,000 nmol/day)
• *postmenopausal females:* less than 20 mcg/24 hours (SI, less than 73 nmol/day)
• *males:* 15 to 40 mcg/24 hours (SI, 55 to 147 nmol/day).

Estrogen's suggestions

Decreased total urine estrogen levels may reflect ovarian agenesis; primary ovarian insufficiency, which can be caused by Stein-Leventhal syndrome, for example; or secondary ovarian insufficiency, which can be caused by pituitary or adrenal hypofunction or metabolic disturbances.

Elevated total estrogen levels in nonpregnant females may indicate tumors of ovarian or adrenocortical origin, adrenocortical hyperplasia, or a metabolic or hepatic disorder. In males, elevated total estrogen levels are associated with testicular tumors. (See *Total urine estrogen test interference.*)

What needs to be done

• Collect the urine over a 24-hour period, using a bottle containing boric acid preservative.

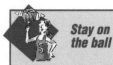

Stay on the ball

Total urine estrogen test interference

Drugs that may influence total urine estrogen levels include:
• hormonal contraceptives
• estrogen therapy
• progesterone therapy
• acetazolamide (during pregnancy).

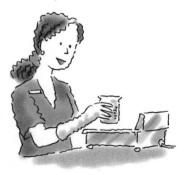

Measuring total urine estrogens helps establish fetoplacental status and can help diagnose ovarian, adrenocortical, and testicular tumors.

- If the patient is pregnant, note the approximate week of gestation on the laboratory slip.
- If the patient is a nonpregnant female, note the stage of her menstrual cycle.
- Refrigerate the specimen or keep it on ice during the collection period.

Urine human chorionic gonadotropin

As a qualitative analysis of urine levels of human chorionic gonadotropin (hCG), this test can detect pregnancy as early as 14 days after ovulation. Quantitative measurements can evaluate suspected hydatidiform mole or hCG-secreting tumors.

The hCG life cycle

Levels of hCG rise steadily and rapidly during the first trimester, peak around week 10 of gestation, and subsequently taper off to less than 10% of peak levels.

What it all means

In qualitative immunoassay analysis, results are reported as negative (nonpregnant) or positive (pregnant) for hCG.

In quantitative analysis, urine hCG levels in the first trimester of a normal pregnancy may be as high as 500,000 International Units/24 hours; in the second trimester, they range from 10,000 to 25,000 International Units/24 hours; and in the third trimester, from 5,000 to 15,000 International Units/24 hours. Levels decline rapidly after delivery and are undetectable within a few days.

With a baby on the way

During pregnancy, elevated urine hCG levels may indicate multiple pregnancy or erythroblastosis fetalis (hemolytic disease of the newborn characterized by anemia, jaundice, and enlargement of the liver and spleen); low levels may indicate threatened abortion or ectopic pregnancy.

Nonpregnant patients

Measurable hCG levels in males and nonpregnant females may indicate choriocarcinoma, ovarian or testicular tumors, melanoma, multiple myeloma, or gastric, hepatic, pancreatic, or breast cancer. (See *Urine hCG test interference*.)

What needs to be done

- Check the patient's recent drug history for use of drugs that may affect hCG levels.

The hCG test is a reliable way to confirm pregnancy.

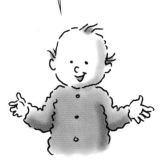

- The patient should restrict fluids for 8 hours before the test.
- The test requires a first-voided morning specimen or a 24-hour urine collection.
- For qualitative analysis, collect a first-voided morning specimen. If this isn't possible, collect a random specimen.
- For quantitative analysis of hCG, collect a 24-hour urine specimen.
- Specify the date of the patient's last menstrual period on the laboratory request. The test should be performed at least 5 days after a missed period.
- Refrigerate the 24-hour specimen or keep it on ice.

Metabolites

Urine 17-hydroxycorticosteroids

This test measures urine levels of 17-hydroxycorticosteroids (17-OHCS)—metabolites of the hormones that regulate glyconeogenesis. More than 80% of all urinary 17-OHCS are metabolites of cortisol, the primary adrenocortical steroid. Because cortisol secretion varies diurnally and in response to stress and many other factors, urine 17-OHCS levels are most accurately determined from a 24-hour specimen.

What it all means

Normal reference values are as follows:
- *men:* 4.5 to 12 mg/24 hours (SI, 12.4 to 33.1 µmol/day)
- *women:* 2.5 to 10 mg/24 hours (SI, 6.9 to 27.6 µmol/day)
- *children ages 8 to 12:* less than 4.5 mg/24 hours (SI, less than 12.4 µmol/day)
- *children younger than age 8:* less than 1.5 mg/24 hours (SI, less than 4.4 µmol/day).

The lowdown on levels

Levels normally increase slightly during the first trimester of pregnancy. Patients who are obese or very muscular may excrete slightly higher amounts of 17-OHCS because of increased cortisol catabolism. Elevated urine 17-OHCS levels may indicate Cushing's syndrome, adrenal carcinoma or adenoma, or a pituitary tumor. Increased levels may also occur in patients with virilism, hyperthyroidism, or severe hypertension. Extreme stress induced by such conditions as acute pancreatitis and eclampsia also increases urine 17-OHCS levels.

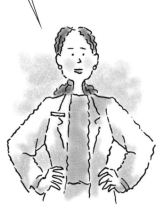

The urine 17-OHCS test assesses adrenocortical function.

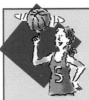

Stay on the ball

Urine 17-OHCS test interference

• Drugs that may elevate levels include meprobamate, phenothiazines, spironolactone, ascorbic acid, chloral hydrate, chlordiazepoxide, penicillin G, hydroxyzine, quinidine, quinine, iodides, and methenamine.
• Drugs that may decrease levels include estrogens, hormonal contraceptives, phenothiazines, hydralazine, phenytoin, thiazide diuretics, nalidixic acid, and reserpine.

Low urine 17-OHCS levels may indicate Addison's disease, hypopituitarism, or myxedema. (See *Urine 17-OHCS test interference*.)

What needs to be done

• Check the patient's history for drugs that may affect 17-OHCS levels.
• Tell the patient he should avoid excessive physical exercise and stressful situations during the collection period, as well as restrict food and fluids that will alter test results (coffee and tea).
• Collect a 24-hour urine specimen in a bottle containing a preservative, discarding the first specimen and retaining the last.
• After the specimen has been collected, tell the patient he can resume activities restricted during the test as well as administration of drugs withheld for testing.
• Refrigerate the specimen or place it on ice during the collection period.

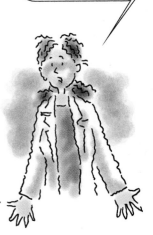

Hey, man...don't stress out! High-stress situations cause 17-OHCS levels to vary.

Urine 17-ketosteroids

This test measures urine levels of 17-ketosteroids (17-KS), which are steroids and steroid metabolites characterized by a ketone group on carbon 17 in the steroid nucleus. They originate primarily in the adrenal glands but can also originate in the testes, which produce one-third of 17-KS in males, and the ovaries, which produce a minimal amount of 17-KS in females.

Androgenic activity

Although not all 17-KS are androgens, all cause androgenic effects. For example, excessive secretion of 17-KS may result in hirsutism (excessive hair growth) and increased clitoral or phallic size; in utero, elevated 17-KS levels may cause a female fetus to develop a male urogenital tract.

Because 17-KS don't include all the androgens, such as testosterone (the most potent androgen), this test provides only a rough estimate of androgenic activity.

What it all means

Normal reference values are as follows:
- *men:* 10 to 25 mg/24 hours (SI, 35 to 87 µmol/day)
- *women:* 4 to 6 mg/24 hours (SI, 4 to 21 µmol/day)
- *children between the ages of 10 and 14:* 1 to 6 mg/24 hours (SI, 2 to 21 µmol/day)
- *children younger than age 10:* less than 3 mg/24 hours (SI, less than 10 µmol/day).

The lowdown on levels

Elevated urine 17-KS levels may result from adrenal hyperplasia, carcinoma or adenoma, or adrenogenital syndrome. In women, elevated levels may also indicate ovarian dysfunction, such as polycystic ovary disease (Stein-Leventhal syndrome), lutein cell tumor of the ovary, or androgenic arrhenoblastoma. In men, elevated 17-KS levels may indicate interstitial cell tumor of the testis. Characteristically, 17-KS levels also rise during pregnancy, severe stress, chronic illness, or debilitating disease.

Depressed urine 17-KS levels may result from Addison's disease, panhypopituitarism, eunuchoidism, or castration and may occur in cretinism, myxedema, and nephrosis. When this test is used to monitor cortisol therapy for adrenogenital syndrome, 17-KS levels typically return to normal with adequate cortisol administration. (See *Urine 17-KS test interference.*)

What needs to be done

- Check the patient's history for drugs that may affect test results.
- If the patient is menstruating, urine collection may have to be postponed.
- The patient should avoid excessive physical exercise and stressful situations during the collection period.
- Collect a 24-hour urine specimen in a bottle containing a preservative to keep the specimen at a pH between 4.0 and 4.5.
- Refrigerate the specimen or place it on ice during collection.

Urine 17-ketogenic steroids

This test determines urine levels of 17-ketogenic steroids (17-KGS), which consist of the 17-OHCS, such as cortisol and its

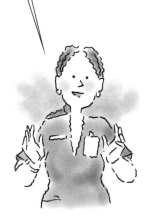

The 17-KS test helps diagnose adrenal and gonadal dysfunction and adrenogenital syndrome.

Stay on the ball

Urine 17-KS test interference

- Meprobamate, phenothiazines, spironolactone, corticotropin, dexamethasone, and antibiotics may elevate levels.
- Estrogens, penicillin, ethacrynic acid, and phenytoin may suppress levels.
- Nalidixic acid and quinine may increase or decrease levels.

metabolites, and other adrenocortical steroids, such as pregnanetriol, that can be oxidized in the laboratory to 17-KS.

For accurate diagnosis of specific disease, 17-KGS must be compared with results of other tests, including plasma corticotropin, plasma cortisol, corticotropin stimulation, single-dose metyrapone, and dexamethasone suppression.

What it all means

Reference values for 17-KGS are as follows:
- *men:* 4 to 14 mg/24 hours (SI, 14 to 49 µmol/day)
- *women:* 2 to 12 mg/24 hours (SI, 7 to 42 µmol/day)
- *children ages 11 to 14:* less than 2 to 9 mg/24 hours (SI, 7 to 31 µmol/day)
- *children younger than age 11:* 0.1 to 4 mg/24 hours (SI, 0.3 to 14 µmol/day).

The lowdown on levels

Elevated 17-KGS levels reflect hyperadrenalism, as in Cushing's syndrome; adrenal carcinoma or adenoma; and some cases of adrenogenital syndrome such as congenital adrenal hyperplasia. Levels also rise with severe physical (burns, infections, or surgery) or emotional stress.

Low levels may reflect hypoadrenalism, as in Addison's disease as well as panhypopituitarism, cretinism, and general wasting. (See *Urine 17-KGS test interference.*)

What needs to be done

- Check the patient's history for drugs that may affect 17-KGS levels.

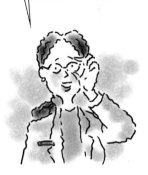

The urine 17-KGS test evaluates adrenocortical function and aids diagnosis of Cushing's syndrome and Addison's disease.

Stay on the ball

Urine 17-KGS test interference

- Corticotropin therapy and drugs, such as meprobamate, phenothiazines, spironolactone, penicillin, and hydralazine, may elevate results.
- Levels may be suppressed by estrogens, quinine, reserpine, thiazide diuretics, and long-term corticosteroid therapy.
- Nalidixic acid, carbamazepine, and dexamethasone may elevate or suppress levels.

- The patient should avoid excessive physical exercise and stressful situations during the collection period.
- Collect a 24-hour urine specimen in a bottle containing a preservative to keep the specimen at a pH between 4.0 and 4.5.
- Refrigerate the specimen or keep it on ice during the collection period.

Proteins and protein metabolites

Urine Bence Jones protein

Bence Jones proteins are abnormal light-chain immunoglobulins of low molecular weight that derive from the clone of a single plasma cell (monoclonal). This globulin appears in the urine of 50% to 80% of patients with multiple myeloma and in most patients with Waldenström's macroglobulinemia.

What it all means

Urine should contain no Bence Jones proteins. The presence of these proteins in urine suggests multiple myeloma or Waldenström's macroglobulinemia. Very low levels in the absence of other symptoms may result from benign monoclonal gammopathy. (See *Bence Jones protein test interference.*)

What needs to be done

- Teach the patient how to collect a midstream clean-catch urine specimen.
- Collect an early-morning urine specimen of at least 50 ml.
- If transport to the laboratory is delayed, refrigerate the specimen. If it isn't analyzed within 24 hours, it must be discarded.

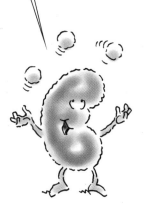

In patients with clinical signs of multiple myeloma, the urine Bence Jones protein test can confirm the diagnosis.

Stay on the ball

Bence Jones protein test interference

- False-positive results may occur in connective tissue disease, renal insufficiency, and certain cancers.

• If a 24-hour urine collection is needed, collect the urine over the period, discarding the first specimen and retaining the last. Keep a 24-hour specimen on ice or in the refrigerator during the collection period.

Urine creatinine

The urine creatinine test measures urine levels of creatinine, the chief metabolite of creatine. Produced in amounts proportional to total body muscle mass, creatinine is removed from the plasma primarily by glomerular filtration and is excreted in the urine.

Because creatinine isn't recycled in the body, it has a relatively high, constant clearance rate, making it an efficient indicator of renal function.

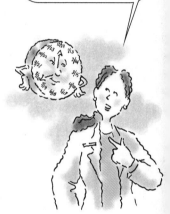

Because creatinine excretion levels are relatively constant, urine creatinine testing can evaluate the accuracy of a 24-hour urine collection.

What it all means

The normal range for urine creatinine levels in males is 14 to 26 mg/kg body weight/24 hours (SI, 120 to 230 µmol/kg body weight/day); in females, 11 to 20 mg/kg body weight/24 hours (SI, 97 to 177 µmol/kg body weight/day).

Decreased levels...renal impairment

Decreased urine creatinine levels may result from impaired renal perfusion (associated with shock, for example) or from renal disease caused by urinary tract obstruction. Chronic bilateral pyelonephritis, acute or chronic glomerulonephritis, and polycystic kidney disease may also depress creatinine levels.

Increased levels...not a problem

Increased urine creatinine levels generally have little diagnostic significance. (See *Urine creatinine test interference.*)

What needs to be done

• Check the patient's history for drugs that may affect creatinine levels.
• Tell the patient not to eat an excessive amount of meat and to avoid strenuous physical exercise during the collection period.
• Collect a 24-hour urine specimen in a refrigerated specimen bottle with a preservative to prevent creatinine degradation, discarding the first specimen and retaining the last.
• Refrigerate the specimen or keep it on ice during the collection period.

Stay on the ball

Urine creatinine test interference

Drugs that may affect urine creatinine levels include corticosteroids, gentamicin, tetracyclines, diuretics, and amphotericin B.

Creatinine clearance

Creatinine is formed and excreted in constant amounts by an irreversible reaction, and it functions solely as the main end product of creatine. Creatinine production is proportional to total muscle mass and is relatively unaffected by normal physical activity, diet, or urine volume.

The rate of clearance is expressed in terms of the volume of blood (in milliliters) that can be cleared of creatinine in 1 minute. Creatinine levels become abnormal when more than 50% of the total nephron units have been damaged.

What it all means

At age 20, creatinine clearance normally ranges from 94 to 140 ml/minute/1.73 m^2 (SI, 0.91 to 1.35 ml/s/m^2) for men and from 72 to 110 ml/minute/1.73 m^2 (SI, 0.69 to 1.06 ml/s/m^2) for women.

When creatinine isn't clearing out

Low creatinine clearance may result from reduced renal blood flow, which is associated with shock or renal artery obstruction; acute tubular necrosis; acute or chronic glomerulonephritis; advanced bilateral chronic pyelonephritis; advanced bilateral renal lesions, such as in polycystic kidney disease, cancer, or renal tuberculosis; or nephrosclerosis. Heart failure and severe dehydration may also cause creatinine clearance to fall below normal. (See *Creatinine clearance test interference.*) High creatinine clearance can suggest poor hydration.

What needs to be done

• Check the patient's history for drugs that may affect creatinine clearance.
• Tell the patient that this test requires a timed urine specimen and at least one blood sample. Be sure to explain how the urine will be collected.
• Tell the patient to avoid strenuous exercise during the testing period.
• Tell the patient he may need to avoid meat, poultry, fish, tea, or coffee for 6 hours before the test.
• Collect a timed urine specimen at 2, 6, 12, or 24 hours in a bottle containing a preservative to prevent degradation of the creatinine.
• Perform a venipuncture anytime during the collection period, and collect the sample in a 7-ml tube without additives, or in a tube volume in accordance with laboratory policy.
• Refrigerate the specimen or keep it on ice during the collection period.

Creatinine levels are proportional to total muscle mass and aren't affected by other variables. So, testing creatinine clearance can assess renal function and monitor progression of renal insufficiency.

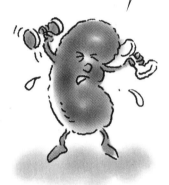

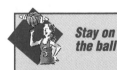

Stay on the ball

Creatinine clearance test interference

• A high-protein diet before the test or strenuous physical exercise during the collection period may alter results.
• Drugs that may decrease levels of creatinine clearance include amphotericin B, thiazide diuretics, furosemide, and aminoglycosides.

• Tell the patient to resume his usual diet, activities, and drugs as ordered.

Urine uric acid

Urine uric acid testing supplements serum uric acid testing to identify disorders that alter production or excretion of uric acid. Derived from dietary purines in organ meats and from endogenous nucleoproteins, uric acid (as urate) is found normally in the blood and in other tissues in amounts totaling about 1 g. Its primary site of formation is the liver, although the intestinal mucosa is also involved in urate production.

As the chief end product of purine catabolism, urate passes from the liver through the bloodstream to the kidneys, where roughly 50% is excreted daily in the urine.

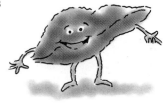

Testing urine uric acid is a good way to detect enzyme deficiencies and metabolic disturbances.

What it all means

Normal urine uric acid values vary with diet but generally range from 250 to 750 mg/24 hours (SI, 1.48 to 4.48 mmol/day). (See *Urine uric acid test interference.*)

Acid elevation

Elevated urine uric acid levels may result from chronic myeloid leukemia, polycythemia vera, multiple myeloma, early remission in pernicious anemia, as well as lymphosarcoma and lymphatic leukemia during radiation therapy. High levels also result from tubular reabsorption defects, such as Fanconi's syndrome and hepatolenticular degeneration (Wilson's disease).

Stay on the ball

Urine uric acid test interference

• A diet high or low in purine may alter results.
• Allopurinol, salicylates, vitamin C, alcohol, phenylbutazone, probenecid, pyrazinamide, and warfarin increase levels.
• Diuretics, such as furosemide, ethacrynic acid, and benzthiazide decrease levels.
• A high-purine diet increases levels; a low-purine diet decreases levels.

Acid depression

Low urine uric acid levels occur in gout and in severe renal damage, as occurs in chronic glomerulonephritis, diabetic glomerulosclerosis, and collagen disorders.

What needs to be done

• Check the patient's history for drugs that may influence uric acid levels.

• Tell the patient that he may need to follow a diet low or high in purines, as ordered, before or during urine collection.

• Collect a 24-hour urine specimen, discarding the first specimen and retaining the last.

Pigments

Urine hemoglobin

Contained in RBCs, hemoglobin combines with oxygen and carbon dioxide to allow RBCs to transport these gases between the lungs and the tissues.

RBC destruction

Aging RBCs are constantly being destroyed by normal mechanisms within the reticuloendothelial system (the system of those cells that can ingest particles). However, when RBC destruction occurs within the circulation instead, as it does in intravascular hemolysis, free hemoglobin enters the plasma and binds with haptoglobin. If the plasma level of hemoglobin exceeds that of haptoglobin, the excess hemoglobin is excreted in the urine. This condition is known as *hemoglobinuria*.

Testing for urine blood pigments can be performed at the patient's bedside. (See *Bedside testing for urine blood pigments*.)

What it all means

Hemoglobin shouldn't be present in urine. Hemoglobinuria may result from severe intravascular hemolysis resulting from a blood transfusion reaction, burns, or a crushing injury; from acquired hemolytic anemias caused by chemical or drug intoxication or malaria; or from the hemolytic anemia known as *paroxysmal nocturnal hemoglobinuria*. Hemoglobinuria may also result from congenital hemolytic anemias, as in hemoglobinopathies or en-

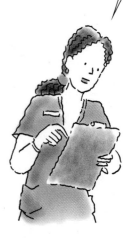

Urine hemoglobin measurement aids diagnosis of hemolytic anemias, infection, or severe intravascular hemolysis from a transfusion reaction.

Bedside testing for urine blood pigments

To test a patient's urine for blood pigments at the bedside, use one of the following methods. Because these methods detect only blood pigments, immunochemical studies are necessary to differentiate hemoglobin from other blood pigments such as myoglobin.

Dipstick, Multistix, or Chemstrips
• Collect a urine specimen.
• Dip the stick into the specimen and withdraw it.
• After 30 seconds, compare the stick to the color chart. Blue indicates a positive reaction; the intensity of color indicates pigment concentration.

Occult tablet
• Collect a urine specimen
• Put one drop of urine on the filter paper. Place the tablet on the urine and then put 2 drops of water on the tablet.
• After 2 minutes, inspect the filter paper around the tablet. Blue indicates a positive reaction; the intensity of color indicates pigment concentration.

Occult solution
• Collect a urine specimen.
• After placing one drop of urine on the filter paper, close the package and turn it over. Open the opposite side and place two drops of solution on the filter paper.
• After 30 seconds, inspect the filter paper. Blue indicates a positive reaction; the intensity of color indicates pigment concentration.

Stay on the ball

Urine hemoglobin test interference

• Large doses of vitamin C or drugs that contain vitamin C as a preservative cause a false-negative test result.
• Nephrotoxic drugs or anticoagulants may cause a positive result for hemoglobinuria or hematuria.
• Specimen contamination with menstrual blood alters test results.

zyme defects and, less commonly, from cystitis, ureteral calculi, or urethritis. Hemoglobinuria and hematuria occur in renal tumor, tuberculosis, or in renal epithelial damage, such as in acute glomerulonephritis or pyelonephritis. (See *Urine hemoglobin test interference.*)

What needs to be done
• Check the patient's history for drugs that may affect free hemoglobin levels.
• If the patient is a female who's menstruating, reschedule the test.
• Collect a random urine specimen.

Urine myoglobin

Myoglobin is a red pigment found in the cytoplasm of cardiac and skeletal muscle cells. The urine myoglobin test measures the level of this pigment in the urine.

The oxygen reservoir

Myoglobin probably serves as a reservoir of oxygen, facilitating its movement within muscle. When muscle cells are extensively damaged, myoglobin is released into the blood, quickly cleared by renal glomerular filtration, and eliminated in the urine.

What it all means

Myoglobin shouldn't appear in the urine. Myoglobinuria occurs in acute or chronic muscular disease, alcoholic polymyopathy, familial myoglobinuria, and extensive myocardial infarction. It also results from severe trauma to the skeletal muscles, such as in a crushing injury, extreme hyperthermia, or severe burns. Transient myoglobinuria, known as "march" myoglobinuria, may follow strenuous or prolonged exercise but disappears after rest. (See *Urine myoglobin test interference*.)

What needs to be done

• Collect a random urine specimen and send it to the laboratory.

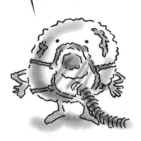

Myoglobin helps muscle cells receive oxygen. Myoglobin testing aids diagnosis of muscle disease or damage.

Stay on the ball

Urine myoglobin test interference

• If performed with Chemstrip or other reagent strips, recent ingestion of large vitamin C amounts can inhibit the reaction.
• Urine contamination with iodine (such as during surgery) causes positive results.
• Extremely dilute urine can reduce test sensitivity.

Sugars, ketones, and mucopolysaccharides

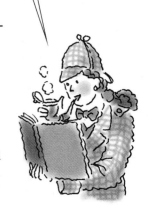

The urine glucose test is an effective diabetes detective.

Urine glucose

The glucose urine test, also called the *glucose oxidase test*, involves the use of commercial, plastic-coated reagent strips (Clinistix, Diastix, or Tes-Tape). It's a specific, qualitative test for glycosuria, which is routinely associated with diabetes mellitus.

Glucose spillover

Normally, nearly all glucose passes into the glomerular filtrate and is reabsorbed by the proximal renal tubule. However, if the blood glucose level exceeds the reabsorption capacity of the tubule, glucose spills into the urine.

What it all means

Glucose shouldn't be present in urine. Glycosuria occurs in diabetes mellitus, adrenal and thyroid disorders, hepatic and CNS diseases, Fanconi's syndrome and other conditions involving low renal threshold, toxic renal tubular disease, heavy metal poisoning, glomerulonephritis, nephrosis, pregnancy, and TPN. It also occurs when administering large amounts of glucose or niacin; because of prolonged use of phenothiazines; and because of use of certain other drugs, such as asparaginase, corticosteroids, carbamazepine, ammonium chloride, thiazide diuretics, dextrothyroxine, and lithium carbonate. (See *Urine glucose test interference*.)

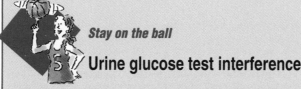

Stay on the ball

Urine glucose test interference

• Reducing substances, such as levodopa, ascorbic acid, phenazopyridine, methyldopa, and salicylates, may cause false-negative results.

What needs to be done

• Have the patient void, then give him a drink of water. After 30 to 45 minutes, collect a second-voided urine specimen, using one of the following procedures:

– *Clinistix test*—Dip the test area of the reagent strip in the specimen for 2 seconds. Remove excess urine by tapping the strip against a clean surface or the side of the container and begin timing. Hold the strip in the air and "read" the color *exactly 10 seconds* after taking the strip out of the urine by comparing it with the reference color blocks on the container label. Ignore color changes that develop after 10 seconds.

– *Diastix test*—Dip the reagent strip in the specimen for 2 seconds. Remove excess urine by tapping the strip against the container and begin timing. Hold the strip in the air and compare the color to the color chart *exactly 30 seconds* after taking the strip out of the urine. Ignore color changes that develop after 30 seconds.

– *Tes-Tape*—Withdraw about 1″ (2.54 cm) of the reagent tape from the dispenser; dip ¼″ (0.6 cm) in the specimen for 2 seconds. Remove excess urine by tapping the strip against the side of the container and begin timing. Hold the tape in the air and compare the color of the darkest part of the tape to the color chart *exactly 60 seconds* after taking the strip out of the urine. If the tape indicates 0.5% or higher, wait an additional 60 seconds to make the final color comparison.

Urine ketones

Ketones are products of fat metabolism not normally found in the urine. However, ketones may be found with excessive fat metabolism, which occurs when the body can't metabolize carbohydrates, carbohydrate intake is inadequate, metabolic demand increases, or excessive carbohydrates are lost. In the urine ketone test, the action of urine on a commercially prepared product (Acetest tablet, Chemstrip K, Ketostix, or Keto-Diastix) measures the urine level of ketone bodies (ketones).

Checking the ketone bodies

Each product measures a specific ketone body. For example, Acetest measures acetone, and Ketostix measures acetoacetic acid. The urine determinations reflect serum concentration.

What it all means

Ketones shouldn't be present in urine. Ketonuria is present in uncontrolled diabetes mellitus and starvation; it also occurs as a

The urine ketone test helps identify diabetic ketoacidosis and carbohydrate deprivation.

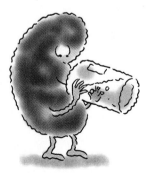

metabolic complication of TPN. (See *Urine ketone test interference.*)

What needs to be done

• Have the patient void; then give him a drink of water. About 30 minutes later, collect a second-voided urine specimen, and use one of the following procedures to test the specimen:

– *Acetest*—Lay the tablet on a piece of white paper and place one drop of urine on the tablet. After 30 seconds, compare the tablet color (white, lavender, or purple) with the color chart.

– *Ketostix*—Dip the reagent stick into the specimen and remove it immediately. After 15 seconds, compare the stick color (buff or purple) with the color chart.

– *Keto-Diastix*—Dip the reagent strip into the specimen and remove it immediately. Tap the edge of the strip against the container or a clean, dry surface to remove excess urine. Hold the strip horizontally to prevent mixing the chemicals from the two areas. Interpret each area of the strip separately. After *exactly 15 seconds,* compare the color of the ketone section (buff or purple) with the appropriate color chart; after 30 seconds, compare the color of the glucose section. Ignore color changes that occur after the specified waiting periods.

Stay on the ball

Urine ketone test interference

• Levodopa, phenazopyridine, and sulfobromophthalein produce inaccurate test results with reagent strips; therefore, Acetest tablets must be used instead.

Minerals

Urine sodium and chloride

The urine sodium and chloride test determines urine levels of sodium, the major extracellular cation, and chloride, the major extracellular anion.

Sodium and chloride—in tandem

Sodium and chloride help maintain osmotic pressure and water and acid-base balance. After these ions are absorbed by the intestinal tract, they're regulated by the kidneys and rise and fall in tandem. The kidneys conserve constant serum levels of sodium and chloride—even at the risk of dehydration or edema—or excrete excessive amounts.

What it all means

Although levels of sodium and chloride in the urine vary greatly with dietary salt intake and perspiration, the normal range in adults for urine sodium excretion is 40 to 220 mEq/24 hours (SI, 40 to 220 mmol/day); in infants and children, from 41 to 115 mEq/L/24 hours (SI, 41 to 115 mmol/day). Urine chloride excretion in adults ranges from 110 to 250 nmol/24 hours (SI, 110 to 250 mmol/day to 40 mmol/day); in children, from 15 to 40 nmol/24 hours (SI, 15 to 40 mmol/day); and in infants, from 2 to 10 mmol/24 hours (SI, 2 to 10 mmol/day).

Out-of-sync levels...

Usually, urine sodium and chloride levels are parallel, rising and falling in tandem. Elevated urine sodium levels may reflect increased salt intake, adrenal failure, salicylate toxicity, diabetic acidosis, salt-losing nephritis, or water-deficient dehydration. Decreased urine sodium levels suggest decreased salt intake, primary aldosteronism, acute renal failure, or heart failure.

...elevated levels...

Elevated urine chloride levels may result from water-deficient dehydration, salicylate toxicity, diabetic acidosis, adrenocortical insufficiency (Addison's disease), or salt-losing renal disease.

...and decreased levels

Decreased levels may result from excessive diaphoresis, heart failure, or hypochloremic metabolic alkalosis caused by prolonged vomiting or gastric suctioning. (See *Urine sodium and chloride test interference.*)

What needs to be done

• Check the patient's drug history for drugs that may influence test results.
• Collect a 24-hour urine specimen, keeping it on ice or in the refrigerator, and send it to the laboratory on completion.

Urine potassium

This quantitative test measures urine levels of potassium, a major intracellular cation (positively charged ion) that helps regulate acid-base balance and neuromuscular function. The kidneys regulate potassium balance through potassium excretion in the urine. Most commonly, this test is done to evaluate hypokalemia when a history and physical examination fail to uncover the cause of altered serum potassium values. If results suggest a renal disorder, additional renal function tests may be ordered.

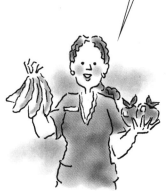

Testing for sodium and chloride can help monitor the effects of a low-salt diet. These minerals help maintain fluid and electrolyte balance.

Stay on the ball

Urine sodium and chloride test interference

• Ammonium chloride and potassium chloride elevate urine chloride levels.
• Sodium bicarbonate and thiazide diuretics raise urine sodium levels; steroids suppress them.

Stay on the ball

Urine potassium test interference

- Potassium-wasting medications, such as ammonium chloride, thiazide diuretics, and acetazolamide, raise levels.
- Excessive vomiting or stomach suctioning produces false results.

What it all means

Normal potassium excretion is 25 to 125 mmol/24 hours (SI, 25 to 125 mmol/day), but varies with diet. In children, potassium excretion is 22 to 57 mmol/24 hours (SI, 22 to 57 mmol/day).

Potassium puzzle

In a patient with hypokalemia and normal kidney function, potassium concentration will be less than 10 mmol/24 hours (SI, 10 mmol/day), indicating that potassium loss is most likely the result of a GI disorder such as malabsorption syndrome.

In a patient with hypokalemia lasting more than 3 days, urine potassium levels above 10 mmol/24 hours (SI, 10 mmol/day) indicate renal losses that may result from such disorders as aldosteronism, renal tubular acidosis, or chronic renal failure. However, extrarenal disorders, such as dehydration, starvation, Cushing's disease, and salicylate intoxication, may also elevate urine potassium levels. (See *Urine potassium test interference*.)

What needs to be done

- Check the patient's history for drugs that may alter test results.
- Collect a 24-hour urine specimen, discarding the first specimen and retaining the last.
- Refrigerate the specimen or place it on ice during the collection period.

Testing urine potassium determines whether hypokalemia stems from renal or extrarenal disorders.

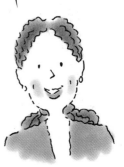

Urine magnesium

The urine magnesium test measures the urine level of magnesium, an important cation absorbed in the intestinal tract and excreted in urine. Measurement of urine magnesium was rarely used in the past, but it's becoming more widely used because magnesium deficiency is detectable earlier in urine than in serum.

Magnesium facts

Magnesium is found primarily in the bones and in intracellular fluid; a small amount is present in extracellular fluid. This element activates many enzyme systems, helps transport sodium and potassium across cell membranes, affects nucleic acid and protein metabolism, and influences intracellular calcium levels through its effect on parathyroid hormone secretion.

What it all means

Normal urinary excretion of magnesium is 6 to 10 mEq/24 hours (SI, 3 to 5 mmol/day).

The lowdown on levels

Low urine magnesium levels may result from malabsorption, acute or chronic diarrhea, diabetic acidosis, dehydration, pancreatitis, advanced renal failure, primary aldosteronism, or decreased dietary intake of magnesium.

Elevated urine magnesium levels may result from early chronic renal disease, adrenocortical insufficiency (Addison's disease), chronic alcoholism, or chronic ingestion of magnesium-containing antacids. (See *Urine magnesium test interference*.)

What needs to be done

• Notify the laboratory and practitioner if the patient is taking drugs that may alter test results.
• Collect a 24-hour urine specimen, discarding the first specimen and retaining the last, and send it to the laboratory upon completion.

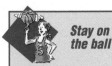

Stay on the ball

Urine magnesium test interference

• Increased calcium intake reduces levels.
• Ethacrynic acid, thiazide diuretics, aldosterone, or magnesium-containing antacids elevate levels.
• Spironolactone lowers levels.

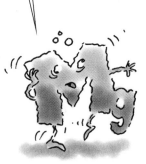

Urine magnesium testing rules out magnesium deficiency in patients with CNS irritation.

Urine calcium and phosphates

This test measures the urine levels of calcium and phosphates, elements essential for the formation and resorption of bone. Urine calcium and phosphate levels generally parallel serum levels.

Normally absorbed in the upper intestine and excreted in stools and urine, calcium and phosphates help maintain tissue and fluid pH, electrolyte balance in cells and extracellular fluids, and permeability of cell membranes. Calcium promotes enzymatic processes, aids blood coagulation, and lowers neuromuscular irritability; phosphates aid carbohydrate metabolism.

What it all means

Normal values depend on dietary intake. In a normal diet, urine calcium levels range from 100 to 300 mg/24 hours (SI, 2.5 to 7.5 mmol/day). Normal excretion of phosphates is less than

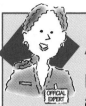

Disorders that affect urine calcium and phosphate levels

These disorders can cause changes in urine calcium or phosphate levels.

Disorder	Urine calcium level	Urine phosphate level
Acute nephritis	Suppressed	Suppressed or normal
Acute nephrosis	Suppressed	Suppressed
Chronic nephrosis	Low	Low
Hyperparathyroidism	Elevated	Elevated
Hypoparathyroidism	Suppressed	Suppressed
Metastatic carcinoma	Elevated	Normal
Milk-alkali syndrome	Low or normal	Low or normal
Multiple myeloma	Elevated or normal	Elevated or normal
Osteomalacia	Low	Low
Paget's disease	Normal	Normal
Renal insufficiency	Suppressed	Suppressed
Renal tubular acidosis	Elevated	Elevated
Sarcoidosis	Elevated	Suppressed
Steatorrhea	Low	Low
Vitamin D intoxication	Elevated	Suppressed

Urine calcium and phosphate test interference

• Thiazide diuretics decrease calcium excretion.
• Prolonged inactivity and use of corticosteroids, sodium phosphate, or calcitonin increase excretion.
• Vitamin D increases phosphate absorption and excretion.
• Parathyroid hormone increases urinary phosphate excretion and decreases urinary calcium excretion.

1,000 mg/24 hours. Many disorders may affect calcium and phosphorus levels. (See *Disorders that affect urine calcium and phosphate levels.*) Likewise, drugs and activity levels can affect levels. (See *Urine calcium and phosphate test interference.*)

> Urine calcium and phosphates testing evaluates calcium and phosphate metabolism and excretion.

What needs to be done

• Note the patient's use of drugs that may alter test results.
• Tell the patient that he needs to be as active as possible before the test.
• As ordered, provide a diet that contains about 130 mg of calcium/24 hours for 3 days before the test, or provide a copy of the diet for the patient to follow at home.
• Collect a 24-hour urine specimen, discarding the first specimen and retaining the last.
• Send the specimen to the laboratory on completion.

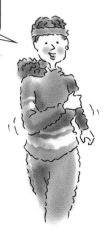

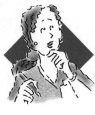

Quick quiz

1. Your patient's urine specific gravity measures 1.001. Based on this finding, your patient may have which disorder?

    A.   Diabetes insipidus

    B.   Heart failure

    C.   Acute glomerulonephritis

    D.   Hepatitis

Answer: A. Low specific gravity (less than 1.005) is characteristic of diabetes insipidus.

2. Before obtaining a specimen for urine amylase testing, the patient should refrain from taking:

    A.   furosemide.

    B.   bumetanide.

    C.   hydrochlorothiazide.

    D.   acetaminophen.

Answer: C. Thiazide diuretics such as hydrochlorothiazide should be withheld for 24 hours before obtaining a specimen for urine amylase testing. Thiazide diuretics may raise urine amylase levels.

3. When teaching the patient about urine aldosterone testing, you should include which instruction?

    A.   Avoid alcohol for 24 hours before the test.

    B.   Avoid sodium-rich foods during the collection period.

    C.   Restrict fluids for 8 hours before the test.

    D.   Fast for 8 hours before the test.

Answer: B. Before urine aldosterone testing, you should instruct the patient to avoid sodium-rich foods, strenuous exercise, and stressful situations during the collection period.

Scoring

☆☆☆   If you answered all three questions correctly, great! "Ur-in" top form!

  ☆☆   If you answered two questions correctly, super! You're 17-KS above the rest!

    ☆   If you answered fewer than two correctly, chin up! A little more practice and you'll be Star of the Bilirubin Ball!

6

Other specimen tests

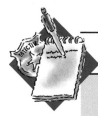

Just the facts

In this chapter, you'll learn:

♦ about other specimen tests

♦ what patient care is associated with these tests

♦ what factors can interfere with test results

♦ what test results may indicate.

A look at other specimen tests

Other specimen tests include pleural fluid analysis, gastric acid stimulation, peritoneal fluid analysis, fecal occult blood, fecal lipids, stool examination for ova and parasite, stool examination for rotavirus antigen, amniotic fluid analysis, Papanicolaou test, semen analysis, cerebrospinal fluid (CSF) analysis, pericardial fluid analysis, and sweat test. Each test is unique and requires its own procedure to collect the specimen. Explain the procedure to the patient in simple terms to allay his anxiety.

Respiratory system

Pleural fluid analysis

In pleural fluid aspiration, also known as *thoracentesis*, the thoracic wall is punctured to obtain a specimen of pleural fluid for analysis or to relieve pulmonary compression and resultant respiratory distress. Locating the fluid before thoracentesis with an X-ray, computed tomography scan, or by ultrasound methods reduces the risk of puncturing the lung, liver, or spleen.

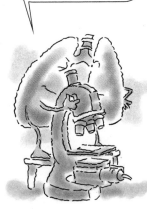

Pleural fluid analysis can help determine the cause of pleural damage, pulmonary compression, and respiratory distress.

What it all means

The pleural cavity should contain less than 20 ml of serous fluid. Pleural effusion results from the abnormal formation or reabsorption of pleural fluid. Certain characteristics classify pleural fluid as either a transudate or an exudate.

Abnormal findings

Pleural effusion results from the abnormal formation or reabsorption of pleural fluid. Transudate and exudate fluids may contain blood (hemothorax), chyl (chylothorax), pus (empyema), or necrotic tissue. Blood-tinged fluid may indicate a traumatic tap; if so, the fluid should clear as aspiration progresses.

Transudate vs. exudate

Transudative effusion generally results from diminished colloidal pressure, increased negative pressure within the pleural cavity, ascites, systemic and pulmonary venous hypertension, heart failure, hepatic cirrhosis, and nephritis. Exudative effusion results from disorders that increase pleural capillary permeability (possibly with changes in hydrostatic or colloid osmotic pressures), lymphatic drainage interference, infections, pulmonary infarctions, and neoplasms. It's associated with depressed glucose levels, elevated lactate dehydrogenase (LD) isoenzymes, and rheumatoid arthritis cells; negative smears, cultures, and cytologic examination may indicate pleurisy associated with rheumatoid arthritis.

Other abnormalities

The most common pathogens that appear in pleural fluid culture studies are *Mycobacterium tuberculosis*, *Staphylococcus aureus*, *Streptococcus pneumoniae* and other streptococci, *Haemophilus influenzae* and, in the case of ruptured pulmonary abscess, anaerobes such as bacteroides.

A high percentage of neutrophils suggests septic inflammation; predominating lymphocytes suggest tuberculosis or fungal or viral effusions. Serosanguineous fluid may indicate pleural extension of a malignant tumor. Elevated LD in a nonpurulent, nonhemolyzed, nonbloody effusion may also suggest malignancy.

Pleural fluid glucose levels that are 30 to 40 mg/dl lower than blood glucose levels may indicate a malignant tumor, bacterial infection, nonseptic inflammation, or metastasis. Increased amylase levels occur with pleural effusions associated with pancreatitis. (See *Characteristics of pulmonary transudate and exudate* and *Pleural fluid analysis interference*.)

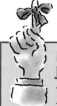

Memory jogger

To remember the difference between transudate and exudate, focus on the prefixes: trans- means "across," and ex- means "out of."

Stay on the ball

Pleural fluid analysis interference

Antimicrobial therapy before aspiration of fluid for culture may decrease the number of bacteria, making isolation of the infecting organism difficult.

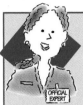

Advice from the experts

Characteristics of pulmonary transudate and exudate

These characteristics help classify pleural fluid as either a transudate or an exudate.

Characteristic	Transudate	Exudate
Appearance	Clear	Cloudy, turbid
Specific gravity	< 1.016	> 1.016
Clot (fibrinogen)	Absent	Present
Protein	< 3 g/dl (SI, < 30 g/L)	> 3 g/dl (SI, > 30 g/L)
White blood cells	Few lymphocytes	Many lymphocytes; may be purulent
Red blood cells	Few	Variable
Glucose level	Equal to serum level	May be less than serum level
Lactate dehydrogenase	Low	High

What needs to be done

- Check the patient's history for bleeding disorders or anticoagulant therapy.
- Explain that a chest X-ray or ultrasound study may precede the test.
- Explain the procedure to the patient and check that an informed consent form has been signed.
- Instruct the patient not to cough, breathe deeply, or move during the test to minimize the risk of lung injury.
- Record the patient's baseline vital signs.
- Clip the hair around the needle insertion site, if necessary, and position the patient properly. (See *Positioning the patient for thoracentesis*, page 224.)

The practitioner does A...

- The practitioner disinfects the skin, drapes the area, injects a local anesthetic, and inserts the thoracentesis needle above the rib. When the needle reaches the pocket of fluid, he attaches the 50-ml syringe and the stopcock and opens the clamps on the tubing to aspirate fluid into the container. The laboratory request and speci-

Positioning the patient for thoracentesis

To prepare the patient for thoracentesis, place him in one of the three positions shown below: sitting on the edge of the bed with his arms on an overbed table, sitting up in bed with his arms on an overbed table, or lying partially on the side, partially on the back with his arms over his head. These positions serve to widen the intercostal spaces and permit easy access to the pleural cavity. Using pillows (as shown) will make the patient more comfortable.

Sitting on edge of bed

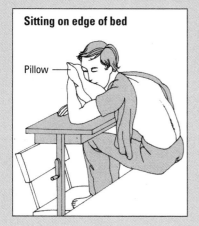

Pillow

Sitting up in bed

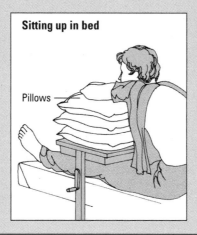

Pillows

Lying partially on unaffected side with head of bed raised 30 to 45 degrees

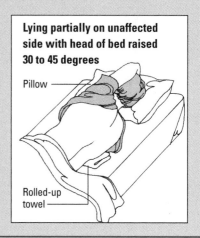

Pillow

Rolled-up towel

men container need to be labeled appropriately (date and time of the test, amount, color, and character of the fluid—such as clear, frothy, purulent, or bloody).

...while you do B, C, and D

- During aspiration, check the patient for signs of respiratory distress, such as weakness, dyspnea, pallor, cyanosis, changes in heart rate, tachypnea, diaphoresis, blood-tinged frothy mucus, and hypotension.
- After the needle is withdrawn, apply slight pressure and a small adhesive bandage to the puncture site.
- Reposition the patient on the unaffected side or as ordered. Tell him to remain on this side for at least 1 hour to seal the puncture site. Elevate the head of the bed to facilitate breathing.

Waiting and watchful

- Monitor vital signs every 30 minutes for 2 hours, then every 4 hours until they're stable.
- Check the puncture site for fluid leakage; a large amount of fluid leakage is abnormal.
- Watch for signs and symptoms of complications. (See *Recognizing complications of thoracentesis.*)

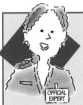

Advice from the experts

Recognizing complications of thoracentesis

You can identify complications of thoracentesis by watching for characteristic signs and symptoms:
- pneumothorax—apprehension, increased restlessness, cyanosis, sudden breathlessness, tachycardia, chest pain
- tension pneumothorax—dyspnea, chest pain, tachycardia, hypotension, absent or diminished breath sounds on the affected side
- subcutaneous emphysema—local tissue swelling, crackling on palpation of site
- infection—fever, rapid pulse rate, pain
- mediastinal shift—labored breathing, cardiac arrhythmias, pulmonary edema.

Gastrointestinal system

Gastric acid stimulation

The gastric acid stimulation test measures gastric acid secretion for 1 hour after subcutaneous injection of pentagastrin or a similar drug that stimulates gastric acid output. It's usually performed if the basal secretion test suggests abnormal gastric secretion.

What it all means

Normally, gastric secretion following stimulation ranges from 8 to 28 mEq/hour for males and from 11 to 21 mEq/hour for females. (See *Gastric acid stimulation test interference.*)

Abnormal findings

Increased gastric secretion may indicate duodenal ulcer; markedly elevated secretion suggests Zollinger-Ellison syndrome. Decreased secretion may indicate gastric carcinoma; achlorhydria may indicate pernicious anemia.

What needs to be done

- Make sure that the patient has signed an appropriate consent form and check for allergies and sensitivities to pentagastrin.
- Tell the patient he must fast from midnight the night before until the test takes place, as well as refrain from smoking.

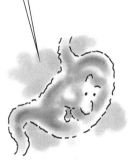

The gastric acid stimulation test helps diagnose duodenal ulcers, Zollinger-Ellison syndrome, pernicious anemia, and gastric carcinoma.

Stay on the ball

Gastric acid stimulation test interference

Gastric acid levels are elevated by cholinergics, adrenergic blockers, and reserpine and depressed by antacids, anticholinergics, hydrogen blockers, and proton pump inhibitors.

- Withhold antacids, anticholinergics, adrenergic-receptor blockers, histamine-2 receptor antagonists, corticosteroids, proton pump inhibitors, and reserpine before the test.
- Tell the patient that the test requires passing a nasogastric (NG) tube and injecting pentagastrin subcutaneously and takes 1 hour.
- During the test, instruct the patient to report adverse effects, such as abdominal pain, nausea, dizziness, and numbness of extremities, immediately.
- After basal gastric secretions have been collected, keep the NG tube in place. Pentagastrin is then injected subcutaneously. Wait 15 minutes and then collect a specimen every 15 minutes for 1 hour.

Read and record

- Record the color and odor of each specimen, and note presence of food, mucus, bile, or blood. Label all specimens "stimulated contents," and number them 1 through 4. If the NG tube will be left in place, clamp it or attach it to low intermittent suction, as ordered.
- Watch for adverse effects after removal of the NG tube, such as nausea, vomiting, abdominal distention, or pain. Watch for adverse effects of pentagastrin, such as rash, hives, nausea, vomiting, abdominal pain, blurred vision, diaphoresis, and shortness of breath.
- Tell the patient to resume his diet and drugs as ordered.

Peritoneal fluid analysis

Peritoneal fluid analysis assesses a sample of peritoneal fluid obtained by paracentesis, a procedure that entails inserting a trocar and cannula through the abdominal wall. For this procedure, the patient receives a local anesthetic. If the sample is removed for therapeutic purposes, the trocar may be connected to a drainage system. However, if only a small amount of fluid is removed for testing, an 18G needle may be used. In a four-quadrant tap, fluid is aspirated from each quadrant to verify trauma and confirm the need for surgery.

What it all means

Peritoneal fluid is normally odorless and clear to pale yellow. (See *Normal findings in peritoneal fluid analysis* and *Peritoneal fluid analysis interference*.)

Judging by looks

Milk-colored peritoneal fluid may result from a malignant tumor, lymphoma, tuberculosis, a parasitic infection, an adhesion, or he-

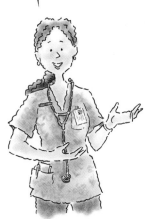

Peritoneal fluid analysis determines the cause of ascites and helps detect abdominal trauma.

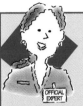

Advice from the experts

Normal findings in peritoneal fluid analysis

Use this chart to determine the normal findings in peritoneal fluid.

Element	Normal value or finding
Alkaline phosphatase	Males > age 18: 90 to 239 units/L (SI, 90 to 239 units/L) Females < age 45: 76 to 196 units/L (SI, 76 to 196 units/L) Females > age 45: 87 to 250 units/L (SI, 87 to 250 units/L)
Ammonia	< 50 mcg/dl (SI, < 29 μmol/L)
Amylase	138 to 404 units/L (SI, 138 to 404 units/L)
Bacteria	None
Cytology	No malignant cells present
Fungi	None
Glucose	70 to 100 mg/dl (SI, 3.5 to 5 mmol/L)
Gross appearance	Sterile, odorless, clear to pale yellow color; scant amount (< 50 ml)
Protein	0.3 to 4.1 g/dl (SI, 3 to 41 g/L)
Red blood cells	None
White blood cells	< 300/μl (SI, < 300 × 10⁹/L)

Stay on the ball

Peritoneal fluid analysis interference

Injury to underlying structures during paracentesis may contaminate the sample with bile, blood, urine, or feces.

patic cirrhosis. Cloudy or turbid fluid may indicate peritonitis. Bloody fluid may result from a benign or malignant tumor, hemorrhagic pancreatitis, or a traumatic tap; however, if the fluid fails to clear on continued aspiration, a traumatic tap isn't the cause. Bile-stained green fluid may indicate a ruptured gallbladder, acute pancreatitis, a perforated intestine, or duodenal ulcer.

The lowdown on levels

A red blood cell (RBC) count over 100/μl (SI, greater than 100/L) indicates a neoplasm or tuberculosis; a count over 100,000/μl (SI, greater than 100,000/L) indicates intra-abdominal trauma.

A white blood cell (WBC) count with more than 25% neutrophils occurs in 90% of patients with spontaneous bacterial peritonitis and in 50% of those with cirrhosis. A high percentage of lymphocytes suggests tuberculous peritonitis or chylous ascites. Numerous mesothelial cells indicate tuberculous peritonitis.

Protein levels rise above 3 g/dl in malignancy (SI, greater than 3 g/L) and above 4 g/dl (SI, greater than 4 g/L) in tuberculosis. Peritoneal fluid glucose levels fall in tuberculous peritonitis and peritoneal carcinomatosis.

Amylase levels rise in pancreatic trauma, pancreatic pseudo-cyst, or acute pancreatitis and may also rise in intestinal necrosis or strangulation. Peritoneal alkaline phosphatase levels rise to more than twice the normal serum levels in a ruptured or strangulated small intestine. Peritoneal ammonia levels also exceed twice the normal serum levels in ruptured or strangulated large and small intestines and in a ruptured ulcer or appendix.

Cytologic examination accurately detects malignant cells. Microbiological examination can reveal bacteria and fungi.

What needs to be done

• Tell the patient this test requires a peritoneal fluid sample and may take up to 45 minutes to perform. Explain that he'll receive a local anesthetic to ease discomfort. Instruct him to urinate just before the test to help prevent accidental bladder injury. Make sure that the patient or a responsible family member has signed an informed consent form.
• Record baseline vital signs, weight, and abdominal girth.
• Position the patient on a bed or in a chair, as ordered, with his feet flat on the floor and his back well supported. If he can't tolerate being out of bed, place him in high Fowler's position.
• Assist with clipping hair at the puncture site as necessary, preparing the skin, and draping the area.

Aspiration station

• A local anesthetic is injected and the needle or trocar and cannula are inserted, usually 1″ to 2″ (2.5 to 5 cm) below the umbilicus. (However, it may also be inserted through the flank, the iliac fossa, the border of the rectus, or at each quadrant of the abdomen.) If a trocar and cannula are used, a small incision is made to facilitate insertion. When the needle pierces the peritoneum, it "gives" with an audible sound. The trocar is removed, and a sample of fluid is aspirated with a 50-ml luer-lock syringe. Label samples in the order they're drawn. If additional fluid is drained, I.V. tubing and a collection bag may be attached to facilitate collection. No more than 1,500 ml should be drained.
• Check the patient's vital signs every 15 minutes during the procedure. Watch for deviations from baseline findings. Observe for dizziness, pallor, perspiration, and increased anxiety. If rapid fluid

aspiration induces shock, reduce the vertical distance between the trocar and the collection bag to slow the drainage rate. If necessary, stop the drainage by turning off the stopcock or clamping the tubing.

Pressure dressing

- If fluid aspiration is difficult, reposition the patient as ordered. After aspiration, the trocar or needle is removed, the wound may be sutured, and a pressure dressing is applied.
- Check the dressing frequently and reinforce or apply a pressure dressing if needed.

On the lookout

- Monitor vital signs, and have the patient maintain bed rest until his vital signs are stable. Monitor his urine output for at least 24 hours and watch for hematuria.
- Weigh the patient and measure abdominal girth; compare these with baseline measurements.
- If a large amount of fluid was aspirated, watch for signs of vascular collapse (color change, elevated pulse and respiratory rates, decreased blood pressure and central venous pressure, mental changes, and dizziness). Administer fluids orally if the patient is alert and can accept them.
- Watch for increasing pain and abdominal tenderness, which may indicate a perforated intestine (or puncture of the inferior epigastric artery), hematoma of the anterior cecal wall, or rupture of the iliac vein or bladder.
- Observe the patient with severe hepatic disease for signs of hepatic coma including mental changes, drowsiness, and stupor.
- Administer I.V. infusions and albumin as ordered. Check electrolyte (especially sodium) and serum protein levels.

Fecal occult blood

Fecal occult blood, invisible because of its minute quantity, can be detected by microscopic analysis or by chemical tests for hemoglobin, such as the guaiac test.

Detection tests

Because small amounts of blood (2 to 2.5 ml/day) normally appear in the feces, tests for occult blood are designed to detect quantities larger than this.

What it all means

The indicator should turn to green, indicating that less than 2.5 ml of blood is present. (See *Fecal occult blood test interference.*)

Stay on the ball

Fecal occult blood test interference

- Iron preparations, bromides, rauwolfia derivatives, indomethacin, colchicine, phenylbutazone, and steroids may cause increase due to association with GI blood loss.
- Ascorbic acid (vitamin C) may cause false-normal results even with significant bleeding.
- Ingestion of 2 to 5 ml of blood (for example, from bleeding gums) can cause abnormal results.
- Active bleeding from hemorrhoids may cause false-positive results.

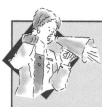

Listen up!

Collecting a stool specimen at home

When teaching the patient how to collect a stool specimen, tell him to:
• collect it in a clean container with a tight-fitting lid
• wrap the container in a brown paper bag
• keep it in the refrigerator (separate from food items) until it can be transported.

Abnormal findings

A positive test indicates GI bleeding, which may result from many disorders. Further tests are necessary to define the site and extent of bleeding.

What needs to be done

Inform the patient that this test requires collection of three stool specimens (occasionally only a random specimen is collected). (See *Collecting a stool specimen at home.*)
• Instruct the patient to maintain a high-fiber diet and to refrain from eating red meat, poultry, fish, turnips, and horseradish for 48 to 72 hours before the test and throughout the collection period.
• Tell the patient that the test requires the collection of three stool specimens. Occasionally, only a random specimen is collected.
• Notify the laboratory and practitioner of drugs the patient is taking that may affect test results. If these drugs must be continued, note this on the laboratory request.
• Wearing gloves, collect three stool specimens or a random specimen, as ordered. Be sure to obtain specimens from two different areas of each stool.
• For the Hemoccult slide test, open the flap on the slide packet and use a wooden applicator to apply a thin smear of the stool specimen to the guaiac-impregnated filter paper exposed in box A. Or, after performing a digital rectal examination, wipe the examination finger on a square of the filter paper. Apply a second smear from another part of the specimen to the filter paper exposed in box B because some parts of the specimen may not contain blood. Allow the specimen to dry for 3 to 5 minutes. Open the flap at the rear of the slide package and place two drops of Hemoccult developing solution on the paper over each smear. A blue reaction will

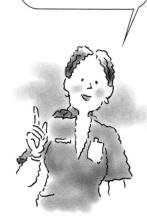

Testing for fecal occult blood detects GI bleeding and aids early diagnosis of colorectal cancer.

appear in 30 to 60 seconds if the test is positive. Record the results and discard the slide package.

• For the Hematest reagent tablet test, the specimen (as collected for the Hemoccult slide test) is placed on the filter paper. The filter paper with the stool smear is placed on a glass plate. Remove a reagent tablet from the bottle, and immediately replace the cap tightly. Place the tablet in the center of the stool smear on the filter paper. Add one drop of water to the tablet, and allow it to soak in for 5 to 10 seconds. Add a second drop, letting it run from the tablet on to the specimen and filter paper. If necessary, tap the plate gently to dislodge any water from the top of the tablet. After 2 minutes the filter will turn blue if the test is positive. Don't read the color that appears on the tablet itself or develops on the filter paper after the 2-minute period. Note the results and discard the paper.

• For the Instant-View fecal occult blood test, add a stool specimen to the collection tube and shake it to mix with the extraction buffer. Dispense four drops into the specimen well of the cassette. Results will appear on the test region and the control region of the cassette in 5 to 10 minutes, indicating whether the level of hemoglobin is greater than 0.05 mcg/ml of stool. Results will also indicate if the device is performing properly.

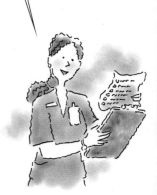

The fecal lipid test can confirm steatorrhea, or excess fat in the stools.

Fecal lipids

Lipids excreted in feces include monoglycerides, diglycerides, triglycerides, phospholipids, glycolipids, soaps (fatty acids and fatty acid salts), sterols, and cholesterol esters.

Lipid origins

These lipids are derived from sloughed intestinal bacterial cells and epithelial cells, unabsorbed dietary lipids, and GI secretions. Normally, dietary lipids emulsified by bile are almost completely absorbed in the small intestine, provided that biliary and pancreatic secretions are adequate. However, excessive excretion of fecal lipids (steatorrhea) occurs in various malabsorption syndromes.

Both qualitative and quantitative tests can detect excessive excretion of lipids; however, only the quantitative test can confirm steatorrhea.

What it all means

Fecal lipids normally make up less than 20% of excreted solids, with excretion of less than 7 g/24 hours. Digestive disorders may affect the production and release of pancreatic lipase or bile; absorptive disorders may affect the intestine's integrity, causing steatorrhea. (See *Fecal lipids test interference*.)

Stay on the ball

Fecal lipids test interference

Azathioprine, bisacodyl, cholestyramine, kanamycin, neomycin, colchicine, aluminum hydroxide, calcium carbonate, alcohol, potassium chloride, and mineral oil may cause increase or decrease due to inhibited absorption or altered chemical digestion.

What needs to be done

• Inform the patient to abstain from alcohol and to maintain a high-fat diet (100 g/day) for 3 days before the test and during the collection period.

• Notify the laboratory and practitioner of drugs the patient is taking that may affect test results; they may need to be restricted. If these drugs must be continued, note this on the laboratory request.

• Teach the patient how to collect a timed stool specimen and provide him with the necessary equipment, as indicated. Tell him to avoid contaminating the stool specimen with toilet tissue or urine.

• Collect a 72-hour stool specimen. Don't use a waxed collection container because the wax may become incorporated in the stools and interfere with test results.

• Refrigerate the collection container and keep it tightly covered.

• After the test, inform the patient to resume his usual diet and drugs withheld, as ordered.

Stool examination for ova and parasites

Examination of a stool specimen can detect several types of intestinal parasites. Some of these parasites live in nonpathogenic symbiosis; others cause intestinal disease. In the United States, the most common parasites include the roundworm *Ascaris lumbricoides* and the hookworm *Necator americanus*; the tapeworms *Diphyllobothrium latum, Taenia saginata* and, rarely, *Taenia solium*; the amoeba *Entamoeba histolytica*; and the flagellates *Giardia lamblia* or *Cyclospora*. Detection of pinworm requires a different collection method. (See *Collection procedure for pinworm.*)

Collection procedure for pinworm

The ova of the pinworm *Enterobius vermicularis* seldom appear in feces because the female migrates to the anus and deposits her ova there. To collect them, place a piece of cellophane tape, sticky side out, on the end of a tongue blade, and press it firmly on the anal area. Then transfer the tape, sticky side down, to a slide (kits with tape and a slide or a sticky paddle are available). Because the female usually deposits her ova at night, collect the specimen early in the morning, before the patient bathes or defecates. Pinworm infection shouldn't be ruled out until five consecutive negative specimens have been obtained.

What it all means

No parasites or ova should appear in stools.

Parasitic presence

The presence of *E. histolytica* confirms amebiasis; *G. lamblia* confirms giardiasis. Because injury to the host is difficult to detect—even when helminth ova or larvae appear—the number of worms is usually correlated with the patient's clinical symptoms to distinguish between helminth infestation and helminth diseases. Eosinophilia may also indicate parasitic infection. (See *Stool ova and parasite test interference*.)

What needs to be done

- Check the patient's history for use of antiparasitic drugs within 2 weeks of the test.
- If the patient has diarrhea, record recent dietary and travel history.
- Instruct the patient to avoid treatments with castor or mineral oil, bismuth, magnesium or antidiarrheal compounds, barium enemas, and antibiotics for 7 to 10 days before the test.
- Tell the patient that the test requires three stool specimens—one every other day or every third day. Up to six specimens may be needed to confirm the presence of *E. histolytica*.
- Collect a stool specimen directly in the container or in a clean, dry bedpan; then, using a tongue blade, transfer it into a properly labeled container.

Contamination cautions

- Don't contaminate the stool specimen with urine or toilet tissue.
- Don't collect stools from a toilet bowl because water is toxic to trophozoites and may contain organisms that interfere with test results.

Immediate action

- Send the specimen to the laboratory immediately. If a liquid or soft stool specimen can't be examined within 30 minutes of passage, place some of it in a preservative; if a formed stool specimen can't be examined immediately, refrigerate it or place it in preservative.
- If the entire stool can't be sent to the laboratory, include macroscopic worms or worm segments as well as bloody and mucoid portions of the specimen.

Stay on the ball

Stool ova and parasite test interference

- Collection of too few specimens may cause false-negative results.
- Stools collected from a toilet bowl may contain organisms that interfere with results.

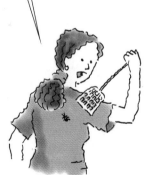

Get off of my back! Stool examination for ova and parasites can confirm or rule out intestinal parasitic infection.

Stool examination for rotavirus antigen

Rotavirus (previously referred to as *orbivirus, reovirus-like agent, duovirus,* and *gastroenteritis virus*) is the most frequent cause of infectious diarrhea in infants and young children.

Virus detection

Human rotaviruses don't replicate efficiently in the usual laboratory cell cultures. Therefore, detection of the typical virus particles in stool specimens by electron microscopy has been replaced by sensitive, specific enzyme immunoassays that can provide results within minutes or a few hours (depending on the assay) after the specimen is received in the laboratory.

What it all means

The detection of rotavirus by enzyme immunoassay is evidence of current infection with the organism. (See *Stool rotavirus antigen test interference.*)

What needs to be done

• Collect the specimens during the prodromal and acute stages of clinical infection to ensure detection of the viral antigens by enzyme immunoassay.
• A stool specimen (1 g in a screw-capped tube or vial) is preferred for detecting rotaviruses. If a microbiologic transport swab is used, it must be heavily stained with feces to be diagnostically productive for rotavirus.
• Avoid using collection containers with preservatives, metal ions, detergents, or serum, which may interfere with the assay.
• Store stool specimens for up to 24 hours at 35.6° to 46.4° F (2° to 8° C). If a longer period of storage or shipment is necessary, freeze the specimens at –4° F (–20° C) or colder.
• Don't store the specimen in a self-defrosting freezer.

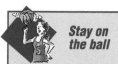

Stay on the ball

Stool rotavirus antigen test interference

Repeated freezing and thawing causes the specimen to deteriorate and yields misleading results.

Reproductive system

Amniotic fluid analysis

Amniocentesis is the transabdominal needle aspiration of 10 to 20 ml of amniotic fluid for laboratory analysis. Amniotic fluid reflects important metabolic changes in the fetus, the placenta, and the mother. Amniocentesis can be performed only when the amniotic fluid level reaches 150 ml, usually after week 16 of pregnancy. It's indicated when a pregnant woman is over age 35; has a family history of genetic, chromosomal, or neural tube defects; or has had a previous miscarriage. Rare complications from this test include spontaneous abortion, trauma to the fetus or placenta, bleeding, premature labor, infection, and Rh sensitization from fetal bleeding into the maternal circulation.

What it all means

Amniotic fluid should be clear but may contain white flecks of vernix caseosa when the fetus is near term. The amount of uric acid in the amniotic fluid increases as the fetus matures, but these levels fluctuate widely and can't accurately predict maturity. Laboratory studies indicate that severe erythroblastosis fetalis, familial hyperuricemia, and Lesch-Nyhan syndrome tend to increase the uric acid level.

Estrone, estradiol, estriol, and estriol conjugates appear in amniotic fluid in varying amounts. Levels of estriol, the most prevalent estrogen, increase substantially at term. Severe erythroblastosis fetalis decreases the estriol level.

Laboratory analysis can identify at least 25 different enzymes (usually in low concentrations) in amniotic fluid. The enzymes have few known clinical implications, although elevated acetylcholinesterase levels may occur with neural tube defects, exomphalos, and other serious malformations. (See *Amniotic fluid analysis findings*, page 236.)

Another method of detecting fetal chromosomal and biochemical disorders in early pregnancy is chorionic villi sampling, which can detect fetal abnormalities up to 10 weeks sooner than amniocentesis. (See *Chorionic villi sampling*, page 237, and *Amniotic fluid analysis interference*.)

What needs to be done

• Explain the procedure to the patient and ensure that an informed consent form has been signed.
• Instruct the patient to urinate just before the test to minimize the risk of puncturing the bladder. However, if the pregnancy is before 20 weeks' gestation, the bladder should be kept full to support the uterus.
• After determining fetal and placental position, usually through palpation and ultrasonography, a practitioner locates a pool of amniotic fluid. After preparing the skin with an antiseptic and alcohol, he injects 1 ml of 1% lidocaine with a 25G needle, first intradermally and then subcutaneously. Then he inserts the 20G to 22G

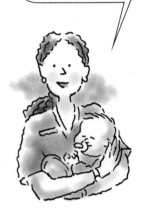

Amniotic fluid analysis detects fetal abnormalities, assesses fetal health, and can determine fetal age and maturity.

Stay on the ball

Amniotic fluid analysis interference

• Blood or meconium in the fluid adversely affects the lecithin-spingomyelin ratio.
• Maternal blood in the fluid may lower creatinine levels.
• Fetal blood in the fluid specimen invalidates alpha-fetoprotein results.

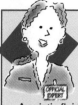

Advice from the experts

Amniotic fluid analysis findings

Amniotic fluid analysis can provide important information about the condition of the mother, fetus, and placenta. This table shows normal findings and abnormal findings and their implications.

Test component	Normal findings	Fetal implications of abnormal findings
Color	Clear, with white flecks of vernix caseosa in a mature fetus	Blood of maternal origin is usually harmless. "Port wine" fluid may indicate abruptio placentae. Fetal blood may indicate damage to the fetal, placental, or umbilical cord vessels.
Bilirubin	Early: < 0.075 mg/dl (SI, < 1.3 µmol/L) Term: < 0.025 mg/dl (SI, < 0.41 µmol/L)	High levels indicate hemolytic disease of the newborn.
Meconium	Absent (except in breach presentation)	Presence indicates fetal hypotension or distress.
Creatinine	More than 2 mg/dl (SI, 177 µmol/L) in a mature fetus	Decrease may indicate fetus at less than 37 weeks.
Lecithin-sphingomyelin ratio	≥ 2:1	Less than 2:1 indicates pulmonary immaturity.
Phosphatidylglycerol	Present	Absence indicates pulmonary immaturity.
Glucose	Less than 45 mg/dl (SI, 2.3 mmol/L)	Excessive increases at term or near term indicate hypertrophied fetal pancreas.
Alpha-fetoprotein	Variable, depending on gestation age and laboratory technique	Inappropriate increases indicate neural tube defects, such as spina bifida or anencephaly; impending fetal death; congenital nephrosis; or contamination of fetal blood.
Bacteria	Absent	Presence indicates chorioamnionitis.
Chromosome	Normal karyotype	Abnormal karyotype indicates fetal chromosome disorders.
Acetylcholinesterase	Absent	Presence may indicate neural tube defects, exomphalos, or other serious malformations.

spinal needle with a stylet into the amniotic cavity and withdraws the stylet. After attaching a 10-ml syringe to the needle, he aspirates the fluid and places it in an amber or foil-covered test tube.

Chorionic villi sampling

Chorionic villi sampling (CVS) is a prenatal test for quick detection of fetal chromosomal and biochemical disorders that's performed during the first trimester of pregnancy. Preliminary results may be available within hours; complete results within a few days. In contrast, amniocentesis can't be performed before week 16 of pregnancy, and the results aren't available for at least 2 weeks. Thus, CVS can detect fetal abnormalities up to 10 weeks sooner than amniocentesis.

Chorionic villi are fingerlike projections that surround the embryonic membrane and eventually give rise to the placenta. Cells obtained from samples are of fetal, rather than maternal, origin and thus can be analyzed for fetal abnormalities. Samples are best obtained between weeks 8 and 12 of pregnancy.

Procedure

To collect a chorionic villi sample, place the patient in the lithotomy position. The practitioner checks the placement of the uterus bimanually, inserts a sterile speculum, and swabs the cervix with an antiseptic solution. If necessary, he may use a tenaculum to straighten an acutely flexed uterus, permitting cannula insertion. Guided by ultrasound, he directs the catheter through the cannula to the villi. He applies suction to the catheter to remove three or more tissue specimens from the villi. Then he withdraws the specimen, places it in a Petri dish, and examines it with a microscope. Part of the specimen is cultured for further testing.

Complications

Possible complications are similar to those for amniocentesis: a small risk of spontaneous abortion, cramps, infection, and bleeding. Studies have found limb malformations in neonates whose mothers underwent CVS.

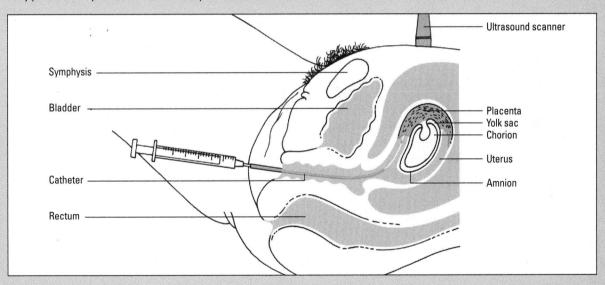

Labels: Symphysis, Bladder, Catheter, Rectum, Ultrasound scanner, Placenta, Yolk sac, Chorion, Uterus, Amnion

After the needle is withdrawn, an adhesive bandage is placed over the needle insertion site.

During the test

- Monitor fetal heart rate and maternal vital signs every 15 minutes for at least 30 minutes.

• If the patient feels faint or nauseated or perspires profusely, position her on the left side to counteract uterine pressure on the vena cava.

After the test

• Before the patient is discharged, instruct her to notify the practitioner immediately if she experiences abdominal pain or cramping, chills, fever, vaginal bleeding or leakage of serous vaginal fluid, or fetal hyperactivity or unusual fetal lethargy.
• Send the specimen to the laboratory immediately.

Papanicolaou test

The Papanicolaou (Pap) test is a cytologic test of the cervix. To perform this test, a practitioner or a specially trained nurse scrapes cells from the patient's cervix and spreads them on a slide. The slide is immersed in a fixative and sent to the laboratory for cytologic analysis.

What it all means

No malignant cells or abnormalities are present in a normal specimen. (See *Pap test interference*.)

Grading the Pap

A Pap smear may be graded in different ways, so check your laboratory's reporting format. In the Bethesda System—the current standardized method—potentially premalignant squamous lesions fall into three categories: atypical squamous cells of undetermined significance, low-grade squamous intraepithelial lesions, and high-grade squamous intraepithelial lesions. The low-grade category includes mild dysplasia and the changes of the human papillomavirus. The high-grade category includes moderate to severe dysplasia and carcinoma in situ.

To confirm a suggestive or positive cytology report, the test may be repeated, followed by a biopsy, or both. (See *ThinPrep for greater accuracy*.)

What needs to be done

• Instruct the patient to avoid having intercourse for 24 hours, douching for 48 hours, and using vaginal creams or drugs for 1 week.
• Just before the test, instruct the patient to empty her bladder. During the procedure, she may experience slight discomfort but no pain from the speculum; however, she may feel some pain

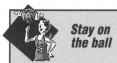

Pap test interference

Exclusive use of a specimen collected from the vaginal fornix and collection during menstruation may alter results.

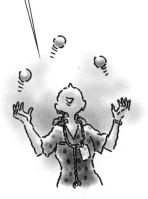

Versatility is a virtue! The Pap test can detect malignant cells, assess inflammatory tissue changes, assess response to chemotherapy and radiation therapy, and detect viral, fungal, and parasitic invasion.

Now I get it!

ThinPrep for greater accuracy

ThinPrep is collected in the same manner as a Papanicolaou (Pap) test using a cytobrush and plastic spatula. Specimens are deposited in a bottle provided with a fixative and sent to a specialized laboratory. A filter is then inserted into the bottle and excess mucus, blood, and inflammatory cells are filtered out by centrifuge. Remaining cells are then placed on a slide in a uniform, thin layer and read as a Pap test. This causes fewer slides to be classified as unreadable, significantly reducing the incidence of false negatives and the need for repeat tests.

when the cervix is scraped. Explain that the procedure takes only 5 to 10 minutes to perform.
• Instruct the patient to disrobe from the waist down and to drape herself. Ask her to lie on the examination table and to place her heels in the stirrups. Tell her to slide her buttocks to the edge of the table.

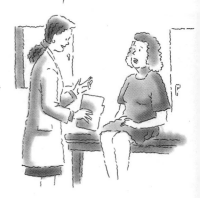

The Pap test shouldn't be scheduled during your menstrual period. The best time to test is midcycle.

The examiner's role

• The examiner puts on gloves and inserts an unlubricated speculum into the vagina. To make insertion easier, he may moisten the speculum with warm water.
• The examiner collects secretions from the cervix and material from the endocervical canal. Then he spreads the specimen on the slide, according to laboratory policy, and immediately immerses the slide in a fixative or sprays it with fixative.

Actions after collection

• Label the specimen appropriately. A bimanual examination may follow removal of the speculum.
• If cervical bleeding occurs, give the patient a sanitary napkin.
• Examine the consistency of the specimen. It should be just thick enough that it isn't transparent. A specimen that's too thin will dry and leave too few cells for adequate screening; if it's too thick, the stain won't penetrate.
• If vaginal or vulval lesions are present, scrapings taken directly from the lesion are preferred.
• In a patient whose uterus is involuting or atrophying from age, use a small pipette, if necessary, to aspirate cells from the squamocolumnar junction and the cervical canal. Use two slides to reduce air-drying artifact.

Semen analysis

Inexpensive, technically simple, and reasonably definitive, semen analysis is usually the first test performed on a male to evaluate fertility.

Volume, motility, morphology

The procedure for analyzing semen for infertility usually includes measuring the volume of seminal fluid, assessing the sperm count, and examining the specimen under a microscope. Sperm are counted in much the same way that red and white blood cells and platelets are counted on an anticoagulated blood sample. Staining and microscopic examination of a drop of semen permits the sperms' motility and morphology to be evaluated.

Some laboratories offer specialized semen tests such as screening for antibodies to spermatozoa.

What it all means

Semen volume normally ranges from 0.7 to 6.5 ml. Liquefied semen is generally highly viscid, translucent, and gray-white, with a musty or acrid odor. After liquefaction, specimens of normal viscosity can be poured in drops. Normally, semen is slightly alkaline, with a pH of 7.3 to 7.9. Other normal characteristics of semen include immediate coagulation and liquefaction within 20 minutes. Normal sperm count ranges from 20 to 150 million/ml, and can be greater; at least 40% of spermatozoa have normal morphology, and at least 20% of spermatozoa show progressive motility within 4 hours of collection.

The normal postcoital cervical mucus test shows 10 to 20 motile spermatozoa per microscopic high-power field and spinnbarkeit (a measure of the tenacity of the mucus) of at least 4″ (10 cm). These findings indicate adequate spermatozoa and receptivity of the cervical mucus. Shaking or dead sperm may indicate antisperm antibodies.

Abnormal findings

Abnormal semen isn't synonymous with infertility. Although a normal sperm count is more than 20 million/ml or more, many males with sperm counts below 1 million/ml have fathered normal children. Only males who can't deliver any viable spermatozoa in their ejaculate during sexual intercourse are absolutely sterile. Nevertheless, subnormal sperm counts, decreased sperm motility, and abnormal morphology are usually associated with decreased fertility. (See *Semen analysis test interference.*)

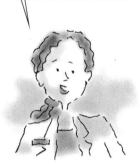

Semen analysis can evaluate male fertility, determine the effectiveness of vasectomy and, in rare cases, rule out paternity on grounds of complete sterility.

Stay on the ball

Semen analysis test interference

• Cigarette smoking, testicular radiation, and certain drugs such as cannabis, cimetidine, cocaine, ketoconazole, sulfasalazine, and vincristine may decrease sperm counts.
• Failure to keep the specimen warm may alter results.

Obtaining semen from a rape victim

When collecting a semen specimen from a rape victim, follow these guidelines:
• Inform the patient that the practitioner will try to obtain a semen specimen from her vagina. Encourage her to express her fears and anxieties, and listen sympathetically. Prepare her for speculum insertion. If she's scheduled for vaginal lavage, tell her to expect a cold sensation when saline solution is instilled to wash out the specimen.
• During the test, she should breathe deeply and slowly through her mouth.
• Handle the patient's clothes as little as possible. If her clothes are moist, put them in a paper bag—not a plastic bag, which causes seminal stains and secretions to mold. Label the bag properly and send it to the laboratory immediately.
• Be aware that the practitioner obtains a specimen from the vagina by direct aspiration, saline lavage, or a direct smear of vaginal contents, using a Papanicolaou stick or, less desirably, a cotton-tipped applicator. Dried smears are usually collected from the skin by gently washing with gauze moistened with physiologic saline solution. Before a postcoital examination, the examiner wipes excess mucus from the external cervix and collects the specimen by direct aspiration of the cervical canal.

Legal precautions

Prepare direct smears on glass microscopic slides after labeling the frosted end. Immediately place the slides in Coplin jars containing 95% ethanol. Use extreme caution in securing, labeling, and delivering specimens to be used for medicolegal purposes. If your facility uses routing slips for such specimens, fill them out carefully, and place them in the permanent medicolegal file.

What needs to be done

• Preparation for semen analysis varies with the test purpose. The following steps refer to fertility evaluation. (For instructions on collecting a semen specimen from a rape victim, see *Obtaining semen from a rape victim*.)

Fertility evaluation

• In most cases, it's helpful to provide written instructions for specimen collection. Inform the patient that the most desirable specimen requires masturbation, ideally in an office or a laboratory.
• The semen should be collected in a clean, plastic specimen container. Instruct the patient to follow orders regarding the period of sexual continence before the test as this may increase his sperm count.
• If the patient prefers to collect the specimen at home, he should deliver the specimen to the laboratory within 1 hour after collection. Warn him not to expose it to extreme temperatures or direct sunlight, which can also increase its temperature. Ideally, it should remain at body temperature until liquefaction is complete (about

20 minutes). If the weather is cold, instruct him to keep the specimen container in a coat pocket to protect it from the cold.

• Alternatives to collection by masturbation include coitus interruptus or the use of a condom or special sheath. For collection by coitus interruptus, instruct the patient to withdraw immediately before ejaculation and to deposit the ejaculate in a suitable specimen container.

• For collection by condom, tell the patient to wash the condom with soap and water, rinse it thoroughly, and allow it to dry completely. (Powders or lubricants applied to the condom may be spermicidal.) Special sheaths that don't contain spermicides are also available for semen collection. After collection, instruct the patient to tie the condom, place it in a glass jar, and deliver it to the laboratory promptly.

• Fertility may also be determined by collecting semen from the woman after coitus (about 2 to 8 hours afterward) to assess the ability of the spermatozoa to penetrate the cervical mucus and remain active. This test to collect semen is done in the office while the woman is in a lithotomy position. The specimen is collected using a 1-ml tuberculin syringe without a cannula or needle.

• All specimens should be delivered to the laboratory promptly and protected from extremes of temperature and direct sunlight.

Miscellaneous specimen tests

Cerebrospinal fluid analysis

CSF, a clear substance that circulates in the subarachnoid space, has many vital functions. It protects the brain and spinal cord from injury and transports products of neurosecretion, cellular biosynthesis, and cellular metabolism through the central nervous system.

Obtaining by puncture

For qualitative analysis, CSF is most commonly obtained by lumbar puncture, usually between the third and fourth lumbar vertebrae; in rare instances, it's obtained by cisternal or ventricular puncture. Specimens of CSF for laboratory analysis are commonly obtained during other neurologic tests such as myelography.

What it all means

Normally, the practitioner records CSF pressure and checks the appearance of the specimen. Three tubes are routinely collected

> CSF analysis measures CSF pressure and circulation; helps diagnose meningitis, brain hemorrhages, tumors, and abscesses; and can be used in the diagnosis of Alzheimer's disease.

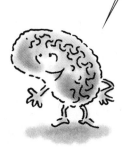

Xpert EV virus test

The Xpert EV test uses molecular biology to help distinguish between viral and bacterial meningitis. Test results are available within 2 hours when compared to regular testing, which could take a few days to a week for results. The fully automated test isolates viral genetic material in cerebrospinal fluid (CSF) using reverse transcription-polymerase chain reaction. It helps identify viruses responsible for about 90% of all viral meningitis cases. This helps minimize delay in treatment as well as prevent unnecessary treatment with antibiotics.

A sample of CSF is added directly to a disposable cartridge and placed into a patented instrument for testing (the GeneXpert DX instrument). In trials, the Xpert EV test correctly identified 96% of patients with viral meningitis. The test is considered valuable when used along with other tests currently available, as it isn't 100% sensitive or 100% specific.

Stay on the ball

CSF analysis interference

- Patient position and activity can alter cerebrospinal fluid (CSF) pressure.
- Crying, coughing, or straining may increase pressure.
- Delay between collection time and laboratory testing may alter results.

and sent to the laboratory for analysis of protein, glucose, RBC and WBC counts as well as for serologic testing, such as the Venereal Disease Research Laboratory test for neurosyphilis. A separate specimen is also sent to the laboratory for culture and sensitivity testing. Electrolyte analysis and Gram stain may be ordered as supplementary tests. (See *Xpert EV virus test*.)

CSF electrolyte levels are of special interest in patients with abnormal serum electrolyte levels or CSF infection and in those receiving hyperosmolar agents. (For the implications of abnormal CSF analysis findings, see *Interpreting CSF analysis findings*, page 244, and *CSF analysis interference*.)

What needs to be done

- Tell the patient this test usually takes at least 15 minutes. Make sure that the patient or a responsible family member has signed an informed consent form.
- Inform the patient that a headache is the most common adverse effect of lumbar puncture, but reassure him that his cooperation during the test helps minimize this reaction.

Assume the position

- Position the patient on his side at the edge of the bed with his knees drawn up to his abdomen and his chin tucked against his chest (fetal position). Provide pillows to support the spine on a horizontal plane. This position allows easy access to the lumbar subarachnoid space. If a sitting position is preferred, have the pa-

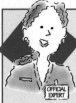

Advice from the experts

Interpreting CSF analysis findings

Obtaining a cerebrospinal fluid (CSF) specimen and interpreting the results helps diagnose various conditions. This table shows normal CSF findings as well as abnormal findings and their implications.

Test	Normal	Abnormal	Implications
Pressure	50 to 180 mm H_2O	Increase	Increased intracranial pressure
		Decrease	Spinal subarachnoid obstruction above puncture site
Appearance	Clear, colorless	Cloudy	Infection
		Xanthochromic or bloody	Subarachnoid, intracerebral, or intraventricular hemorrhage; spinal cord obstruction; traumatic lumbar puncture (usually only in initial specimen)
		Brown, orange	Elevated protein levels, red blood cell (RBC) breakdown (blood present for at least 3 days)
Protein	15 to 50 mg/dl (SI, 0.15 to 0.5 q/L)	Marked increase	Tumors, trauma, hemorrhage, diabetes mellitus, polyneuritis, blood in CSF
		Marked decrease	Rapid CSF production
Gamma globulin	3% to 12% of total protein	Increase	Demyelinating disease, neurosyphilis, Guillain-Barré syndrome
Glucose	50 to 80 mg/dl (SI, 2.8 to 4.4 mmol/L)	Increase	Systemic hyperglycemia
		Decrease	Systemic hypoglycemia, bacterial or fungal infection, meningitis, mumps, postsubarachnoid hemorrhage
Cell count	0 to 5 white blood cells; no RBCs	Increase	Active disease: meningitis, acute infection, onset of chronic illness, tumor, abscess, infarction, demyelinating disease
	No RBCs	RBCs	Hemorrhage or traumatic lumbar puncture
VDRL test for syphilis and other serologic tests	Negative	Positive	Neurosyphilis
Chloride	118 to 130 mEq/L (SI, 118 to 130 mmol/L)	Decrease	Infected meninges
Gram stain	No organisms	Gram-positive or gram-negative organisms	Bacterial meningitis

tient sit up and bend his chest and head toward his knees. Help him maintain this position throughout the procedure.

Puncture, pain...

- After the skin is prepared for injection, the area is draped. Instruct the patient to remain still and breathe normally; movement and hyperventilation can alter pressure readings or cause injury.
- The anesthetic is injected, and the spinal needle is inserted in the midline between the spinous vertebral processes, usually between the third and fourth lumbar vertebrae. When the stylet is removed from the needle, CSF drips from it if the needle is properly positioned. A stopcock and manometer are attached to the needle to measure initial (opening) CSF pressure.

...and postpunctural procedures

- After the specimen is collected, label the containers in the order in which they were filled and record specific instructions for the laboratory. A final pressure reading is taken, and the needle is removed. Clean the puncture site with an antiseptic solution, and apply a small adhesive bandage. Send the form and labeled specimens to the laboratory immediately.

Resting reminders

- In most cases, you'll be instructed to keep the patient lying flat for 8 hours after lumbar puncture, but some allow a 30-degree elevation. Encourage him to drink fluids.

Red alert

- Check the puncture site for redness, swelling, and drainage every hour for the first 4 hours, then every 4 hours for the next 24 hours. Watch for complications, such as a reaction to the anesthetic, meningitis, bleeding into the spinal canal, and cerebellar tonsillar herniation and medullary compression. Observe closely for signs of an adverse reaction, such as elevated pulse rate, pallor, or clammy skin. Alert the practitioner immediately to significant changes.
- Infection at the puncture site contraindicates removal of CSF; in a patient with increased intracranial pressure, CSF should be removed with extreme caution because the rapid reduction in pressure that follows withdrawal of fluid can cause cerebellar tonsillar herniation and medullary compression.

In case of elevation

- If CSF pressure is elevated, assess neurologic status every 15 minutes for 4 hours. If the patient is stable, assess every hour for 2 hours, then every 4 hours or according to the pretest schedule.

Pericardial fluid analysis

Pericardial fluid analysis involves the needle aspiration—pericardiocentesis—and analysis of pericardial fluid. Both therapeutic and diagnostic, it's most useful as an emergency measure to relieve cardiac tamponade. It can also provide a fluid sample to confirm and identify the cause of pericardial effusion (excess pericardial fluid).

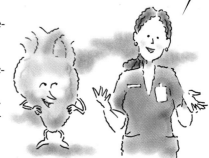

Pericardial fluid analysis helps identify the cause of pericardial effusion and helps determine appropriate therapy.

Possible complications

Pericardiocentesis should be performed cautiously because of the risk of potentially fatal complications, such as laceration of a coronary artery or the myocardium; other possible complications include ventricular fibrillation or vasovagal arrest, pleural infection, and accidental puncture of the lung, liver, or stomach. To minimize the risk of complications, echocardiography should precede pericardiocentesis to determine the effusion site. Generally, surgical drainage and biopsy are safer than pericardiocentesis.

What it all means

The pericardium normally contains 10 to 50 ml of sterile fluid. Pericardial fluid is clear and straw-colored, without evidence of pathogens, blood, or malignant cells. The WBC count in the fluid is usually less than 1,000/µl (SI, less than 1×10^9/L). Its glucose concentration should approximate the glucose levels in whole blood.

Transudates and exudates

Pericardial effusions are typically classified as transudates or exudates. Transudates are protein-poor effusions that usually arise from mechanical factors altering fluid formation or resorption, such as increased hydrostatic pressure, decreased plasma oncotic pressure, or obstruction of the pericardial lymphatic drainage system by a tumor.

Most exudates result from inflammation and contain large amounts of protein. Inflammation damages the capillary membrane, allowing protein molecules to leak into the pericardial fluid. Exudate effusions occur in pericarditis, neoplasms, acute myocardial infarction, tuberculosis, rheumatoid disease, and systemic lupus erythematosus. Turbid or milky effusions may result from lymph or pus accumulation in the pericardial sac or from tuberculosis or rheumatoid disease. Bloody pericardial fluid may indicate hemopericardium, hemorrhagic pericarditis, or a traumatic tap. Hemorrhagic effusions may indicate a malignant tumor, closed chest trauma, Dressler's syndrome, or postcardiotomy syndrome. (See *Pericardial fluid analysis interference*.)

What needs to be done

• Check the patient's history for current use of antimicrobial drugs and make sure an informed consent form has been signed. Let him know that the test takes 10 to 20 minutes and he need not restrict food or fluids.

• Explain the procedure to the patient. Inform him that an I.V. line will be started and he'll receive I.V. sedation as ordered.

• Place the patient in a supine position with the thorax elevated 60 degrees and tell him to remain still during the procedure. After the skin is prepared, a local anesthetic is administered at the insertion site.

Stay on the ball

Pericardial fluid analysis interference

Antimicrobial therapy can prevent isolation of the causative organism.

How it's done

• With the three-way stopcock open, a 50-ml syringe is attached to one end and the cardiac needle to the other. The patient is connected to the monitor, which is set to read lead V_1. (Make sure resuscitation equipment is nearby.) The needle is inserted through the chest wall into the pericardial sac, maintaining gentle aspiration until fluid appears in the syringe. The needle is angled 35 to 45 degrees toward the tip of the right scapula between the left costal margin and the xiphoid process.

• When the needle is properly positioned, a Kelly clamp is attached at the skin surface so the needle won't advance further. During aspiration, fluid specimen tubes are labeled and numbered. When the needle is withdrawn, pressure is applied to the site *immediately* with sterile gauze pads for 3 to 5 minutes. Then a bandage is applied. (See *Aspirating pericardial fluid*, page 248.)

• Watch for grossly bloody aspirate—a sign of inadvertent puncture of a cardiac chamber.

Fill 'er up! By the end of this test, I'll be filled with pericardial fluid.

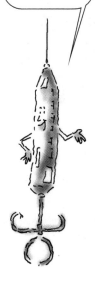

On alert

• Check vital signs and heart sounds every 15 minutes until stable, then every half hour for 2 hours, every hour for 4 hours, and every 4 hours thereafter.

• Be alert for respiratory or cardiac distress. Watch especially for signs of cardiac tamponade.

Collection technique

• Clean the top of the culture and sensitivity tube with an antiseptic solution to reduce the risk of extrinsic contamination.

• If bacterial culture and sensitivity tests are scheduled, record on the laboratory request any antimicrobial drugs the patient is re-

Aspirating pericardial fluid

In pericardiocentesis, a needle and syringe assembly is inserted through the chest wall into the pericardial sac (as illustrated below). Electrocardiographic (ECG) monitoring, with a leadwire attached to the needle and electrodes placed on the limbs (right arm [RA], right leg [RL], left arm [LA], and left leg [LL]), helps ensure proper needle placement and avoids damage to the heart.

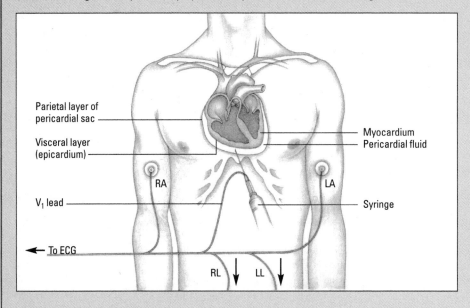

ceiving. If anaerobic organisms are suspected, consult the laboratory about proper collection technique to avoid exposing the aspirate to air.
• Send all specimens to the laboratory immediately.

Sweat test

The sweat test quantitatively measures electrolyte concentrations—primarily sodium and chloride—in sweat, usually through pilocarpine iontophoresis (pilocarpine is a sweat inducer). This test is used almost exclusively in children to confirm cystic fibrosis (CF); it's also performed in adults to determine if they're homozygous or heterozygous for CF.

What it all means

Normal sodium values in sweat range from 10 to 30 mEq/L (SI, 10 to 30 mmol/L). Normal chloride values range from 10 to 35 mEq/L

(SI, 10 to 35 mmol/L). In women, sweat electrolyte levels fluctuate cyclically; chloride levels usually peak 5 to 10 days before onset of menses, and most women retain fluid before menses. Men also show fluctuations up to 70 mEq/L (SI, 70 mmol/L).

Abnormal findings

Sodium levels of 50 to 60 mEq/L (SI, 50 to 60 mmol/L) strongly suggest CF. Concentrations above 60 mEq/L (SI, greater than 60 mmol/L) with typical clinical features confirm the diagnosis. Only a few conditions other than CF cause elevated sweat electrolyte levels—most notably, untreated adrenal insufficiency as well as type I glycogen storage disease, vasopressin-resistant diabetes insipidus, meconium ileus, and renal failure. However, only CF raises sweat electrolyte levels above 80 mEq/L (SI, above 80 mmol/L). (See *Sweat test interference.*)

What needs to be done

• Tell the patient he may feel a slight tickling sensation but won't feel pain. Stay with him during the test to help minimize anxiety.
• With distilled water, wash the test area; then dry it. The flexor surface of the right forearm is commonly used; if the patient's arm is too small to secure electrodes, the right thigh is used. Never perform iontophoresis on the chest, especially in a child, because the current can induce cardiac arrest.
• Place a gauze pad saturated with premeasured pilocarpine solution on the positive electrode; place a gauze pad saturated with normal saline solution on the negative electrode. Apply both electrodes to the area to be tested and secure them with straps.

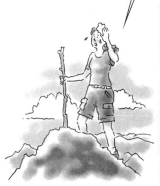

The sweat test confirms CF.

Electro-precautions

• Leadwires to the analyzer are given a current of 4 mA in 15 to 20 seconds. This process (iontophoresis) is continued at 15- to 20-second intervals for 5 minutes. After iontophoresis, remove both electrodes. Discard the pads, clean the patient's skin with distilled water, and then dry it. (Always perform iontophoresis on the right arm or right thigh.)

Halt!

• Stop the test immediately if the patient complains of a burning sensation, which usually indicates that the positive electrode is exposed or positioned improperly. Adjust the electrode and then continue the test.

Sweat collection

- Using forceps, place a dry gauze pad or filter paper (previously weighed on a gram scale) on the area where the pilocarpine was used. Cover the pad or filter paper with a slightly larger piece of plastic and seal the edges of the plastic with waterproof adhesive tape. Leave the gauze pad or filter paper in place for about 30 to 40 minutes. Make sure that at least 100 mg of sweat is collected for analysis. (Droplets on the plastic usually indicate induction of an adequate amount of sweat.)
- Remove the pad or filter paper with the forceps, place it immediately in the weighing bottle, and insert the stopper in the bottle. Send the bottle to the laboratory immediately. The difference between the first and second weights indicates the weight of the sweat specimen collected.

After collection

- Wash the tested area with soap and water and dry it thoroughly.
- If the area looks red, reassure the patient that this is normal and that the redness will disappear within a few hours.
- Tell the patient he may resume his usual activities.

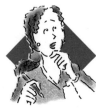

Quick quiz

1. Which symptoms are adverse effects of gastric acid stimulation testing?

　　A.　Tachycardia, cyanosis, and chest pain
　　B.　Abdominal pain, nausea, and dizziness
　　C.　Fever, tachycardia, and sudden breathlessness
　　D.　Bradycardia, flushing and shortness of breath

Answer: B. Adverse effects of gastric acid stimulation testing include abdominal pain, nausea, dizziness, and numbness of the extremities. Report these findings immediately.

2. When preparing a patient for fecal occult blood testing, you should instruct him to refrain from consuming which foods for 48 to 72 hours before testing?

　　A.　Horseradish, turnips, fish, and red meat
　　B.　Alcohol, high-fiber foods, and high-sodium foods
　　C.　High-fat foods, alcohol, and foods containing vanilla
　　D.　High-sugar foods, high-fiber foods, and high-potassium foods

Answer: A. The patient should maintain a high-fiber diet and refrain from eating red meat, poultry, fish, turnips, and horseradish for 48 to 72 hours before the fecal occult blood test and throughout the collection period.

3. Amniocentesis can be performed only when the amniotic fluid level reaches 150 ml. This typically occurs after which week of gestation?

    A.   6
    B.   12
    C.   16
    D.   24

Answer: C. Amniocentesis can be performed only when the amniotic fluid level reaches 150 ml, usually after week 16 of pregnancy.

4. Which factor may alter Pap test results?

    A.   Douching within 72 hours of the test
    B.   Collecting the specimen immediately after menstruation
    C.   Having intercourse within 24 hours of the test
    D.   Taking a shower before the test

Answer: C. Douching within 48 hours or having intercourse within 24 hours of a Pap test can wash away cellular deposits, altering results.

5. Which disorder does a sweat test confirm?

    A.   Renal failure
    B.   Hyperkalemia
    C.   Hypothyroidism
    D.   Cystic fibrosis

Answer: D. A sweat test is used almost exclusively in children to confirm cystic fibrosis.

6. A pleural fluid analysis that reveals predominantly lymphocytes most likely suggests:

    A.   septic inflammation.
    B.   tuberculosis.
    C.   tumor extension.
    D.   malignancy.

Answer: B. A pleural fluid analysis that reveals predominantly lymphocytes suggests tuberculosis or viral or fungal effusions.

Scoring

☆☆☆ If you answered all six questions correctly, superb! You're one heck of a specimen!

☆☆ If you answered four or five questions correctly, terrific! You're testing your way to perfection!

☆ If you answered fewer than four questions correctly, don't worry! Your specimen-collecting skills will be perfect in no time!

Cultures

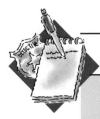

Just the facts

In this chapter, you'll learn:

♦ about cultures

♦ what patient care is associated with cultures

♦ what factors can interfere with these tests

♦ what culture results may indicate.

A look at cultures

Cultures are performed to isolate organisms and determine the cause of infection. Each culture requires its own specimen collection technique. Explain the procedure to the patient to ensure proper collection and avoid inadvertent specimen contamination.

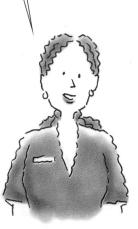

A urine culture diagnoses UTI and monitors microorganism colonization after urinary catheter insertion.

Urine cultures

Although urine in the kidneys and bladder is normally sterile, a small number of bacteria are usually present in the urethra and, consequently, may pass into the urine. A single negative culture doesn't always rule out infection; some infections, such as chronic low-grade pyelonephritis, may go undetected this way.

Colony count

Significant results of urine culture are possible only after quantitative examination. To distinguish between true bacteriuria and contamination, it's necessary to know the number of organisms in a milliliter of urine, estimated by a culture technique known as a *colony count*. In addition, a quick centrifugation test can determine where a urinary tract infection (UTI) originates. (See *Quick centrifugation test*, page 254.)

Clean-voided midstream collection is the method of choice for obtaining a urine specimen.

What it all means

Culture results of sterile urine are normally reported as "no growth," which usually indicates the absence of UTI.

Overpopulation problem

Bacterial counts of 100,000 or more organisms of a single microbe species per milliliter indicate probable UTI. Counts under 100,000/ml may be significant, depending on the patient's age, sex, history, and other individual factors. All growths from catheterized urine or suprapubic aspirations are considered significant and are investigated by using susceptibility tests to identify the causative organism. Isolation of more than two species of organisms or of vaginal or skin organisms usually suggests contamination and requires a repeat culture. Urine cultures also identify pathogenic fungi. (See *Urine culture test interference.*)

What needs to be done

• Check the patient's history for current use of antimicrobial drugs. Explain to the patient that this test requires the collection of a clean-voided urine specimen. (See *Collecting a clean-voided urine specimen.*)
• Collect a urine specimen as ordered.
• When obtaining a specimen from an indwelling urinary catheter, clamp the tubing below the collection port to collect a specimen in the tubing. Then use an alcohol pad to clean the port. Using a sterile needle and syringe, aspirate a 4-ml specimen from the port and transfer it into a sterile specimen cup. Remember to unclamp the catheter when you're finished with the procedure.
• Record current antimicrobial therapy and fluid- or drug-induced diuresis on the laboratory request.
• Seal the cup with a sterile lid and send it to the laboratory at once.

Now I get it!

Quick centrifugation test

The quick centrifugation test can determine whether the source of a urinary tract infection (UTI) is in the lower tract (bladder) or the upper tract (kidneys). The test involves urine centrifugation in a test tube, followed by staining of the sediment with fluorescein. If at least one-fourth of the bacteria fluoresce when viewed under a fluorescent microscope, an upper tract UTI is present; lack of fluorescence means a lower tract UTI.

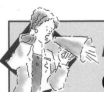

Listen up!

Collecting a clean-voided urine specimen

To teach a patient how to collect a clean-catch midstream urine specimen, tell him to:
• clean the periurethral area with antiseptic towelettes
• after cleaning, begin voiding in the toilet
• then stop and continue to urinate into the sterile cup, without touching the inside of the cup.

Stay on the ball

Urine culture test interference

Fluid- or drug-induced diuresis and antimicrobial therapy may alter the results.

• If transport is delayed for more than 30 minutes, store the specimen at 39.2° F (4° C) or place it on ice, unless a urine transport tube containing preservative is used.

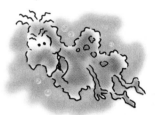

A stool culture identifies pathogenic organisms causing GI disease, detects viruses, and identifies carrier states.

Stool culture

Normally, feces contain many species of bacterial flora and several potentially pathogenic organisms. Identifying these organisms is vital to treatment to prevent possibly fatal complications (especially in a debilitated patient), and to confine these severe infectious diseases. A sensitivity test may follow pathogen isolation.

Stool culture may also detect viruses, such as enterovirus, which can cause aseptic meningitis.

What it all means

More than 95% of normal fecal flora consist of anaerobes, including non-spore-forming bacilli, clostridia, and anaerobic streptococci. The remainder consist of aerobes, including gram-negative bacilli (predominantly *Escherichia coli* and other *Enterobacteriaceae*, plus small amounts of *Pseudomonas*), gram-positive cocci (mostly enterococci), and a few yeasts.

Abnormal findings

Isolation of some pathogens indicates bacterial infection or other disorders. (See *Pathogens of the GI tract*, page 256.)

If a stool culture shows no unusual growth, detection of viruses by immunoassay or electron microscopy may diagnose nonbacterial gastroenteritis. (See *Stool culture test interference*.)

What needs to be done

• Check the patient's history for dietary patterns, recent antimicrobial therapy, exposure to lake or river water, and recent travel that might suggest an endemic infection or infestation.
• Collect the specimen before antimicrobial therapy is started.
• Explain to the patient that this test may require the collection of a stool specimen on three consecutive days.
• Collect a stool specimen directly in the container. If the patient isn't ambulatory, collect it in a clean, dry bedpan. Using a tongue blade, transfer the specimen to the container. If the specimen is collected by rectal swab, insert the swab past the anal sphincter, rotate it gently, and withdraw it. Then place the swab in the appropriate container.
• Use gloves when handling the specimen; put the specimen container in a leakproof bag.

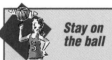

Stay on the ball

Stool culture test interference

Antimicrobial therapy may decrease bacterial growth in the specimen. Contamination of the specimen by urine causes possible injury to or destruction of enteric pathogens. Recent barium studies may cause interference in detecting parasites.

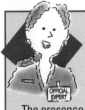

Advice from the experts

Pathogens of the GI tract

The presence of these pathogens in a stool culture may indicate certain disorders:
• *Aeromonas hydrophila:* gastroenteritis, which causes diarrhea, especially in children
• *Campylobacter jejuni:* gastroenteritis
• *Clostridium botulinum:* food poisoning and infant botulism (a possible cause of sudden infant death syndrome)
• Toxin-producing *Clostridium difficile:* pseudomembranous enterocolitis
• *Clostridium perfringens:* food poisoning
• Enterotoxigenic *Escherichia coli:* gastroenteritis (resembles cholera or shigellosis)
• *Salmonella:* gastroenteritis, typhoid fever, nontyphoidal salmonellosis, paratyphoid fever, enteric fever
• *Shigella:* shigellosis, bacillary dysentery
• *Staphylococcus aureus:* food poisoning, suppression of normal bowel flora from antimicrobial therapy
• *Vibrio cholerae:* cholera
• *V. parahaemolyticus:* food poisoning, especially seafood
• *Yersinia enterocolitica:* gastroenteritis, enterocolitis (resembles appendicitis), mesenteric lymphadenitis, ileitis.

• Check with the laboratory for the collection procedure for a virus test.
• Send the specimen to the laboratory immediately; be sure to include mucoid and bloody portions and always represent the first, middle, and last portion of the feces passed. If a specimen can't be transported to the laboratory within 1 hour, refrigerate it or place it in transport media.
• Indicate the suspected cause of the patient's GI disorder and his current antimicrobial therapy on the laboratory request.

Throat culture

A throat culture requires swabbing the throat, streaking a culture plate, and allowing the organisms to grow to enable isolation and identification of pathogens. A Gram-stained smear may provide preliminary identification, which may guide clinical management and determine the need for further tests. Culture results must be interpreted in light of clinical status, recent antimicrobial therapy, and the amount of normal flora.

What it all means

Throat flora normally include nonhemolytic and alpha-hemolytic streptococci, *Neisseria* species, staphylococci, diptheroids, some *Haemophilus* species, pneumococci, yeasts, enteric gram-negative organisms, spirochetes, *Veillonella* species, and *Micrococcus* species.

Abnormal findings

Possible pathogens cultured include group A beta-hemolytic streptococci (*Streptococcus pyogenes*), which can cause scarlet fever or pharyngitis; *Candida albicans*, which can cause thrush; *Corynebacterium diphtheriae*, which can cause diphtheria; and *Bordetella* pertussis, which can cause whooping cough. Other cultured bacteria include *Legionella* species, *Mycoplasma pneumoniae*, *Staphylococcus aureus*, *Streptococcus pneumoniae*, and *H. influenzae*. It's also used to screen for carriers of *N. meningitidis*. Fungi include *Histoplasma capsulatum*, *Coccidioides immitis*, and *Blastomyces dermatitidis*. Viruses include adenovirus, enterovirus, herpesvirus, rhinovirus, influenza virus, and parainfluenza virus. (See *Throat culture test interference*.)

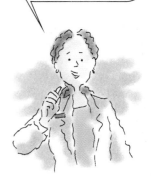

Throat cultures isolate and identify pathogens, particularly group A beta-hemolytic streptococci, and screen asymptomatic carriers of pathogens, especially *Neisseria meningitidis*.

What needs to be done

• Check for a recent history of antimicrobial therapy, and obtain the throat specimen before beginning antimicrobial therapy.
• Explain to the patient that this test helps identify the microorganisms and takes about 30 seconds. Tell him he may gag during swabbing.
• Use gloves when performing the procedure and handling specimens.
• Have the patient tilt his head back and close his eyes. With the throat well illuminated, check for inflamed areas, using a tongue blade.

Swab the deck

• Swab the tonsillar areas from side to side; include inflamed or purulent sites. Don't touch the tongue, cheeks, or teeth with the swab.
• Immediately place the swab in the culture tube. If a commercial sterile collection and transport system is used, crush the ampule and force the swab into the medium to keep it moist. In addition to the traditional throat culture, a rapid strep test may be done which provides faster results (See *Rapid strep test*, page 258.)

Special delivery

• Note recent antimicrobial therapy on the laboratory request. Also indicate the suspected organism.

Stay on the ball

Throat culture test interference

Failure to report recent or current antimicrobial therapy may alter test results.

Rapid strep test

The rapid strep test is a fast diagnostic test to determine the presence of Group A streptococcal bacteria in the throat. The traditional test for a strep throat is a throat culture; however, results aren't available for 2 to 3 days, possibly causing a delay in treatment. The rapid strep test is much quicker, producing results within minutes. The specimen is obtained by rubbing a cotton swab against the back of the throat; this swab is then tested for a protein produced by the strep bacteria. Most rapid strep test methods have a sensitivity of 75% to 80%. A positive test indicates infection with Group A streptococcal bacteria, requiring antibiotic treatment. If the rapid strep screen is negative, a throat culture may be done as well, due to the possibility of a false-negative result. Typically, both specimens are taken at once, in case the culture is needed.

• Send the specimen to the laboratory immediately; keep the container upright during transport. Don't refrigerate specimens.

Nasopharyngeal culture

Direct microscopic inspection of a Gram-stained smear of the nasopharyngeal specimen provides preliminary identification of organisms, which may guide clinical management and determine the need for additional testing. Streaking a culture plate with the swab, allowing any organisms present to grow, permits isolation and identification of pathogens. Cultured pathogens may require susceptibility testing to determine the appropriate antimicrobial agent.

What it all means

Flora commonly found in the nasopharynx include nonhemolytic streptococci, alpha-hemolytic streptococci, *Neisseria* species (except *N. meningitidis* and *N. gonorrhoeae*), *Staphylococcus epidermidis* and, occasionally, *S. aureus*. (See *Nasopharyngeal culture test interference*.)

Abnormal findings

Pathogens may include group A beta-hemolytic streptococci; occasionally groups B, C, and G beta-hemolytic streptococci; *B. pertussis*; *C. diphtheriae*; *S. aureus*; large numbers of pneumococci; *H. influenzae*; *Myxovirus influenzae*; paramyxoviruses; *C. albicans*; *Mycoplasma* species; *Mycobacterium tuberculosis*; *B. per-*

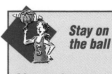

Stay on the ball

Nasopharyngeal culture test interference

Recent antimicrobial therapy decreases bacterial growth.

Obtaining a nasopharyngeal specimen

When the swab passes into the nasopharynx, gently but quickly rotate it to collect a specimen. Then remove the swab, taking care not to injure the nasal mucous membrane.

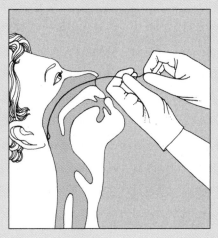

A nasopharyngeal culture can identify pathogens that can cause upper respiratory tract symptoms.

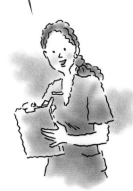

tussis; and *N. meningitidis.* Viruses can be isolated, especially carriers of influenza virus A and B.

What needs to be done

• Inform the patient of how and where the specimen will be obtained and that he may experience slight discomfort and may gag.
• Put on gloves. Moisten the swab with sterile water or saline. Ask the patient to cough before you begin collecting the specimen, and then position the patient with his head tilted back.
• Using a penlight and a tongue blade, inspect the nasopharyngeal area. Next, without touching the sides of the patient's nostril or his tongue, gently pass the swab through the nostril and into the nasopharynx, keeping the swab near the septum and floor of the nose. (See *Obtaining a nasopharyngeal specimen.*)
• If *B. pertussis* is suspected, Dacron or calcium alginate mini-tipped swabs should be used for collection.

Lab notes

• If the specimen is for isolation of a virus, verify the laboratory's recommended collection and refrigeration techniques.
• Note recent antimicrobial therapy or chemotherapy on the laboratory request.
• Tell the laboratory if *Corynebacterium diphtheriae* or *B. pertussis* is suspected; these organisms need special growth media.
• Keep the container upright.

Sputum culture

Bacteriologic examination of sputum—material raised from the lungs and bronchi during deep coughing—is an important aid in managing lung disease.

The usual method of specimen collection is expectoration. Other methods include tracheal suctioning and bronchoscopy. A Gram stain of expectorated sputum must be examined to ensure that it's representative of secretions from the lower respiratory tract rather than contaminated by oral flora. Careful examination of an acid-fast sputum smear may provide presumptive evidence of a mycobacterial infection, such as tuberculosis.

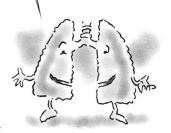

A sputum culture isolates and identifies the cause of a pulmonary infection.

What it all means

Flora commonly found in the respiratory tract include alpha-hemolytic streptococci, *Neisseria* species, diptheroids, some *Haemophilus* species, pneumococci, staphylococci, and yeasts such as *Candida*. However, the presence of normal flora doesn't rule out infection. A culture isolate must be interpreted in light of the patient's overall clinical condition.

On-site organisms

Pathogenic organisms most commonly found in sputum include *Streptococcus pneumoniae*, *Mycobacterium tuberculosis*, *Klebsiella pneumoniae* (and other Enterobacteriaceae), *H. influenzae*, *Staphylococcus aureus*, and *Pseudomonas aeruginosa*. Other pathogens such as *Pneumocystis carinii*, *Legionella* species, *Mycoplasma pneumoniae*, and respiratory viruses may exist in the sputum and can cause lung disease, but they usually require serologic or histologic diagnosis rather than diagnosis by sputum culture. (See *Sputum culture test interference*.)

What needs to be done

• Explain to the patient that this test requires sputum, not saliva. Instruct him to brush his teeth and gargle with water immediately before obtaining the specimen and teach him how to expectorate.
• For expectoration: Put on gloves and a mask. Instruct the patient to cough deeply and expectorate into the container. If the cough is nonproductive, use chest physiotherapy or nebulization to induce sputum, as ordered. Using sterile technique, close the container securely and place it in a leakproof bag before sending it to the laboratory.
• For tracheal suctioning: Administer oxygen to the patient, as necessary. Using sterile gloves, lubricate the catheter with normal saline solution and pass the catheter through the nostril, without

Stay on the ball

Sputum culture test interference

• Failure to report current or recent antimicrobial therapy may alter results.
• Sputum collected over an extended period may cause pathogens to deteriorate or become overgrown, producing false-negative or false-positive results.

Using an in-line trap

- Put on sterile gloves. Push the suction tubing onto the male adapter of the in-line trap.
- Insert the suction catheter into the rubber tubing of the trap. Then suction the patient.
- After suctioning, disconnect the in-line trap from the suction tubing and catheter.
- To seal the container, connect the rubber tubing to the female adapter of the trap.

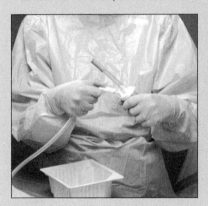
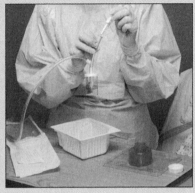
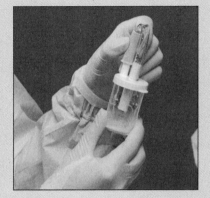

suction. (The patient will cough when the catheter passes through the larynx.) Advance the catheter into the trachea. Apply suction for no longer than 15 seconds to obtain the specimen. Stop suction and gently remove the catheter. Discard the catheter and gloves. Then detach the in-line sputum trap from the suction apparatus and cap the opening. If the patient becomes hypoxic or cyanotic, remove the catheter immediately and administer oxygen. (See *Using an in-line trap*.)

- For bronchoscopy: After a local anesthetic is sprayed into the patient's throat or he gargles with a local anesthetic, the bronchoscope is inserted through the pharynx and trachea into the bronchus. Secretions are then collected with a bronchial brush or aspirated through the inner channel of the scope, using an irrigating solution, such as normal saline solution, if necessary. After the specimen is obtained, the bronchoscope is removed.

- After bronchoscopy, observe the patient carefully for signs of hypoxemia, laryngospasm, bronchospasm, pneumothorax, perforation of the trachea or bronchus (subcutaneous crepitus), or trauma to respiratory structures. Check for difficulty breathing or swallowing. Don't give liquids until the gag reflex returns. In a patient with asthma or chronic bronchitis, watch for aggravated bronchospasms.

- Include on the laboratory request the nature and origin of the specimen, the date and time of collection, the initial diagnosis, and any current antimicrobial therapy.

- Send the specimen to the laboratory immediately.

Blood culture

A blood culture involves inoculating a culture medium with a blood sample and incubating it for isolation and identification of the causative pathogens in bacteremia (bacterial invasion of the bloodstream) and septicemia (systemic spread of such infection). Blood cultures can identify about 67% of pathogens within 24 hours and up to 90% within 72 hours. Blood cultures are ideally performed on 2 consecutive days.

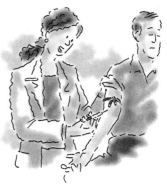

A blood culture confirms bacteremia and identifies the causative organism in bacteremia and septicemia.

Time factor

Bacteremia may be transient, intermittent, or continuous. The timing of sample collection for blood cultures varies; it usually depends on the type of suspected bacteremia—either intermittent or continuous—and on whether drug therapy needs to be started regardless of test results.

What it all means

Blood normally has no pathogenic organisms.

Common pathogens

Common blood pathogens include *Neisseria meningitidis*, *Streptococcus pneumoniae* and other *Streptococcus* species, *Haemophilus influenzae*, *Staphylococcus aureus*, *Pseudomonas aeruginosa*, *Brucella*, and organisms classified as Bacteroidaceae and Enterobacteriaceae.

Immunodeficiency issues

Debilitated or immunocompromised patients may have isolates of *Candida albicans*. In patients with human immunodeficiency virus infection, *Mycobacterium tuberculosis* and *M. avium complex* may be isolated as well as other *Mycobacterium* species on a less frequent basis. (See *Blood culture test interference*.)

What needs to be done

• Inform the patient of the number of samples required and that some discomfort may be felt from the needle punctures and the pressure of the tourniquet. Let him know that dietary restrictions aren't necessary before the test.
• Put on gloves. After cleaning the venipuncture site with an alcohol swab, clean it again with a povidone-iodine swab, starting at the site and working outward in a circular motion. Wait at least 1 minute for the skin to dry, and then remove the residual iodine with an alcohol swab. Apply the tourniquet.

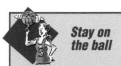

Stay on the ball

Blood culture test interference

• Previous or current antimicrobial therapy may give false-negative results.
• Removing the culture bottle cap (instead of injecting through it) or using incorrect culture media may prevent proper specimen growth.

Venipuncture procedures

- Perform a venipuncture and draw 10 to 20 ml of blood for an adult or 2 to 6 ml for a child. Draw the blood directly into a special collection-processing tube if the lysis-centrifugation technique (Isolator) is being used. Whenever possible, blood cultures should be collected before administering antimicrobial agents.
- Clean the diaphragm tops of the culture bottles with alcohol or povidone-iodine, and change the needle on the syringe. If broth is being used, add blood to each bottle until a 1:5 or 1:10 dilution is achieved. For example, add 10 ml of blood to a 100 ml bottle. The size of the bottle varies depending on facility procedure.
- If a special resin is being used, add blood to the resin in the bottles and invert gently to mix.
- Note current or recent antimicrobial therapy on the laboratory request slip, as well as a tentative diagnosis.
- Send each sample to the laboratory immediately after collection.

Wound culture

A wound culture consists of microscopic analysis of a specimen from a lesion to confirm infection.

Aerobic and anaerobic

Wound cultures may be aerobic (for detection of organisms that usually require oxygen to grow and typically appear in a superficial wound) or anaerobic (for organisms that need little or no oxygen and appear in areas of poor tissue perfusion, such as postoperative wounds, ulcers, or compound fractures.

Indications for wound culture include fever as well as inflammation and drainage in damaged tissue.

What it all means

A clean wound has no pathogenic organism. (See *Wound culture test interference.*)

Abnormal findings

The most common aerobic pathogens in wounds are *Staphylococcus aureus*, group A beta-hemolytic streptococci, *Proteus* species, *Escherichia coli* and other Enterobacteriaceae, and some *Pseudomonas* species; the most common anaerobic pathogens are some *Clostridium*, *Bacteroides*, *Peptococcus*, and *Streptococcus* species.

Stay on the ball

Wound culture test interference

Failure to report recent or current antimicrobial therapy may affect culture and sensitivity reporting.

What needs to be done

• Using gloves, prepare a sterile field and clean the area around the wound with antiseptic solution.

Culture differences

• For aerobic culture: Express the wound and swab as much exudate as possible, or insert the swab deep into the wound and gently rotate. Obtain exudate from the entire wound, using more than one swab. Immediately place the swab in the aerobic culture tube.

• For anaerobic culture: Insert the swab deep into the wound, gently rotate it, and immediately place it in the anaerobic culture tube; or insert the needle into the wound, aspirate 1 to 5 ml of exudate, and immediately inject the exudate into the anaerobic culture tube. (See *Anaerobic specimen collector.*)

Completing the culture

• Dress the wound as ordered.

Memory jogger

To remember the difference between aerobic and anaerobic, think of jogging. When you jog, an aerobic activity, your body requires oxygen—aerobic means oxygen is required. Anaerobic means without oxygen.

Anaerobic specimen collector

Some anaerobes die when they're exposed to the slightest bit of oxygen. To facilitate anaerobic collection and culturing, tubes filled with carbon dioxide (CO_2) or nitrogen are used for oxygen-free transport.

The anaerobic specimen collector shown here consists of a rubber-stoppered tube filled with CO_2, a small inner tube, and a swab attached to a plastic plunger. The drawing on the left shows the tube before specimen collection. The small inner tube containing the swab is held in place by the rubber stopper.

After specimen collection (right), the swab is quickly replaced in the inner tube and the plunger depressed. This separates the inner tube from the stopper, forcing it into the larger tube and exposing the specimen to the CO_2-rich environment. Keep the tube upright.

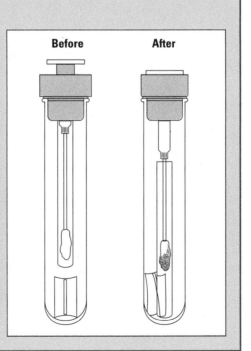

Before   **After**

• Record on the laboratory request recent antimicrobial therapy, the source of the specimen, and the suspected organism.
• If the needle is covered with a rubber stopper, the aspirate may be sent to the laboratory in the syringe.
• Send the specimen to the laboratory within 15 minutes to prevent growth or deterioration of microbes.

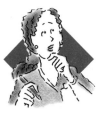

Quick quiz

1. What's the *least* amount of urine required to perform a urine culture?
    A.   60 ml
    B.   30 ml
    C.   10 ml
    D.   3 ml

Answer: D. When collecting a urine specimen for urine culture, at least 3 ml of urine is required; don't fill the specimen cup more than halfway.

2. How should you position a patient when collecting a nasopharyngeal specimen?
    A.   With his head tilted toward the left side
    B.   With his head tilted toward the right side
    C.   With his head tilted forward
    D.   With his head tilted back

Answer: D. Ask the patient to cough before you begin collecting the specimen; then position him with his head tilted back.

3. What's the usual method for collecting a sputum culture?
    A.   Tracheal suctioning
    B.   Expectoration
    C.   Bronchoscopy
    D.   Laryngeal suctioning

Answer: B. The usual method for sputum specimen collection is expectoration; other methods include tracheal suctioning and bronchoscopy.

4. Which aerobic pathogen is commonly found in wounds?
    A.   *Clostridium*
    B.   *Bacteroides*
    C.   *Staphylococcus aureus*
    D.   *Haemophilus influenzae*

Answer: C. The most common aerobic pathogens in wounds are
S. aureus, group A beta-hemolytic streptococci, *Proteus* species,
Escherichia coli and other Enterobacteriaceae, and some
Pseudomonas species.

Scoring

☆☆☆   If you answered all four questions correctly, wow! You represent
the *highest* of cultures!

☆☆   If you answered three questions correctly, great! You'll have a
cult(ure) following in no time!

☆   If you answered fewer than three questions correctly, don't fret!
You'll be cruising through cultures before you know it!

Biopsy

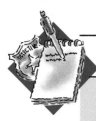

Just the facts

In this chapter, you'll learn:

♦ about biopsies and how they're performed
♦ what patient care is associated with these tests
♦ what factors can interfere with these tests
♦ what biopsy results may indicate.

A look at biopsy

Typically, a biopsy is performed to confirm cancer when other tests point to that diagnosis. In a biopsy, tissue specimens are examined microscopically. The specimen may be obtained during surgery, from a local excision or needle aspiration, or with special instruments (such as tissue punches or curettes). Common biopsy sites include the lung, breast, prostate gland, cervix, and skin.

Because of the possible cancer diagnosis, expect the patient to be anxious. Explain the procedure in terms he can understand, and provide emotional support to ease his anxiety.

> Lung biopsy helps confirm lung lesions and diseases.

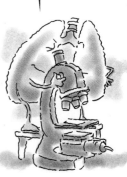

Respiratory system

Lung biopsy

In a lung biopsy, a specimen of pulmonary tissue is excised for examination, using either the closed or open technique. The closed technique, performed under local anesthesia, includes both needle and transbronchial biopsies. The open technique, performed under general anesthesia in the operating room, includes both limited and standard thoracotomies.

Easy access

Needle biopsy is appropriate when the lesion is readily accessible. This procedure provides a much smaller specimen than the open technique. Transbronchial biopsy, the removal of multiple tissue specimens through a fiber-optic bronchoscope, is appropriate for some lung abnormalities or when the patient's condition won't tolerate an open biopsy.

What it all means

Examination of lung tissue specimens can reveal squamous cell or oat cell carcinoma and adenocarcinoma.

What needs to be done

• Describe the test to the patient and tell him that the test takes 30 to 60 minutes. Instruct him to fast for 8 hours before the procedure. Sometimes the patient is permitted to have clear liquids the morning of the test.
• Make sure the patient has signed an informed consent form. Check his history for hypersensitivity to the local anesthetic.
• Tell the patient that chest X-ray and blood studies (prothrombin time, partial thromboplastin time, and platelet count) will be performed before the test.

You're getting verrry sleepy

• Administer a mild sedative, as ordered, 30 minutes before the biopsy to help the patient relax.
• After the biopsy site is selected, lead markers are placed on the patient's skin, and X-rays are ordered to verify the markers' correct placement.
• Place the patient in a sitting position, with arms folded on a table in front of him; instruct him to remain as still as possible and to refrain from coughing.
• During biopsy, observe for signs of respiratory distress—shortness of breath, elevated pulse rate, and cyanosis (late sign); if such signs develop, report them immediately.

Damage control

• The skin over the biopsy site is prepared, and the area is draped. To prevent damage to intercostal nerves and vessels, a local anesthetic is injected with a 25G needle just above the lower rib.
• Using a 22G needle, the examiner anesthetizes the intercostal muscles and parietal pleura, makes a small incision (2 to 3 mm) with a scalpel, and introduces the needle through the incision, chest wall, and pleura, into the tumor or pulmonary tissue.

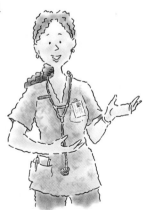

Needle biopsy provides a smaller specimen than open biopsy.

- When the needle is in the tumor or pulmonary tissue, the specimen is obtained and the needle is withdrawn. The specimen is divided immediately. The tissue for histology is placed in a properly labeled bottle containing 10% neutral buffered formalin solution; the tissue for microbiology is placed in a sterile container.
- Pressure is exerted on the biopsy site to stop the bleeding, and a small bandage is applied.

Distress signals

- Check vital signs every 15 minutes for 1 hour, every hour for 4 hours, and then every 4 hours for 24 hours. Watch for bleeding, shortness of breath, increased pulse, diminished breath sounds on the biopsy side and, eventually, cyanosis. Make sure the chest X-ray is repeated immediately after the biopsy, as ordered.

Pleural biopsy

Pleural biopsy is the removal of pleural tissue, by needle biopsy or open biopsy, for examination. Performed under local anesthesia, pleural biopsy usually follows thoracentesis—aspiration of pleural fluid—which is performed when the cause of the effusion is unknown. However, it can be performed separately.

Open pleural biopsy, performed in the absence of pleural effusion, permits direct visualization of the pleura and the underlying lung. It's performed in the operating room.

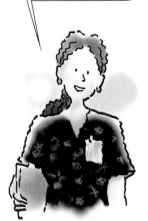

Pleural biopsy helps differentiate between nonmalignant and malignant disease. It also helps diagnose viral, fungal, parasitic, and collagen vascular disease.

What it all means

Microscopic examination of the tissue specimen can reveal malignant disease, tuberculosis, or viral, fungal, parasitic, or collagen vascular disease. Primary tumors of the pleura are commonly fibrous and epithelial.

What needs to be done

- Explain the procedure to the patient. Let him know that blood studies will be necessary before the biopsy and that chest X-rays will be taken before and after the biopsy.
- Make sure the patient has signed an informed consent form. Check the patient history for hypersensitivity to the local anesthetic. Just before the procedure, record vital signs.
- Seat the patient on the side of the bed, with his feet resting on a stool and his arms supported by the overbed table or his upper body. If he can't sit up, place him in a side-lying position with the side to be biopsied facing up.
- Tell him to remain still during the procedure. Prepare the skin and drape the area.

• The local anesthetic is then administered.

Long John Silverman

• If your patient is having a Vim-Silverman needle biopsy, the needle is inserted through the appropriate intercostal space into the biopsy site, with the outer tip distal to the pleura and the central portion pushed in deeper and held in place. The outer case is inserted about ⅜″ (1 cm), the entire assembly is rotated 360 degrees, and the needle and tissue specimen are withdrawn.

Cope-ing with a needle biopsy

• When the biopsy is performed using a Cope's needle, a trocar is introduced through the appropriate intercostal space into the biopsy site. The sharp obturator is then removed, and a hooked stylet is inserted through the trocar. The opened notch is directed against the pleura, along the intercostal space, and is slowly withdrawn. While the outer tube is held stationary, the inner tube is twisted to cut off the tissue specimen and the assembly is withdrawn. (See *Scoping out a Cope's needle.*)

Scoping out a Cope's needle

Used to obtain a pleural biopsy specimen, a Cope's needle consists of three parts: a sharp obturator (A) and a cannula (B), which when fitted together are called a *trocar,* and a blunt-ended, hooked stylet (C). The trocar is used to gain access to the pleural cavity. Then the obturator is removed, leaving the cannula in place. The stylet is passed through the cannula to excise a tissue specimen, as shown below.

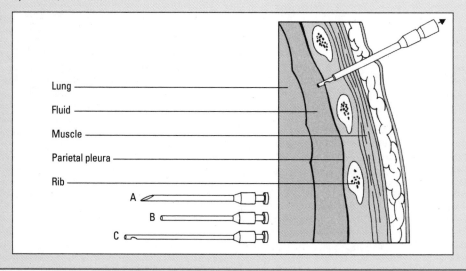

Lung

Fluid

Muscle

Parietal pleura

Rib

A

B

C

Specimen treatment

- The specimen is immediately put in a special solution in a labeled specimen bottle. Then the skin around the biopsy site is cleaned, and an adhesive bandage is applied.

Close attention

- After the biopsy, check the patient's vital signs every 15 minutes for 1 hour and then every hour for 4 hours or until his condition is stable. Make sure the chest X-ray is repeated immediately after the biopsy. Instruct the patient to lie on his unaffected side to promote healing of the biopsy site.
- Watch for signs of respiratory distress (shortness of breath), shoulder pain, and such other complications as pneumothorax (immediate) and pneumonia (delayed).
- Send the specimen to the laboratory immediately.
- Pleural biopsy is contraindicated in patients with severe bleeding disorders.

Reproductive system

Breast biopsy

Breast biopsy is necessary to confirm or rule out cancer. Needle biopsy or fine-needle biopsy can provide a core of tissue or a fluid aspirate, but needle biopsy should be restricted to fluid-filled cysts and advanced malignant lesions. Both methods have limited diagnostic value because of the small and perhaps unrepresentative specimens they provide. Open biopsy, or incisional biopsy, provides a complete tissue specimen, which can be sectioned to allow more accurate evaluation. All techniques require only a local anesthetic and commonly are performed on outpatients.

Stereotactic biopsy immobilizes the breast and allows the computer to calculate the exact location of the mass based on X-rays from two angles. (See *Making breast biopsy more accurate*, page 272.)

An excisional biopsy may be done under general anesthesia. If sufficient tissue is obtained and the mass is found to be a malignant tumor, specimens are sent for estrogen and progesterone receptor assays to assist in determining future therapy and the prognosis. (See *MammaPrint test*, page 273.)

Because breast cancer remains the most prevalent cancer in women, genetic researchers are continually working to identify women at risk.

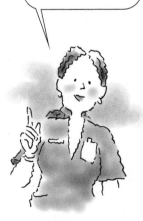

Breast biopsy helps differentiate benign and malignant tumors but may be inconclusive.

Making breast biopsy more accurate

Numerous medical centers offer improved accuracy of breast biopsies, using computers linked to X-rays. The procedure causes less pain and carries a lower risk of deformity than conventional biopsies. It requires only local anesthesia and can be completed in about 1 hour.

To be exact...
In the past, practitioners had to rely on two-dimensional X-rays to locate calcium deposits for biopsy, and they couldn't make sure they were cutting into the correct area. Using computer co-ordinates, a probing tube is inserted into the breast to remove a tissue specimen as the patient lies facedown on a raised operating table. A rotating camera under the table takes X-rays of the breast from every angle. The practitioner then matches up the coordinates to make sure the specimen comes from the correct area.

Test results usually take less than 2 days and are 100% accurate, pinpointing the exact three-dimensional location of calcium deposits.

What it all means

Breast tissue normally consists of cellular and noncellular connective tissue, fat lobules, and various lactiferous ducts. It's normally pink, more fatty than fibrous, and shows no abnormal development of cells or tissue elements.

Abnormal breast tissue may exhibit a wide range of malignant or benign pathology.

Tumor evaluation

The receptor assays evaluate tumors for estrogen and progesterone protein and assign a positive or negative value to the estrogen and progesterone receptors. This positive or negative value assists in the prognosis and treatment of breast cancer.

What needs to be done

• Before the test, obtain a complete medical history.
• Explain how the test is done and that it permits a microscopic examination of a breast tissue specimen. Tell the patient the biopsy will take 15 to 30 minutes. If she's to receive a general anesthetic, advise her to fast from midnight before the test until after the biopsy. Explain that pretest studies, such as blood tests, urine tests, and chest X-rays may be required.
• Make sure the patient has signed an informed consent form. Check her history for hypersensitivity to anesthetics. Offer her emotional support, and assure her that breast masses don't always indicate cancer.

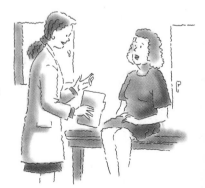

I know you're scared, but breast masses don't always indicate cancer.

MammaPrint test

The Food and Drug Administration recently approved the MammaPrint test, a gene-based test that helps tell early-stage breast cancer patients whether they need chemotherapy after surgery. From looking at the signature of 70 cancer-related genes in a breast tumor, the test determines whether the person is at high or low risk for recurrence after surgery. Low risk means that she has a 95% chance of remaining cancer-free after five years and a 90% chance of remaining cancer-free after 10 years without chemotherapy. High risk indicates a 23% chance of recurrence within five years and a 29% chance of reoccurrence after 10 years; these women are more likely to need chemotherapy. This suggests that the number of women undergoing breast cancer chemotherapy can be reduced. Test results are available in about two days.

What's your type?

• The procedure varies with the type of biopsy your patient requires. She may require a needle biopsy or an open biopsy.

Needle biopsy

• Instruct your patient to undress to the waist.
• After guiding her to a sitting or recumbent position with her hands at her sides, tell her to remain still.
• The practitioner then prepares the biopsy site, administers a local anesthetic, and introduces the syringe (luer-lock syringe for aspiration, Vim-Silverman needle for tissue specimen) into the lesion.
• Fluid aspirated from the breast is expelled into a properly labeled, heparinized tube; the tissue specimen is placed in a labeled specimen bottle containing normal saline solution or formalin.
• Send both specimens to the laboratory immediately. (With fine-needle aspiration, a slide is made and viewed immediately under a microscope.)
• Because breast fluid aspiration isn't diagnostically accurate, some practitioners aspirate fluid only from cysts. If such fluid is clear yellow and the mass disappears, the aspiration is both diagnostic and therapeutic, and the aspirate is discarded. If aspiration yields no fluid or if the lesion recurs two or three times, an open biopsy is then considered appropriate.
• After the procedure, pressure is exerted on the biopsy site and, after bleeding has stopped, an adhesive bandage is applied.

Open biopsy

• Incisional biopsy generally provides an adequate specimen for analysis. After administering a general or local anesthetic, the practitioner makes an incision in the breast to expose the mass.

He may then incise a portion of tissue or excise the entire mass. If the mass is smaller than 2 cm in diameter and appears benign, it's usually excised. If it's larger or appears malignant, a specimen is usually incised before the mass is excised.

• The specimen is placed in a properly labeled specimen bottle containing 10% formalin solution. Tissue that appears malignant is sent for frozen section and receptor assays. Receptor assay specimens must not be placed in the formalin solution. Specimens must be sent to the laboratory immediately.

• After the procedure, the wound is sutured and an adhesive bandage is applied.

Aftercare

• If the patient has received a local anesthetic during needle or open biopsy, check her vital signs and provide drugs for pain, as ordered. Watch for and report bleeding, tenderness, or redness at the biopsy site.

• If the patient received a general anesthetic, check vital signs every 30 minutes for the first 4 hours, every hour for the next 4 hours, and then every 4 hours. Give an analgesic as ordered. Watch for and report bleeding, tenderness, or redness at the biopsy site.

• An ice bag at the biopsy site may provide comfort. Instruct the patient to wear a support bra at all times until healing is complete.

• Provide emotional support to the patient who's awaiting diagnosis.

Prostate gland biopsy

Prostate gland biopsy is the needle excision of a prostate tissue specimen for examination. A perineal, transrectal, or transurethral approach may be used; the transrectal approach is usually used for high prostatic lesions. Indications include potentially malignant prostatic hypertrophy and prostatic nodules.

What it all means

The prostate gland normally consists of a thin, fibrous capsule surrounding the stroma, which is made up of elastic and connective tissues and smooth-muscle fibers. The epithelial glands, found in these tissues and muscle fibers, drain into the chief excreting ducts. Microscopic tissue examination can confirm cancer.

What needs to be done

• Before the biopsy, describe the procedure to the patient.

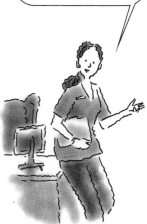

Prostate biopsy can help confirm prostate cancer or determine the cause of prostatic hyperplasia.

• Make sure the patient has signed an informed consent form. Check his history for hypersensitivity to the anesthetic or to other drugs. For a transrectal approach, prepare the bowel by administering enemas until the return is clear. Give an antibacterial agent, as ordered, to minimize the risk of infection. Just before the biopsy, check vital signs and give a sedative, as ordered.

• The practitioner may choose the perineal, transurethral, or transrectal approach. An alternative method to the transrectal approach is the automated cone biopsy.

Perineal approach

• Place the patient in the proper position (left lateral, knee-chest, or lithotomy), and clean the perineal skin.

• After giving the local anesthetic, the practitioner makes a 2-mm incision into the perineum. He immobilizes the prostate by inserting a finger into the rectum and inserts the needle into a prostate lobe. He rotates the needle gently, pulls it out about 5 mm, and reinserts it at another angle, repeating the procedure in several areas.

• Specimens are placed immediately in a labeled specimen bottle containing 10% formalin solution. Pressure is exerted on the puncture site, which is then bandaged.

Transurethral approach

• Position the patient on a special table. Place his legs in stirrups and drape him to maintain privacy.

• The practitioner passes an endoscopic instrument through the urethra, permitting direct viewing of the prostate and passage of a cutting loop. The loop is rotated to chip away pieces of tissue and is then withdrawn.

• The specimen is placed immediately in a labeled specimen bottle containing 10% formalin solution.

Transrectal approach

• Place the patient in a left lateral position.

• The practitioner attaches a curved needle guide to the finger palpating the rectum and pushes the biopsy needle along the guide, into the prostate. As the needle enters the prostate, the patient may experience pain. The practitioner rotates the needle to cut off the tissue and then withdraws it.

• The specimen is placed immediately in a bottle containing 10% formalin solution.

• An alternative to transrectal detection is the automated cone biopsy, in which the practitioner uses a spring-powered device with an inner trocar needle to cut through prostatic tissue. This technique is quick and reportedly painless.

Aftercare

• Check vital signs immediately after the procedure, every 2 hours for 4 hours, and then every 4 hours.
• Observe the biopsy site for a hematoma and signs of infection, such as redness, swelling, and pain.
• Watch for urine retention, urinary frequency, and hematuria.

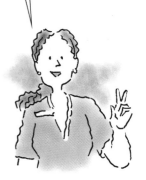

Cervical punch biopsy is used to evaluate suspicious cervical lesions and to diagnose cervical cancer.

Cervical punch biopsy

Cervical punch biopsy is the excision by sharp forceps of a cervical tissue specimen for microscopic examination. Generally, multiple biopsies are done to obtain specimens from different areas.

What it all means

Cervical tissue should have no dysplasia or abnormal cell growth. Microscopic examination of a cervical tissue specimen identifies abnormal cells and differentiates the tissue as intraepithelial neoplasia or invasive cancer.

Cone biopsy

If cervical biopsy doesn't show the cause of an abnormal Papanicolaou test or if the specimen shows advanced dysplasia (abnormal tissue changes) or carcinoma in situ (malignant cell changes in the epithelial tissue that don't extend beyond the basement membrane), a cone biopsy is done in the operating room under general anesthesia. A cone biopsy collects a larger tissue specimen and allows more accurate evaluation of dysplasia.

What needs to be done

• Explain the procedure to the patient. Tell her that the biopsy provides a cervical tissue specimen for microscopic study.
• Make sure the patient has signed an informed consent form, and instruct her to void just before the biopsy. If she's an outpatient, she should have someone accompany her home after the biopsy.
• Biopsy sites are selected by direct visualization of the cervix with a colposcope (the most accurate method) or by Schiller's test, which stains normal squamous epithelium a dark mahogany but fails to color abnormal tissue.

Direct visualization

• Place the patient in the lithotomy position, and tell her to relax as the unlubricated speculum is inserted.
• For direct visualization, the practitioner inserts the colposcope through the speculum, locates the biopsy site, and cleans the

cervix with a swab soaked in 3% acetic acid solution. He then inserts the biopsy forceps through the speculum or the colposcope and removes tissue from any lesion or from selected sites, starting from the posterior lip to avoid obscuring other sites with blood.

• The practitioner immediately places each specimen in 10% formalin solution in a labeled bottle.

• To control bleeding after biopsy, the practitioner swabs the cervix with 5% silver nitrate solution (cautery or sutures may be used instead). If bleeding persists, the practitioner may insert a tampon.

Schiller's test

• With this test, the practitioner inserts an applicator stick saturated with iodine solution through the speculum. This stains the cervix to identify lesions for biopsy.

Make your request

• Record the patient's and practitioner's names and the biopsy sites on the laboratory request and send the specimens immediately.

• Instruct the patient in aftercare. (See *Recovering from cervical punch biopsy*.)

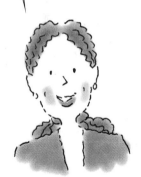

Two's company! Make sure someone accompanies the outpatient home after the biopsy.

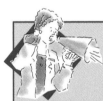

Listen up!

Recovering from cervical punch biopsy

After a cervical punch biopsy, encourage the outpatient to rest briefly before leaving the office. To help her recover from the procedure, provide these instructions:

• Avoid strenuous exercise for 24 hours.

• If a tampon was inserted after the biopsy, leave it in place for 8 to 24 hours, as ordered.

• Know that some bleeding may occur, but report bleeding that's heavier than menstrual bleeding.

• Avoid using additional tampons, according to the practitioner's directions, because tampons can irritate the cervix and provoke bleeding.

• If you had cryotherapy or laser treatment during the procedure, avoid douching and refrain from intercourse for up to 2 weeks, or as directed.

• Be aware that a foul-smelling, gray-green vaginal discharge is normal for several days after the biopsy and may persist for 3 weeks.

Other organ-specific biopsies

Bone marrow aspiration and biopsy

Bone marrow, the soft tissue contained in the medullary canals of long bone and the interstices of cancellous bone, may be removed by aspiration or needle biopsy under local anesthesia. In aspiration biopsy, a fluid specimen in which pustulae of marrow are suspended is removed. In needle biopsy, a core of marrow—cells, not fluid—is removed. These methods are commonly used concurrently to obtain the best possible marrow specimens.

What it all means

Yellow marrow contains fat cells and connective tissue; red marrow contains hematopoietic cells, fat cells, and connective tissue. Special stains that detect hematologic disorders produce these normal findings: the iron stain, which measures hemosiderin (storage iron), has a +2 level; the Sudan black B (SBB) stain, which shows granulocytes, is negative; and the periodic acid–Schiff (PAS) stain, which detects glycogen reactions, is negative.

Abnormal findings

Histologic examination of a bone marrow specimen can help detect myelofibrosis, granulomas, lymphomas, or cancer. Hematologic analysis, including the differential count and the myeloid-erythroid ratio, can implicate a wide range of disorders. (See *Bone marrow: Normal values.*)

In an iron stain, decreased hemosiderin levels may indicate a true iron deficiency. Increased levels may accompany other anemias or blood disorders. A positive SBB stain can distinguish acute myelogenous leukemia from acute lymphoblastic leukemia (negative SBB), or it may indicate granulation in myeloblasts. A positive PAS stain may mean acute or chronic lymphocytic leukemia, amyloidosis, thalassemia, lymphoma, infectious mononucleosis, iron deficiency anemia, or sideroblastic anemia.

What needs to be done

• Explain the procedure to the patient. A mild sedative will be given 1 hour before the test, if ordered. Tell the patient the test usually takes only 5 to 10 minutes and that more than one bone marrow specimen may be required. Let him know a blood sample will be collected before the biopsy for laboratory testing.

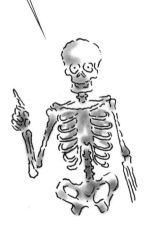

Bone marrow aspiration and biopsy helps diagnose hematologic disorders and metastatic tumors. It also can determine the cause of infection and monitor the effectiveness of chemotherapy.

Bone marrow: Normal values

Cell types	Adults	Children	Infants
Basophils	0.01%	0.06%	0.07%
Eosinophils	3.1%	3.6%	2.6%
Lymphocytes	16.2%	16%	49%
Megakaryocytes	0.1%	0.1%	0.05%
Myeloid:erythroid ratio	2:1 to 4:1	2.9:1	4.4:1
Neutrophils, total	56.5%	57.1%	32.4%
Myeloblasts	0.2% to 1.5%	1.2%	0.62%
Promyelocytes	2.1% to 4.1%	1.4%	0.76%
Myelocytes	8.2% to 15.7%	18.3%	2.5%
Metamyelocytes	9.6% to 24.6%	23.3%	11.3%
Bands	9.5% to 15.3%	0	14.1%
Segmented	6% to 12%	12.9%	3.6%
Normoblasts, total	25.6%	23.1%	8%
Pronormoblasts	0.2% to 1.3%	0.5%	0.1%
Basophilic	0.5% to 2.4%	1.7%	0.34%
Polychromatic	17.9% to 29.2%	18.2%	6.9%
Orthochromatic	0.4% to 4.6%	2.7%	0.54%
Plasma cells	1.3%	0.4%	0.02%

History and consent

• Make sure the patient has signed an informed consent form. Check his history for hypersensitivity to the local anesthetic. After checking with the practitioner, tell the patient which bone—sternum, anterior or posterior iliac crest, vertebral spinous process, rib, or tibia—will be used as the biopsy site. (See *Common bone marrow aspiration and biopsy sites.*) A child requires additional steps. (See *Preparing a child for bone marrow biopsy.*)

• A bone marrow specimen can be collected by bone marrow aspiration or needle biopsy. For both procedures position the patient and instruct him to remain as still as possible.

• During the biopsy, talk to the patient quietly, describe what's being done, and answer questions.

Aspiration biopsy

• The practitioner prepares the biopsy site and injects a local anesthetic. He then inserts the needle through the skin, the subcutaneous tissue, and the cortex of the bone. The practitioner removes the stylet from the needle and attaches a 10- to 20-ml syringe. He aspirates 0.2 to 0.5 ml of marrow and withdraws the needle.

• Pressure is applied to the site for 5 minutes while the marrow slides are being prepared. If the patient has thrombocytopenia, pressure is applied for 10 to 15 minutes.

• The biopsy site is cleaned again, and a sterile adhesive bandage is applied.

• If the practitioner doesn't obtain an adequate marrow specimen on the first attempt, he may reposition the needle or remove and reinsert it in another site within the anesthetized area. If the second attempt fails, a needle biopsy may be necessary.

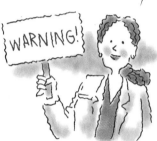

Bone marrow biopsy is contraindicated in patients with severe bleeding disorders.

Needle biopsy

• With a needle biopsy, the site is prepared and the skin is marked at the site with an indelible pencil or marking pen.

• The practitioner then injects a local anesthetic intradermally, subcutaneously, and at the surface of the bone.

• He inserts the biopsy needle into the periosteum and sets the needle guard as indicated.

• He advances the needle until the outer needle passes through the cortex of the bone, and then inserts the inner needle into the outer needle and removes the stylet.

• Alternately rotating the inner needle clockwise and counterclockwise, the practitioner directs the needle into the marrow cavity and removes a tissue plug. He withdraws the needle assembly and places the marrow in a labeled bottle containing a Zenker's acetic acid solution.

• After the biopsy site is cleaned, a sterile adhesive bandage or a pressure dressing is applied.

Common bone marrow aspiration and biopsy sites

These illustrations show commonly used sites for bone marrow aspiration and biopsy.

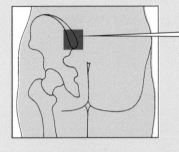

Usually, the posterior superior iliac spine is preferred for bone marrow aspiration because no vital organs or vessels are located nearby.

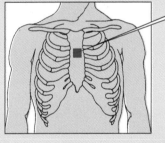

The sternum involves the greatest risk. However, it's commonly used for marrow aspiration because it's near the surface, the cortical bone is thin, and the marrow cavity contains numerous cells and relatively little fat or supporting bone.

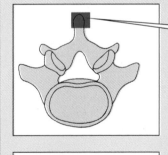

The spinous process is the preferred site if multiple punctures are necessary, marrow is absent at other sites, or the patient objects to sternal puncture.

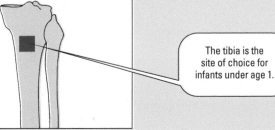

The tibia is the site of choice for infants under age 1.

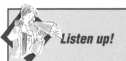

Listen up!

Preparing a child for bone marrow biopsy

To prepare a child for bone marrow biopsy, give him his own biopsy kit: a syringe without a needle, cotton balls, and adhesive bandages. Act out the procedure by using a doll or stuffed animal as a model. This will help you gain the child's confidence and answer questions he may have. Be sure to describe the kinds of pressure and discomfort he'll feel during the procedure.

Show and tell

Before the biopsy, show the child the equipment on the tray and explain what it's for in simple terms. Encourage the parents to get involved by helping you hold the child still and reassuring him. Tell the child that he'll feel some pain when the practitioner aspirates the bone marrow and that it's okay to cry or yell if he wants to. Reassure him that the pain will go away quickly.

Aftercare

- Check the biopsy site for bleeding and inflammation.
- Observe the patient for signs of hemorrhage and infection, such as rapid pulse rate, low blood pressure, and fever.
- Send the specimen or slides to the laboratory immediately.

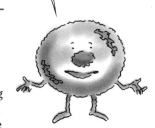

Thyroid biopsy differentiates various thyroid diseases.

Thyroid biopsy

Thyroid biopsy—excision of a thyroid tissue specimen for microscopic examination—is indicated for patients with thyroid enlargement or nodules (even if serum triiodothyronine [T_3] and serum thyroxine [T_4] levels are normal), breathing and swallowing difficulties, vocal cord paralysis, weight loss, hemoptysis, or a full sensation in the neck. It's commonly performed when noninvasive tests, such as thyroid ultrasonography, are abnormal or inconclusive.

Needle versus open biopsy

A thyroid tissue specimen may be obtained with a hollow needle under local anesthesia or during open biopsy under general anesthesia. Fine-needle aspiration with a microscopic examination can aid diagnosis and replace an open biopsy. Open biopsy, performed in the operating room, is more complex and provides more direct information; the surgeon obtains a tissue specimen from the exposed thyroid and sends it to the laboratory for rapid analysis. Open biopsy also permits immediate excision of suspicious thyroid tissue. Coagulation studies should precede thyroid biopsy.

What it all means

Examination of normal tissue shows fibrous networks dividing the gland into pseudolobules that consist of follicles and capillaries. Cuboidal epithelium lines the follicle walls and contains the protein thyroglobulin, which stores T_3 and T_4. Malignant tumors appear as well-encapsulated, solitary nodules of uniform but abnormal structure. Papillary carcinoma is the most common type of thyroid cancer. Follicular carcinoma, a less common form, strongly resembles normal cells.

Benign distinctions

Such benign conditions as nontoxic nodular goiter demonstrate hypertrophy, hyperplasia, and hypervascularity. Distinct histologic patterns characterize subacute granulomatous thyroiditis, Hashimoto's disease, and hyperthyroidism.

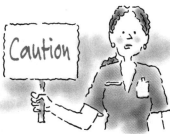

Thyroid biopsy should be used cautiously in patients with coagulation defects.

Caution

Missed malignancy

Because many malignant thyroid tumors are multicentric and small, a negative report doesn't necessarily rule out cancer.

What needs to be done

• Explain the procedure to the patient. If he'll receive a general anesthetic, explain that he needs to restrict food and fluids.
• Make sure the patient has signed an informed consent form. Check for hypersensitivity to anesthetics or analgesics.
• For needle biopsy, place the patient in the supine position with a pillow under his shoulder blades.
• Prepare the skin over the biopsy site. As the practitioner prepares to inject the local anesthetic, warn the patient not to swallow.
• After the anesthetic is injected, the carotid artery is palpated and the biopsy needle is inserted parallel to the thyroid cartilage to prevent damage to the deep structures and the larynx. When the specimen is obtained, the needle is removed and the specimen is immediately placed in formalin.

When the biopsy is over

• Apply pressure to the biopsy site to stop bleeding. If bleeding continues for more than a few minutes, press on the site for up to 15 minutes more. Apply an adhesive bandage.
• To make the patient more comfortable, place him in semi-Fowler's position. Tell him that to avoid strain on the biopsy site he should put both hands behind his neck when he sits up.
• Observe for difficulty breathing. Check the back of the neck and the patient's pillow for bleeding every hour for 8 hours. Report bleeding immediately.
• Keep the biopsy site clean and dry.

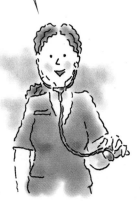

Lymph node biopsy can distinguish between benign and malignant tumors and stage metastatic cancer.

Lymph node biopsy

Lymph node biopsy is the surgical excision of an active lymph node or needle aspiration of a nodal specimen for histologic examination. Both techniques usually use local anesthesia and sample superficial nodes in the cervical, supraclavicular, axillary, or inguinal region. Excision, the preferred technique, provides a larger specimen.

What it all means

Microscopic examination of the tissue specimen distinguishes malignant from nonmalignant causes of lymph node enlargement.

Lymph node malignancy may also result from metastatic cancer. When histologic results aren't clear or nodular material isn't involved, mediastinoscopy or laparotomy can provide another nodal specimen.

What needs to be done

• Describe the procedure to the patient. For excisional biopsy, instruct him to restrict food from midnight on and to drink only clear liquids. For a needle biopsy, instruct that he doesn't need to restrict food and fluids.
• Make sure the patient has signed an informed consent form. Check his history for hypersensitivity to the anesthetic. Just before the biopsy, record baseline vital signs.

Excisional biopsy

• For excisional biopsy, prepare the skin over the biopsy site, and drape the area for privacy.
• The practitioner administers the anesthetic. He then makes an incision, removes an entire node, and places it in a properly labeled bottle containing normal saline solution.
• After the biopsy, he sutures the wound and applies a sterile dressing.

Needle biopsy

• For needle biopsy, the practitioner prepares the site and administers a local anesthetic.
• The practitioner grasps the node between thumb and forefinger, inserts the needle directly into the node, and obtains a small core specimen.
• He then removes the needle and places the specimen in a properly labeled bottle containing normal saline solution.
• Pressure is exerted on the biopsy site to control bleeding, and an adhesive bandage is applied.

Aftercare

• Check vital signs and watch for bleeding, tenderness, and redness at the biopsy site.
• Tell the patient that he may resume his usual diet.

Skin biopsy

Skin biopsy is the removal of a small piece of tissue, under local anesthesia, from a lesion suspected of being malignant.

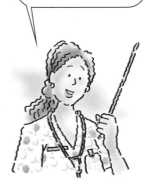

Skin biopsy can differentiate among skin cancers and benign growths. It's also useful for diagnosing chronic bacterial or fungal skin infections.

Three techniques

A specimen may be secured by one of three techniques: shave, punch, or excision. A shave biopsy cuts the lesion above the skin line and leaves the lower layers of dermis intact, permitting further biopsy at the site. A punch biopsy removes an oval core from the center of a lesion. An excisional biopsy, the procedure of choice, removes the entire lesion. It's indicated for rapidly expanding lesions; sclerotic, bullous, or atrophic lesions; and examination of a lesion's border and surrounding normal skin.

What it all means

Normal skin consists of squamous epithelium (epidermis) and fibrous connective tissue (dermis). Microscopic examination of the tissue specimen may reveal a benign or malignant lesion.

Growths may be benign...

Benign growths include cysts, seborrheic keratoses, warts, keloids, pigmented nevi, dermatofibromas, and multiple neurofibromas.

...or malignant

Malignant skin cancers include basal cell carcinoma, squamous cell carcinoma, and malignant melanoma. Basal cell carcinoma occurs on hair-bearing skin, the most common location being the face, including the nose and its folds. Squamous cell carcinoma most commonly appears on the lips, mouth, and genitalia. Malignant melanoma, the most deadly skin cancer, can spread throughout the body by way of the lymphatic system and the blood vessels.

What needs to be done

• Describe the procedure to the patient. Tell the patient he doesn't need to restrict food and fluids.
• Make sure the patient has signed an informed consent form. Check his history for hypersensitivity to the local anesthetic.
• Position the patient comfortably and clean the biopsy site before the practitioner administers a local anesthetic.

Shave biopsy

• During a shave biopsy, the practitioner cuts off the protruding growth at the skin line with a #15 scalpel and immediately places the tissue in a specimen bottle containing 10% formalin solution.
• Pressure is applied to the area to stop the bleeding.

Punch biopsy

• With a punch biopsy, the practitioner pulls taut the skin surrounding the lesion, firmly introduces the punch into the lesion, and rotates to obtain a tissue specimen. He then lifts the plug with forceps or a needle and severs as deeply into the fat layer as possible.
• The specimen is placed in specimen bottle containing 10% formalin solution or, if indicated, in a sterile container.
• The practitioner then closes the wound, using sutures as indicated by size of the wound.

Excisional biopsy

• For excisional biopsy, the practitioner uses a #15 scalpel to excise the lesion completely.
• He removes the tissue specimen and immediately places it in a specimen bottle containing 10% formalin solution.
• Pressure is applied to the site to stop the bleeding.
• The practitioner typically closes the wound using 4-0 sutures.

Finishing up

• Check the biopsy site for bleeding.
• Administer drugs for pain as needed and ordered.
• Advise the patient with sutures to keep the area as clean and dry as possible. Facial sutures are removed in 3 to 5 days; trunk sutures, in 7 to 14 days. Instruct him to leave adhesive strips in place for 14 to 21 days or until they fall off.
• Send the specimen to the laboratory immediately.

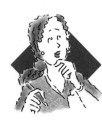

Quick quiz

1. During lung biopsy, you should monitor the patient for such complications as:

    A.   respiratory distress.
    B.   shoulder pain.
    C.   abdominal pain.
    D.   calf pain.

Answer: A. During lung biopsy, you should monitor for signs of respiratory distress, such as shortness of breath, elevated pulse rate, and cyanosis.

2. During a needle biopsy of the thyroid, the patient is placed in:
   A.   supine position.
   B.   supine position with the neck extended.
   C.   supine position with a pillow under the shoulder blades.
   D.   prone position.

Answer: C. The supine position with a pillow under the shoulder blades pushes the trachea and thyroid forward and allows neck veins to fall backward.

3. Which procedure is preferred for skin biopsy?
   A.   Shave biopsy
   B.   Punch biopsy
   C.   Scrape biopsy
   D.   Excisional biopsy

Answer: D. Excisional biopsy is the procedure of choice because it removes the entire lesion.

4. What's the site of choice for a bone marrow aspiration and biopsy in an infant under age 1?
   A.   Sternum
   B.   Tibia
   C.   Iliac spine
   D.   Spinous process

Answer: B. The tibia is the site of choice for a bone marrow aspiration and biopsy in an infant under age 1.

5. A positive Sudan black B stain can distinguish acute myelogenous leukemia from:
   A.   acute lymphoblastic leukemia.
   B.   acute lymphocytic leukemia.
   C.   chronic lymphocytic leukemia.
   D.   amyloidosis.

Answer: A. A positive Sudan black B stain can distinguish acute myelogenous leukemia from acute lymphoblastic leukemia.

6. Which type of breast biopsy allows exact computerized location of the breast mass?
   A.   Fine needle
   B.   Open
   C.   Stereotactic
   D.   Incisional

Answer: C. Stereotactic biopsy allows exact computerized location of the breast mass.

Scoring

☆☆☆   If you answered all six questions correctly, congratulations! You've just been inducted to the Biopsy Hall of Fame!

☆☆   If you answered four or five questions correctly, way to go! You're an official Biopsy Buff!

☆   If you answered fewer than four questions correctly, don't worry! You'll be winning the biopsy game in no time!

Endoscopy

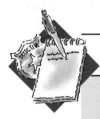

Just the facts

In this chapter, you'll learn:

♦ about endoscopic procedures and how they're performed

♦ the patient care associated with these tests

♦ factors that can interfere with these tests

♦ what endoscopic results may indicate.

A look at endoscopy

Endoscopy, which allows direct visualization using a fiber-optic scope, helps diagnose abnormalities of the GI tract, lungs, and reproductive system. When explaining the procedure to your patient, be sure to use terms he can understand. Ask him if he has any allergies, and tell him he'll receive a sedative beforehand to help him relax.

Gastrointestinal system

Colonoscopy

Colonoscopy is the visual examination of the lining of the large intestine using a flexible fiber-optic endoscope. This test is indicated for patients with a history of constipation and diarrhea, persistent rectal bleeding, or lower abdominal pain when results of proctosigmoidoscopy and a barium enema test prove negative or inconclusive.

Although usually a safe procedure, colonoscopy can cause perforation of the large intestine, excessive bleeding, and retroperi-

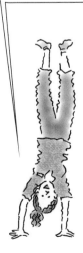

Colonoscopy is versatile! It can diagnose inflammatory and ulcerative bowel disease, locate the origin of lower GI bleeding, and diagnose colonic strictures, polyps, and lesions.

Virtual colonoscopy

Virtual colonoscopy combines computed tomography (CT) scanning and X-ray images with sophisticated image processing computers to generate three-dimensional (3-D) images of the patient's colon. These images are interpreted by a skilled radiologist to recreate and evaluate the colon's inner surface. Although this procedure isn't as accurate as a routine colonoscopy, it's less invasive and is useful in screening the patient with small polyps. The colon must be free from residue and fecal material. Bowel preparation consists of following a clear liquid diet for 24 hours before the procedure; also, the patient performs GoLYTELY bowel preparation the evening before and takes a rectal suppository on the morning of the test.

Before performing the CT scan, a thin red rectal tube is placed, and air is introduced into the colon to distend the bowel. This may produce mild cramping. The CT scan is done with the patient in the supine position and again while prone. The scans are then shipped over a network to a 3-D image processing computer, and a radiologist evaluates the images obtained. If polyps are identified, a colonoscopy may be scheduled to remove them.

Stay on the ball

Colonoscopy interference

These factors may interfere with test results by inhibiting visual examination or colonoscope passage:

• barium retained in the intestine from previous diagnostic studies
• blood from acute colonic hemorrhage
• sigmoid colon fixation from inflammatory bowel disease, surgery, or radiation therapy
• consuming liquids with red dye (such as red gelatin dessert), which may appear like blood in the large intestine and may produce false results.

toneal emphysema. The test may be performed on an inpatient or an outpatient basis.

Colonoscopy is contraindicated in patients with a near-term pregnancy, a recent history of acute myocardial infarction or abdominal surgery, ischemic bowel disease, acute diverticulitis, peritonitis, fulminant granulomatous colitis, fulminant ulcerative colitis, or a perforated viscus. For these cases or for screening purposes, a virtual colonoscopy may be an option to help visualize polyps early before they become concerns. (See *Virtual colonoscopy*.)

What it all means

The normal mucosa of the large intestine beyond the sigmoid colon appears light pink-orange and is marked by semilunar folds and deep tubular pits. Blood vessels are visible beneath the intestinal mucosa, which glistens from mucus secretions.

Abnormal findings

Colonoscopy, along with microscopic test results, may reveal proctitis, granulomatous and ulcerative colitis, Crohn's disease, and malignant or benign lesions. Colonoscopy alone can detect diverticular disease or the site of lower GI bleeding. (See *Colonoscopy interference*.)

What needs to be done

• Explain to the patient that this test permits examination of the lining of the large intestine by inserting a flexible instrument

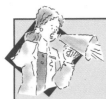

Listen up!

Following a clear liquid diet

You'll need to teach your patient about following a clear liquid diet before certain intestinal tests. The diet consists of transparent foods that are liquid or that will liquefy at room temperature. This diet reduces stool volume in the bowels, letting the practitioner see the inside of the bowels more easily.

Listed below are the only foods and beverages your patient should eat or drink when following a clear liquid diet:
- water
- ice chips
- clear tea (no milk or lemon)
- strained, clear fruit juices, such as apple, grape, and cranberry (no pulp)
- decaffeinated coffee (may vary with facility)
- clear carbonated beverages
- plain fruit gelatin (no fruit added)
- chicken or beef broth (fat-free only)
- chicken or beef bouillon
- frozen ice pops (no fruit or pulp)
- clear, fruit-flavored drink mixes.

through his anus. Instruct him to maintain a clear liquid diet for 24 to 48 hours before the test and to take nothing by mouth after midnight the night before the procedure. (See *Following a clear liquid diet.*)
- Inform the patient not to take aspirin products starting 5 days before the procedure, as ordered. Unless advised not to, the patient may take the usual medications in the morning of the procedure with a sip of water. Withhold medications as ordered.

Quick cleaning

- Inform the patient that the large intestine must be thoroughly cleaned to be clearly visible. Give him a laxative, such as 10 oz (296 ml) of magnesium citrate, 3 tbs of castor oil, or a gallon of GoLYTELY solution in the evening. Phospho-soda may also be used (usually two 45 ml bottles mixed with equal amounts of ginger ale; the day before the test, one is consumed in the morning and one in the evening). Chill the solution to make it more palatable. If you're using GoLYTELY, instruct the patient to drink the preparation quickly, drinking 8 oz (236.6 ml) every 10 minutes un-

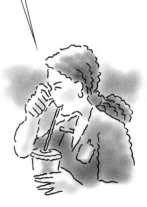

After drinking all these liquids to prepare for colonoscopy, I may never be thirsty again!

til the entire gallon is consumed. This laxative produces watery diarrhea in 30 to 60 minutes and clears the bowel in 4 to 5 hours.
• If fecal results still aren't clear, the patient will receive a laxative, suppository, or tap-water enema. Don't administer a soapsuds enema because this irritates the mucosa and stimulates mucous secretions that may hinder the examination.

Sedate and consent

• Tell the patient an I.V. line will be started before the procedure and he may receive a sedative to help him relax. Tell the patient he must arrange for transportation home because he shouldn't drive for 12 hours afterward.
• Make sure the patient or responsible family member has signed a consent form. Check the patient's vital signs 30 minutes before the test; if they're stable, give the sedative as ordered.

Baselines and other basics

• Obtain baseline vital signs, and monitor vital signs throughout the procedure. Attach the patient to a continuous electrocardiogram monitor and pulse oximeter.
• Place the patient on his left side, with his knees flexed, and drape him. Instruct him to breathe deeply and slowly through his mouth as the practitioner inserts his gloved, lubricated index finger into the anus and rectum and palpates the mucosa. After a water-soluble lubricant has been applied to the patient's anus and to the tip of the colonoscope, tell the patient the colonoscope is about to be inserted.

Scoping out the situation

• After the colonoscope is inserted through the patient's anus, a small amount of air is blown in to locate the bowel lumen. The scope is advanced through the rectum into the sigmoid colon under direct vision. When the instrument reaches the descending sigmoid junction, assist the patient to a supine position to aid the scope's advance, if necessary. After the scope has passed the splenic flexure, it's advanced through the transverse colon and hepatic flexure, into the ascending colon and cecum.
• Biopsy forceps or a cytology brush may be passed through a channel in the colonoscope to obtain specimens for microscopic examination; a special instrument may used to remove polyps. If tissue specimen is removed, immediately place it in a specimen bottle containing 10% formalin; immediately place cytology smears in a Coplin jar containing 95% ethyl alcohol.
• If a tissue or cell specimen is obtained during the procedure, send it to the appropriate laboratory immediately.

A safe watch

• Observe the patient closely for signs of bowel perforation, including malaise, rectal bleeding, abdominal pain and distention, fever, and mucopurulent drainage. Notify the practitioner immediately if such signs develop.
• Check vital signs until they're stable.
• Watch closely for adverse effects of the sedative, such as respiratory depression, hypotension, excessive diaphoresis, bradycardia, and confusion. Have emergency resuscitation equipment available and an opioid antagonist such as naloxone ready for I.V. use, if necessary. Monitor his level of consciousness (LOC).

Resuming and recovering

• Provide a safe environment until the patient has recovered from sedation; then tell him he may resume his usual diet.
• Tell the patient he may pass large amounts of flatus resulting from the air blown into the colon during the procedure. Provide privacy to minimize embarrassment.
• If a polyp has been removed, inform the patient that there may be some blood in his stools and that he should report excessive bleeding immediately.
• Outpatients may be discharged when fully awake. Make sure the patient has transportation home.
• Advise the patient to avoid alcohol for 24 hours after being sedated.

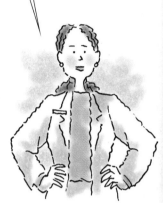

After colonoscopy, immediately report rectal bleeding, abdominal pain, and other signs of bowel perforation.

Capsule endoscopy

Capsule endoscopy is an imaging system that consists of a tiny video camera with a light source and transmitter inside a capsule, allowing recording of images along its path. The capsule endoscope measures about 11 x 30 mm and is propelled along the digestive tract by peristalsis. The clear end records images of the stomach walls and, particularly, the small intestine, where many other diagnostic techniques may not reach or otherwise visualize. (See *Detecting disorders in the stomach and small intestine*, page 294.)

The images are transmitted to a data recorder on a belt placed around the patient's waist. After swallowing the pill, the patient can leave the facility and return to work or other activities of daily living. This test is useful in detecting causes of bleeding and anemia, as well as detecting polyps or cancer. The procedure is contraindicated in the patient with a suspected obstruction, fistula, or stricture, and in the patient who can't swallow (an infant, a young child, or someone with a swallowing impairment). It's also con-

Now I get it!

Detecting disorders in the stomach and small intestine

In capsule endoscopy, after the patient swallows the capsule, it travels through the body by the natural movement of the digestive tract. A receiver worn outside the body records the images. The strength of the signal indicates the capsule's location.

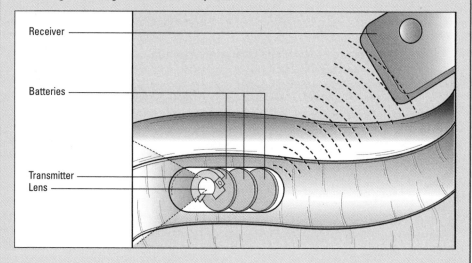

Receiver

Batteries

Transmitter

Lens

Picture this! Capsule endoscopy is an imaging system that consists of a tiny video camera. This test is useful in detecting causes of bleeding and anemia, as well as detecting polyps or cancer.

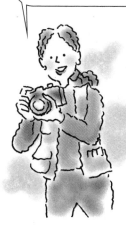

traindicated in a patient with cardiac pacemakers or other implanted medical devices.

What it all means

The camera illustrates normal anatomy of the stomach and small intestine. The battery is short-lived, so images of the large intestine are unobtainable.

Bowels and bleeding

The camera may detect bleeding sites or abnormalities of the stomach and small bowel, such as erosions, Crohn's disease, celiac disease, benign and malignant tumors of the small intestine, vascular disorders, medication-related small-bowel injuries, and pediatric small-bowel disorders. The pill can't be used to stop bleeding, take tissue specimens, remove growths, or repair any problems detected. Other invasive studies may be needed. (See *Capsule endoscopy interference.*)

What needs to be done

• Inform the patient that he may need to fast for 12 hours before the test, but is allowed fluids for up to 2 hours before the test unless ordered otherwise. (Usually no preparation is involved, but some patients may benefit from it.)
• Explain to the patient that he'll need to swallow the camera pill and that it will send information to a receiver he'll wear on his belt. Tell him that the procedure is painless and after swallowing the pill he can go home or go to work. Explain that walking helps facilitate movement of the pill.
• Tell the patient that he'll need to return to the facility in 24 hours (or as directed) so the recorder can be removed from his belt.
• Check to see if an informed consent form has been signed.

Then what happens?

• The patient ingests the camera pill, as ordered, and a receiver is attached to his belt. The pill records images for up to 6 hours along its path of the stomach, small intestine, and mouth of the large intestine, transmitting the information to the receiver.
• The patient returns to the facility, as ordered, so the images can be transmitted into the computer, where they're displayed on the screen.
• Tell the patient that he may resume his usual diet after the images are obtained and that the pill will be excreted normally in his stools in 8 to 72 hours.

Stay on the ball

Capsule endoscopy interference

• Narrowing or obstruction of the intestine can cause the pill to become lodged.
• Barium retained from a previous study or inadequate cleansing or failure to remain in nothing-by-mouth status before the study may impair clear imaging.

Endoscopic ultrasound

Endoscopic ultrasound (EUS) combines ultrasonography with endoscopy to visualize the GI wall and adjacent structures. Incorporation of the ultrasound probe at the distal end of the ultrasonic endoscope allows ultrasound imaging that provides a detailed picture.

What it all means

EUS usually reveals normal anatomy with no evidence of tumor.

Abnormal EGD EUS findings

If endoscopic ultrasonography is used in combination with an esophagogastroduodenoscopy (EGD), results may reveal acute or chronic ulcers, benign or malignant tumors, or inflammatory disease, including gastritis, esophagitis, and duodenitis. They may also show diverticula, varices, Mallory-Weiss syndrome, esophageal and pyloric stenosis, and esophageal hiatal hernia.

Check me out! Endoscopic ultrasound is used to stage certain GI tract cancers and evaluate bile duct abnormalities.

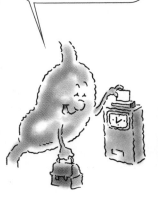

Abnormal colonoscopy EUS findings

When combined with colonoscopy, EUS findings may indicate ulcerative colitis, Crohn's disease, diverticular disease, or malignant or benign lesions of the colon. They may also isolate the site of lower GI bleeding.

Abnormal sigmoidoscopy EUS findings

EUS findings when combined with sigmoidoscopy may reveal benign or malignant tumors. (See *Endoscopic ultrasound interference*.)

What needs to be done

• Explain the procedure to the patient. Check his history for allergies, medications, and information pertinent to his current complaint. Instruct him to fast for 6 to 8 hours before the test. If he's undergoing colonoscopy or sigmoidoscopy, tell him he may have to take a laxative the evening before the procedure and may need to follow a clear liquid diet, as ordered.
• Inform the patient that he may receive an I.V. sedative to help him relax before the endoscope is inserted. If the patient is an outpatient, advise him to arrange for someone to drive him home. Make sure he or a responsible family member has signed the consent form.
• Obtain baseline vital signs, and leave the blood pressure cuff in place for monitoring throughout the procedure, according to your facility's policy. Throughout the procedure, observe the patient's skin and temperature. Monitor his LOC and pain tolerance, and observe for abdominal distention.

Esophageal approach

• With an EGD EUS, tell the patient to hold his breath while his mouth and throat are sprayed with a local anesthetic.
• Let him know that the anesthetic spray will cause him to lose some control of his secretions. Encourage him to let saliva drain from the side of his mouth to decrease the risk of aspiration.

Scope advancement

• After placing the patient in a left lateral position, ask him to bend his head forward and to open his mouth.
• The practitioner inserts his finger into the mouth and guides the tip of the endoscope alongside his finger to the back of the throat. As the endoscope passes through the throat, the patient's head is slowly extended to aid scope advancement. The patient's chin must be kept at midline. The endoscope is then passed along the esophagus under direct vision. When the endoscope is about 12″

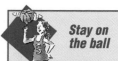

Stay on the ball

Endoscopic ultrasound interference

The following factors may inhibit visual examination or endoscope passage:
• esophageal stricture
• barium retained in the intestine from previous diagnostic studies
• blood from acute colonic hemorrhage
• sigmoid colon fixation from inflammatory bowel disease, surgery, or radiation therapy.

(30.5 cm) into the esophagus, position the patient's head with his chin toward the table so saliva can drain from his mouth.
• When examination of the esophagus and the cardiac sphincter is complete, the endoscope is rotated clockwise, with the tip angled upward, and advanced into the stomach. After examining the stomach lining, the endoscope is advanced into the duodenum. Then the practitioner slowly withdraws the endoscope and reexamines suspicious areas of the gastric and esophageal lining.

Just passing through

• During the examination, air may be instilled into the GI tract to open the bowel lumen and flatten tissue folds, or water may be instilled to rinse material or fluids from the lens. The practitioner may apply suction to remove unnecessary insufflated air or secretions. Biopsy forceps may be passed through the scope to obtain a tissue specimen, or a cytology brush may be passed through to obtain cells.
• Tissue specimens are immediately placed in a specimen bottle containing 10% formaldehyde solution; cell specimens are smeared on glass slides and placed in a Coplin jar containing 95% ethyl alcohol.

Keeping a close watch

• Observe the patient for possible perforation. Perforation in the cervical area of the esophagus produces pain on swallowing and with neck movement; thoracic perforation causes substernal or epigastric pain that increases with breathing or trunk movement; diaphragmatic perforation produces shoulder pain and dyspnea; gastric perforation causes abdominal or back pain, cyanosis, fever, or pleural effusion.
• Observe the patient for evidence of aspiration of gastric contents, which could precipitate aspiration pneumonia.
• For inpatients, check vital signs every 15 minutes for 4 hours, every hour for 4 hours, and then every 4 hours. Observe outpatients for a 30- to 60- minute recovery period, monitoring vital signs every 15 minutes. When fully awake, outpatients may be discharged if the gag reflex has returned.
• Provide a safe environment for the patient until he has recovered from the sedative. Keep his bed's side rails up.
• Withhold food and fluids until the gag reflex returns, which is usually within 1 hour. Test the gag reflex by touching the back of the throat with a tongue blade.
• Tell the patient he may burp some insufflated air and may have a sore throat for 3 to 4 days.
• Instruct the patient to watch for persistent difficulty swallowing and for pain, fever, black stools, or bloody vomitus. Tell him to notify the practitioner immediately if any of these complications de-

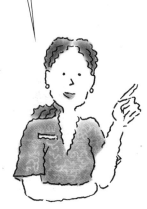

A camera may be attached to the endoscope to photograph areas for later study, or a measuring tube may be passed through the endoscope to determine the size of a lesion.

velop. Also, instruct him to avoid alcohol for 24 hours and driving
for 12 hours.

Opposite-end approach

• If your patient requires a colonoscopic or sigmoidoscopic EUS,
place him on his left side, with his knees flexed, and drape him.
Instruct him to breathe deeply and slowly through his mouth as
the practitioner inserts his gloved, lubricated index finger into the
anus and rectum and palpates the mucosa. After a water-soluble
lubricant has been applied to the patient's anus and to the tip of
the scope, tell the patient the scope is about to be inserted.

• After the scope is inserted through the patient's anus, a small
amount of air is blown into the bowel to locate the bowel lumen.
The practitioner advances the scope through the rectum into the
sigmoid colon. When the instrument reaches the descending sigmoid junction, assist the patient to a supine position to aid the
scope's advance, if necessary. After the scope has passed the
splenic flexure, it's advanced through the transverse colon and
hepatic flexure into the ascending colon and cecum, if a colonoscopy is being performed.

Specimen collection

• Biopsy forceps or a cytology brush may be passed through a
channel in the endoscope to obtain specimens for microscopic examination; a special instrument may be used to remove polyps. If
a tissue specimen is removed, immediately place it in a specimen
bottle containing 10% formalin; immediately place cytology
smears in a Coplin jar containing 95% ethyl alcohol.

• If a tissue or cell specimen is obtained, send it to the appropriate laboratory immediately.

Check, check, and recheck

• For inpatients, check vital signs every 15 minutes for 4 hours,
every hour for 4 hours, and then every 4 hours. Observe outpatients for a 30- to 60-minute recovery period, monitoring vital
signs every 15 minutes. When fully awake, outpatients may be discharged. Because of sedation, outpatients shouldn't drive for 12
hours. Make sure these patients have transportation home.

Reproductive system

Colposcopy

In colposcopy, the cervix and vagina are visually examined by means of a colposcope—an instrument that contains a magnifying lens and a light. Colposcopy is primarily used to evaluate abnormal cytology or grossly suspicious lesions and to examine the cervix and vagina after a positive Papanicolaou (Pap) test. During the examination, a biopsy may be performed and photographs taken of suspicious lesions, using the colposcope and attachments. Biopsy risks include bleeding (especially during pregnancy) and infection.

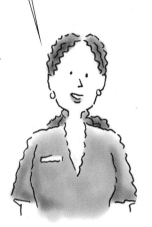

Colposcopy helps confirm abnormal cervical tissue growth after a positive Pap test. It also helps evaluate vaginal and cervical lesions.

What it all means

Surface contour of the cervical vessels should be smooth and pink; columnar epithelium should appear grapelike. Different tissue types should have definite borders.

Abnormal colposcopy findings include white epithelium or punctuation and mosaic patterns, which may indicate underlying cervical tissue abnormalities, indicating possible invasive cancer or precancerous tissue changes. Abnormal findings also include atypical vessels, which may indicate invasive cancer. Other abnormalities visible during colposcopy include inflammatory changes, atrophy, erosion, papilloma (benign epithelial tumor), and condyloma (wart-like growth). (See *Colposcopy interference*.)

What needs to be done

• Explain the procedure to the patient. Tell her the procedure is safe and painless and takes 10 to 15 minutes. Advise her that a biopsy may be performed at the time of examination and may cause minimal but easily controlled bleeding and mild cramping.
• The practitioner puts on gloves and, with the patient in the lithotomy position, inserts the speculum and, if indicated, performs a Pap test. Then he swabs the cervix with acetic acid solution to remove mucus. After examining the cervix and vagina, he performs a biopsy on areas that appear abnormal. Finally, he stops bleeding by applying pressure or hemostatic solutions or by cautery.

Brief abstinence

After a biopsy, instruct the patient to abstain from intercourse and avoid inserting anything in her vagina, including a tampon, until

Stay on the ball

Colposcopy interference

Failure to clean the cervix of foreign materials, such as creams and medications, may impair visualization. Active untreated infection interferes with an accurate assessment and causes procedural discomfort.

biopsy site healing is confirmed (approximately 10 days). Inform the patient that spotting and minimal discharge can be expected for 24 to 48 hours after the procedure; heavy vaginal bleeding, lower abdominal pain, or signs of infection (fever, unusual discharge) should be reported.

Laparoscopy

Laparoscopy permits visualization of the peritoneal cavity by the insertion of a small fiber-optic telescope (laparoscope) through the anterior abdominal wall.

Laparoscopy has largely replaced laparotomy because it requires a smaller incision, is faster, and reduces the risk of postoperative adhesions. Nevertheless, laparotomy is usually preferred when extensive surgery is indicated. Potential laparoscopy risks include a punctured visceral organ, which can cause bleeding or spilling of intestinal contents into the peritoneum.

Laparoscopy is contraindicated in the patient with advanced abdominal wall cancer, advanced pulmonary or cardiovascular disease, intestinal obstruction, palpable abdominal mass, large abdominal hernia, chronic tuberculosis, or a history of peritonitis.

What it all means

Normal findings include mobile uterus and fallopian tubes of normal size and shape and with no adhesions. The ovaries are of normal size and shape; cysts and endometriosis are absent.

Cyst sightings

An ovarian cyst appears as a bubble on the surface of the ovary. The cyst may be clear, filled with follicular fluid or serous or mucous material, or red, blue, or brown, if filled with blood. Adhesions appear as sheets or strands of tissue that may be almost transparent or thick and fibrous. Endometriosis resembles small, blue powder burns on the peritoneum or the serous membrane of any pelvic or abdominal structure. Fibroids (fibrous, encapsulated connective tissue tumors) appear as lumps on the uterus; hydrosalpinx (distention of the fallopian tube caused by fluid), as an enlarged fallopian tube; ectopic pregnancy, as an enlarged or ruptured fallopian tube. In pelvic inflammatory disease, infection or abscess is evident. (See *Laparoscopy interference.*)

What needs to be done

• Explain the procedure to the patient. Instruct her to fast after midnight before the test or for at least 8 hours before surgery. Tell

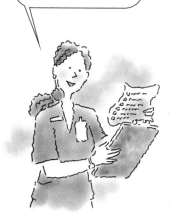

> Laparoscopy can detect cysts, adhesions, fibroids, and infection. As a treatment it can be used for adhesion destruction, tubal sterilization, and foreign body removal.

Stay on the ball

Laparoscopy interference

Adhesions, marked obesity, or tissue or fluid that attaches to the lens may obstruct the field of vision.

the patient she may experience pain at the puncture site and in the shoulder.
• Inform the patient that she'll receive a local or general anesthetic, and tell her whether the procedure will require an outpatient visit or overnight hospitalization.

Don't know much about history?

• Make sure the patient or a responsible family member has signed an informed consent form. Check the patient history for hypersensitivity to the anesthetic. Make sure all laboratory work is completed and results reported before the test. Instruct the patient to empty her bladder just before the test.
• The patient is anesthetized and placed in the lithotomy position. The practitioner catheterizes the bladder and then performs a bimanual examination of the pelvic area to detect abnormalities that may contraindicate the test and to ensure that the bladder is empty.
• The practitioner makes an incision at the inferior rim of the umbilicus. He inserts a special needle into the peritoneal cavity and insufflates 2 to 3 L of carbon dioxide or nitrous oxide. Next, he removes the needle and inserts a trocar and sheath into the peritoneal cavity. After removing the trocar, he inserts the laparoscope through the sheath to examine the pelvis and abdomen.
• To evaluate tubal patency, dye is infused through the cervix and the fimbria (the fringelike extremity of the fallopian tubes) is observed for spillage.
• After the examination, he may perform minor surgical procedures such as ovarian biopsy. He may insert a second trocar at the pubic hairline to provide a channel for inserting other instruments.

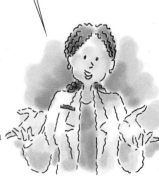

Laparoscopy is commonly performed in place of laparotomy. It requires a smaller incision, which allows a faster recovery.

Aftercare

• Monitor vital signs and urine output. Immediately report sudden changes; they may indicate complications.
• After administration of a general anesthetic, check for an allergic reaction and monitor electrolyte balance and hemoglobin level and hematocrit, as ordered. Help the patient ambulate after recovery as ordered.
• Tell the patient she may resume her normal diet as ordered.
• Instruct the patient to restrict activity for 2 to 7 days as ordered.
• Reassure the patient that some abdominal and shoulder pain is normal and should disappear within 24 to 36 hours. Provide analgesics as ordered. If pain continues or worsens, notify the practitioner immediately because this may be a sign of bowel perforation.

Other endoscopies

Bronchoscopy

Bronchoscopy is the direct visualization of the larynx, trachea, and bronchi through a standard metal or fiber-optic broncho-scope, a slender flexible tube with mirrors and a light at its distal end. A brush, biopsy forceps, or a catheter may be passed through the bronchoscope to obtain specimens for cytologic examination.

A flexible fiber-optic bronchoscope is used most commonly be-cause it's smaller, allows a better view of the smaller bronchial structures, and carries less risk of trauma than a rigid broncho-scope. However, a large, rigid bronchoscope must be used to re-move foreign objects, excise endobronchial lesions, and control massive hemoptysis.

Possible complications of bronchoscopy include hypoxemia, cardiac arrhythmias, bleeding, infection, bronchospasm, and pneumothorax.

What it all means

The trachea normally consists of smooth muscle containing C-shaped rings of cartilage at regular intervals. The bronchi appear structurally similar to the trachea, with the right bronchus slightly larger and more vertical than the left bronchus. Smaller segmental bronchi branch off from the main bronchi.

Abnormalities

Abnormalities of the bronchial wall include inflammation, swelling, protruding cartilage, ulceration, tumors, and enlarge-ment of the mucous gland orifices or submucosal lymph nodes.

Abnormalities that originate in the trachea include stenosis, compression, ectasia (dilation of tubular vessel), irregular bronchial branching, and abnormal separation into two branches resulting from a diverticulum.

Abnormal substances in the trachea or bronchi include blood, secretions, and foreign bodies.

Small findings...big consequences

Results of tissue and cell studies may indicate interstitial pul-monary disease, lung cancer, tuberculosis, or other pulmonary in-fections. Lung cancers include squamous cell carcinoma, small-cell (oat cell) carcinoma, adenocarcinoma, and large-cell (undif-ferentiated) carcinoma. Bronchoscopy findings must be

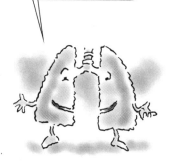

Bronchoscopy allows visual examination and removal of a tumor or a foreign body in the tracheobronchial tree. It also helps diagnose cancer, tuberculosis, or other infections by obtaining a specimen for examination.

correlated with X-ray and microscopic findings as well as with the patient's signs and symptoms.

What needs to be done

• Describe the procedure to the patient, and explain that this test allows examination of the lower airways. Instruct the patient to fast for 6 to 12 hours before the test. Tell him that the room will be darkened and that the procedure takes 45 to 60 minutes. Advise him that test results are usually available in 1 day, except for a tuberculosis report, which may take up to 6 weeks.

• Tell the patient that a chest X-ray and blood studies, such as partial thromboplastin time, platelet count and, possibly, arterial blood gas analysis, will precede the bronchoscopy.

Expect the anesthetics

• Advise him that he may receive a sedative I.V. to help him relax.

• Make sure the patient or a responsible family member has signed the informed consent form. Check the patient history for hypersensitivity to the anesthetic, and obtain baseline vital signs. Administer the preoperative sedative as ordered. If the patient is wearing dentures, instruct him to remove them just before the test.

Ventilation station

• A patient with severe respiratory failure who can't breathe adequately by himself should be put on a ventilator before bronchoscopy.

• Place the patient in the supine position on a table or bed. Tell him to remain relaxed, with his arms at his sides, and to breathe through his nose. Provide supplemental oxygen by nasal cannula, if ordered. Make sure a handheld resuscitation bag with face mask is readily available.

• After the local anesthetic is sprayed into the patient's throat and takes effect, the practitioner introduces the bronchoscope through the patient's mouth or nose. When the bronchoscope is just above the vocal cords, lidocaine is flushed through the inner channel of the scope to the vocal cords to anesthetize deeper areas. (See *Features of the bronchoscope*, page 304.)

Detective work

• The practitioner inspects the trachea and bronchi, observes the color of the mucosal lining, and notes masses or inflamed areas. Biopsy forceps may be used to remove a tissue specimen from a suspect area, a bronchial brush to obtain cells from the surface of a lesion, or a suction apparatus to remove foreign bodies or mucus plugs. Lavage may be performed to diagnose the infectious

Features of the bronchoscope

The bronchoscope, inserted through the nostril into the bronchi, has four channels (see inset): two light channels (A), which provide a light source; one visualizing channel (B) to see through; and one open channel (C), which accommodates biopsy forceps, a cytology brush, suction apparatus, a lavage device, anesthetic, or oxygen.

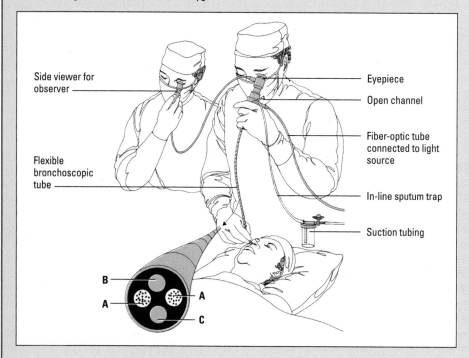

Side viewer for observer

Flexible bronchoscopic tube

Eyepiece

Open channel

Fiber-optic tube connected to light source

In-line sputum trap

Suction tubing

B

A

A

C

Trouble signs

Bronchoscopy can be a risky procedure. After your patient undergoes bronchoscopy, watch him carefully for the following complications:
• laryngeal edema or laryngospasm, such as laryngeal stridor and dyspnea
• hypoxemia
• pneumothorax (dyspnea, cyanosis, diminished breath sounds on the affected side)
• bronchospasm (dyspnea, wheezing) and bleeding (hemoptysis)
• tracheal or bronchial perforation (subcutaneous crepitus around the face and neck).

causes of infiltrates or to remove thickened secretions. After the tissue, mucus, or secretion is collected, place the specimens in appropriate containers and label them properly.

Powers of observation

• Monitor vital signs. Notify the practitioner immediately if the patient has an adverse reaction to the anesthetic or sedative. (See *Trouble signs.*)
• As ordered, place the conscious patient in semi-Fowler's position; place the unconscious patient on his side with the head of the bed slightly elevated to prevent aspiration.
• Provide an emesis basin, and instruct the patient to spit out saliva rather than swallow it. Observe sputum for blood, and notify the practitioner immediately if excessive bleeding occurs.

Refrain, restrict, and reassure

- Tell the patient who has had a biopsy to refrain from clearing his throat and coughing, which could dislodge the clot at the biopsy site and cause hemorrhaging.
- Restrict food and fluids until the gag reflex returns (usually in 2 hours). Then let the patient resume his usual diet, beginning with sips of clear liquid or ice chips. Smoking should be avoided for 24 hours.
- Reassure the patient that hoarseness, loss of voice, and sore throat after this procedure are only temporary. The patient should seek medical attention for difficulty breathing, fever, and increased hemoptysis.
- Send the specimens to the laboratory immediately.

Arthroscopy

Most commonly used to examine the knee, arthroscopy is the visual examination of the interior of a joint with a specially designed fiber-optic endoscope. Unlike radiographic studies, arthroscopy permits concurrent surgery or biopsy using a technique called *triangulation*, in which instruments are passed through a separate cannula. Thus, arthroscopy provides a safe, convenient alternative to open surgery and separate biopsy.

Although arthroscopy is commonly performed under a local anesthetic, it may also be performed under a spinal or general anesthetic, particularly when surgery is anticipated. Arthroscopy complications include infection, hematoma, thrombophlebitis, and joint injury.

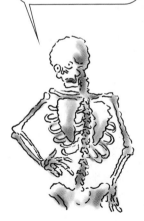

Arthroscopy can be a real saving grace. It can diagnose joint diseases and monitor their progression and therapy. Surgeons also use the technique to perform joint surgery.

What it all means

The knee is a typical diarthrodial joint surrounded by muscles, ligaments, cartilage, and tendons and lined with synovial membrane. In children, the menisci (crescent-shaped cartilage) are smooth and opaque, with thick outer edges attached to the joint capsule and inner edges lying snugly against the condylar (the rounded portion at the end of the bone) surfaces, unattached. Articular cartilage appears smooth and white; ligaments and tendons appear cablelike and silvery. The synovium (the membrane that lines the joint capsule) is smooth and marked by a fine vascular network. Degenerative changes begin during adolescence.

Arthroscopic abnormalities

Arthroscopic examination can reveal a torn meniscus, chondromalacia (softening of the cartilage); dislocation; subluxation (partial or incomplete dislocation); fracture; degenerative articular

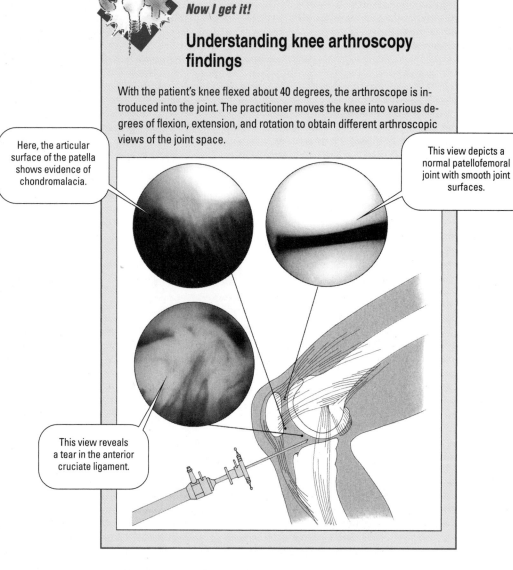

Now I get it!

Understanding knee arthroscopy findings

With the patient's knee flexed about 40 degrees, the arthroscope is introduced into the joint. The practitioner moves the knee into various degrees of flexion, extension, and rotation to obtain different arthroscopic views of the joint space.

Here, the articular surface of the patella shows evidence of chondromalacia.

This view depicts a normal patellofemoral joint with smooth joint surfaces.

This view reveals a tear in the anterior cruciate ligament.

cartilage; torn anterior cruciate or tibial collateral ligaments; Baker cyst (cyst that contains synovial fluid) and ganglion cyst; synovitis; rheumatoid and degenerative arthritis; and foreign bodies associated with gout, pseudogout, and osteochondromatosis.

Depending on test findings, appropriate treatment or surgery can follow arthroscopy. If arthroscopic surgery can't be performed, arthrotomy (incision into the joint) is the procedure of choice. (See *Understanding knee arthroscopy findings*.)

What needs to be done

• Describe the procedure to the patient. Instruct him to fast after midnight before the procedure.

Razor sharp

• Make sure the patient or a responsible family member has signed an informed consent form. Check the patient history for hypersensitivity to the anesthetic. Just before the procedure, shave the area 5″ (12.7 cm) above and below the joint; then administer a sedative as ordered.

Technique time

• Arthroscopic techniques vary with the surgeon and the type of arthroscope used. In most cases, as much blood as possible is drained from the leg by wrapping it in an elastic bandage and elevating it, or by instilling a mixture of lidocaine with epinephrine and sterile normal saline solution into the knee to distend the knee and help reduce bleeding. Then the surgeon anesthetizes the joint, makes a small incision, and passes a cannula through the incision and positions it in the joint cavity. Next, he inserts the arthroscope through the cannula and examines the knee structures. If necessary, he takes photographs for further study.
• When the examination is complete, a synovial biopsy or appropriate surgery is performed. After the surgery, the arthroscope is removed, the joint is irrigated, and an adhesive strip and compression bandage are applied to the site.
• Watch for fever and swelling, increased pain, and localized inflammation at the incision site. If the patient reports discomfort, administer analgesics as ordered.
• Monitor the patient's circulation and sensation in his leg.

Crucial (and cruciate) instruction

• Instruct the patient to report fever, bleeding, drainage, or increased joint swelling or pain.
• If an immobilizer is ordered, teach the patient how to apply it.
• Tell the patient that showering is permitted after 48 hours, but a tub bath should be avoided until after the postoperative visit.
• Tell the patient that he may resume his usual diet.

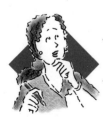

Quick quiz

1. Before colonoscopy, the patient should avoid:
    A.   a soap-suds enema.

B. GoLYTELY.
C. castor oil.
D. water.

Answer: A. A soap-suds enema irritates the mucosa and stimulates mucus secretions that may hinder the examination.

2. A patient is scheduled for an EGD in the morning. When preparing him, you should explain that:
A. he may have liquids before the procedure.
B. he must remove his dentures before the procedure.
C. he may drive home after the procedure.
D. he'll need to stay overnight.

Answer: B. The endoscope passes through the mouth into the esophagus. Therefore, the patient must remove his dentures before the procedure to prevent airway obstruction.

3. After a bronchoscopy that required a biopsy, you should instruct the patient to:
A. refrain from clearing his throat.
B. perform coughing and deep breathing every 4 hours.
C. resume his diet immediately.
D. swallow any secretions.

Answer: A. The patient must refrain from clearing his throat and coughing because these actions could dislodge the clot at the biopsy site and cause hemorrhaging.

4. After arthroscopy, you should instruct the patient to:
A. elevate his leg, apply ice, and bear full weight.
B. elevate his leg, apply warm soaks, and bear partial weight.
C. keep his leg straight with a knee brace.
D. elevate his leg, apply ice, and bear partial weight.

Answer: D. After arthroscopy, the patient should elevate the affected leg and apply ice for 24 hours to reduce swelling. He should bear only partial weight, using crutches, a walker, or a cane, for 48 hours.

Scoring

☆☆☆ If you answered all four questions correctly, awesome! You're an endoscopy expert!

☆☆ If you answered three questions correctly, terrific! The end of endoscopic study is just around the corner!

☆ If you answered fewer than three questions correctly, don't worry! With a little more work, you'll end up acing endoscopy!

Ultrasonography

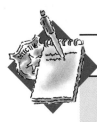

Just the facts

In this chapter, you'll learn:

♦ about ultrasonographic procedures and how they're performed

♦ the patient care associated with these tests

♦ factors that can interfere with these tests

♦ what ultrasonographic results may indicate.

A look at ultrasonography

Ultrasonography uses high-frequency sound waves to obtain diagnostic information. The sound waves are directed into the targeted tissue and reflected back to a transducer. A computer interprets the waves, some of which appear on a screen for immediate visualization while others convert to audible sounds. Some waves are recorded for a permanent test record, called a *sonogram* or *echogram*.

Before ultrasonography, explain the procedure to the patient in terms he can understand to ease his anxiety.

Cardiovascular system

Echocardiography

Echocardiography examines the size, shape, and motion of cardiac structures using a transducer placed at an acoustic window (an area where bone and lung tissue are absent) on the patient's chest. The transducer directs sound waves toward cardiac structures, which reflect these waves. The transducer picks up the echoes, converts them to electrical impulses, and relays them to an echocardiography machine for display on a screen and for recording on a strip chart or videotape.

On the move with M-mode

The most commonly used echocardiographic techniques are M-mode (motion-mode) and two-dimensional (cross-sectional). In M-mode echocardiography, a single, pencil-like ultrasound beam strikes the heart, producing a vertical view of cardiac structures. This method is useful for precisely recording the motion and dimensions of intracardiac structures.

2-D echo

In two-dimensional echocardiography, the ultrasound beam rapidly sweeps through an arc, producing a cross-sectional, or fan-shaped, view of cardiac structures; this technique is useful for recording lateral motion and providing the correct spatial relationship between cardiac structures. In many cases, both techniques are performed to complement each other. (See *Comparing two types of echocardiography*.)

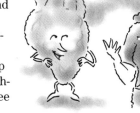

Echocardiography helps diagnose and evaluate valvular abnormalities and atrial tumors, and it measures the size of the heart's chambers.

What it all means

A normal echocardiogram reveals normal position, size, and movement of the cardiac valves and heart muscle wall and shows normal directional flow of blood within the heart chambers.

Detect heart valve abnormalities

The echocardiogram may detect valvular abnormalities, such as mitral stenosis, mitral valve prolapse, aortic insufficiency, and aortic stenosis. Chamber or valvular abnormalities may indicate a congenital disorder. In coronary artery disease, ischemia or infarction may cause motion abnormalities in the ventricular walls. The echocardiogram is especially sensitive in detecting pericardial effusion. (See *Echocardiography interference*.)

What needs to be done

• Explain the procedure to the patient. If the patient is to have cardiac stress testing, explain the procedure and how to prepare for the test. (See *Teaching about cardiac stress testing*, page 312.)
• Inform the patient that he may be asked to inhale a gas with a slightly sweet odor (amyl nitrite) while changes in heart function are recorded; describe the possible adverse effects (dizziness, flushing, and tachycardia), but assure him that such symptoms quickly subside.

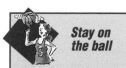

Stay on the ball

Echocardiography interference

Thickened chest muscles, chronic obstructive pulmonary disease, and chest wall abnormalities may alter test results.

Now I get it!

Comparing two types of echocardiography

This illustration shows how M-mode and two-dimensional echocardiography differ. The shaded areas beneath the transducer identify cardiac structures that intercept and reflect the transducer's ultrasonic waves.

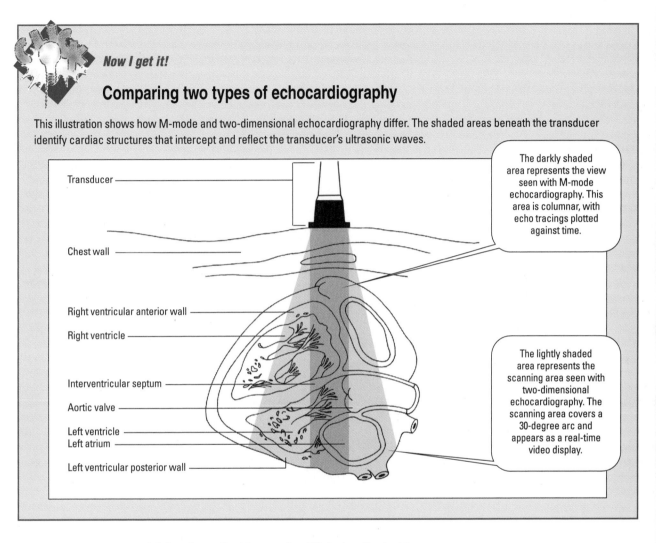

Transducer

Chest wall

Right ventricular anterior wall

Right ventricle

Interventricular septum

Aortic valve

Left ventricle
Left atrium

Left ventricular posterior wall

The darkly shaded area represents the view seen with M-mode echocardiography. This area is columnar, with echo tracings plotted against time.

The lightly shaded area represents the scanning area seen with two-dimensional echocardiography. The scanning area covers a 30-degree arc and appears as a real-time video display.

- Advise the patient to remain still during the test because movement may distort results.

Position is everything

- The patient is placed in the supine position. Conductive gel is applied to the third or fourth intercostal space to the left of the sternum, and the transducer is placed over it. The transducer is systematically angled to direct ultrasonic waves at specific heart regions. For a different view of the heart, the transducer is placed beneath the xiphoid process or directly above the sternum.
- During the test, the oscilloscope screen, which displays the returning echoes, is observed; significant findings are recorded on a strip chart recorder (in M-mode echocardiography) or videotape recorder (in two-dimensional echocardiography).

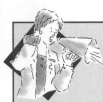

Listen up!

Teaching about cardiac stress testing

Exercise echocardiography and dobutamine stress echocardiography are types of cardiac stress testing that detect changes in heart wall motion through the use of two-dimensional echocardiography with exercise or a dobutamine infusion. Imaging is done before and after either exercise or dobutamine administration. Usually, these tests are performed to:
• identify the cause of chest pain
• detect heart abnormalities, obstructions, or damage
• determine the heart's functional capacity after myocardial infarction or cardiac surgery
• evaluate myocardial perfusion
• measure the heart chambers
• set limits for an exercise program.

Preparing your patient
When preparing your patient for these tests, cover the following points:
• Explain that this test will evaluate how his heart performs, and how specific heart structures work, under stress.
• Instruct him not to eat, smoke, or drink alcohol or caffeinated beverages for at least 4 hours before the test.
• Advise him to ask his practitioner whether he should withhold current medications before the test.
• Tell him to wear a two-piece outfit because he'll be removing all clothing above the waist and will wear a hospital gown. Instruct him to wear comfortable sneakers or soft-soled shoes. Advise female patients to wear a support bra.
• Explain that electrodes will be placed on his chest and arms to obtain an initial electrocardiogram (ECG). Mention that the areas where electrodes are placed will be cleaned with alcohol and the skin will be abraded for optimal electrode contact.
• Tell him that an initial echocardiogram will be performed while he's lying down. Conductive gel, which feels warm, will be placed on his chest. Then a special transducer will be placed at various angles on his chest to visualize different parts of his heart. Emphasize that he must remain still to prevent distorting the images.
• Inform the patient that the entire procedure should take 60 to 90 minutes. Explain that the practitioner will compare the echocardiograms to diagnose his heart condition.

Explaining exercise echocardiography
If the patient will have an exercise stress test after the initial echocardiogram, cover these teaching points:
• Tell him he'll walk on the treadmill at a prescribed rate for a predetermined time to raise his heart rate. After he reaches the prescribed heart rate, he'll lie down and a second echocardiogram will be done.
• Explain that he may feel tired, sweaty, and slightly short of breath during the test. If his symptoms are severe or chest pain develops, the test will be stopped.
• Reassure him his blood pressure will be monitored during the test. After the test is complete, his ECG and blood pressure will be monitored for 10 minutes.

Describing the dobutamine stress test
If the patient will undergo a dobutamine stress test after the initial echocardiogram, cover these teaching points:
• Explain that an I.V. line will be inserted into his vein for the dobutamine infusion. Tell him this drug will increase his heart rate without exercise. Tell him to expect initial discomfort when the I.V. line is inserted. Mention that during the infusion, he may feel palpitations, shortness of breath, and fatigue.
• Inform the patient that a second echocardiogram will be done during the dobutamine infusion. After the drug is infused and his heart rate reaches the desired level, a third echocardiogram will be obtained.
• Reassure the patient that his blood pressure will be monitored during the test.

A different view

- For a left lateral view of the heart, the patient may be on his left side. To record heart function under various conditions, he's asked to inhale and exhale slowly, hold his breath, or inhale amyl nitrite.
- Doppler echocardiography may also be used in this examination. This technique assesses heart sounds and murmurs as they relate to cardiac hemodynamics.
- After the procedure, remove the conductive gel from the skin.

Transesophageal echocardiography

In transesophageal echocardiography (TEE), ultrasonography is combined with endoscopy to provide a better view of the heart's structures. A small transducer is attached to the end of a gastro-scope and inserted into the esophagus, allowing images to be taken from the posterior aspect of the heart. This causes less tissue penetration and interference from chest wall structures and produces high-quality images of the thoracic aorta (except for the superior ascending aorta, which is shadowed by the trachea).

This test is appropriate for inpatients and outpatients, for patients under general anesthesia, and for critically ill, intubated patients on ventilators.

What it all means

TEE can reveal thoracic and aortic disorders, endocarditis, congenital heart disease, intracardiac thrombi, and tumors; it can also evaluate valvular disease or repairs. Findings may include aortic dissection or aneurysm, mitral valve disease, or congenital defects such as patent ductus arteriosus. (See *Transesophageal echocardiography interference*, page 314.)

What needs to be done

- Explain the procedure to the patient. Tell him he'll need to fast for 6 hours before the test.
- Before the test, have the patient remove dentures or oral prostheses, and note loose teeth. Tell him he'll receive an I.V. sedative before the procedure. Ask the patient about any allergies, and note them on the chart. Make sure the patient or a responsible family member signs an informed consent form, if required.
- Have resuscitation equipment, including a suction apparatus, readily available.
- Connect the patient to monitors so his blood pressure, heart rate, and pulse oximetry values can be assessed.

Is there an echo in here? Transesophageal echocardiography evaluates aortic disorders, valvular heart disease, and problems with prosthetic devices.

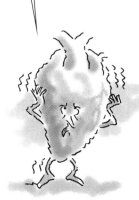

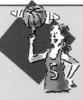

Stay on the ball

Transesophageal echocardiography interference

• Inability of the patient to cooperate or remain still may impair clear imaging.
• Improper adjustment of the equipment to accommodate obese or thin patients may impair clear imaging.
• Patients with chronic obstructive pulmonary disease and those on mechanical ventilators aren't good candidates for this test because excessive air in the lungs impedes movement of ultrasound waves.

TEE should be avoided in patients with esophageal obstruction or varices, GI bleeding, previous mediastinal radiation therapy, or severe cervical arthritis.

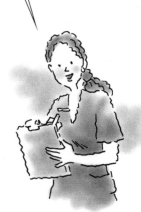

• Help the patient lie down on his left side, and administer the ordered sedative. Then the back of his throat is sprayed with a topical anesthetic. A bite block is placed in his mouth, and he's instructed to close his lips around it.
• The practitioner introduces the gastroscope and advances it. Ultrasound images are recorded and reviewed after the procedure.
• Monitor the patient's vital signs and oxygenation. Observe the cardiac monitor closely for a vasovagal response, which may occur with gagging.

TEE-time is over

• Keep the patient in a supine position until the sedative wears off.
• Encourage the patient to cough after the procedure, while lying on his side or sitting upright.
• Don't give the patient food or water until his gag reflex returns.
• Advise the outpatient to have someone drive him home.

Doppler ultrasonography

Doppler ultrasonography evaluates blood flow in the major blood vessels of the arms and legs and in the extracranial cerebrovascular system. A handheld transducer directs high-frequency sound waves to the artery or vein being tested. The sound waves strike moving red blood cells and are reflected back to the transducer at frequencies that correspond to blood-flow velocity through the vessel. The transducer then amplifies the sound waves to permit direct listening and graphic recording of blood flow. Measurement of systolic pressure helps detect the presence, location, and ex-

Now I get it!

How the Doppler probe works

The Doppler ultrasonic probe directs high-frequency sound waves through layers of tissue. When these waves strike red blood cells (RBCs) moving through the bloodstream, their frequency changes in proportion to the flow velocity of the RBCs. Recording these waves permits detection of arterial and venous obstruction but not quantitative blood flow measurement.

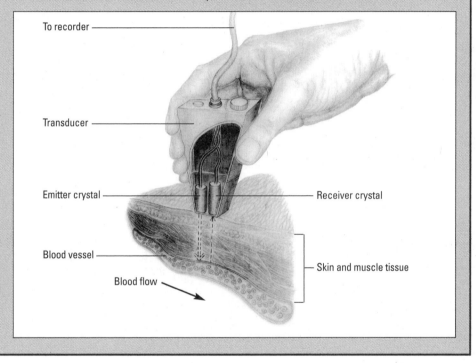

To recorder

Transducer

Emitter crystal

Receiver crystal

Blood vessel

Skin and muscle tissue

Blood flow

tent of peripheral arterial occlusive disease. (See *How the Doppler probe works.*)

Pulse volume recorder testing may be performed along with Doppler ultrasonography to yield a quantitative recording of changes in blood volume or flow in an extremity or organ.

What it all means

Arterial waveforms of the arms and leg are triphasic, with a prominent systolic component and one or more diastolic sounds. The ankle-arm pressure index (also called *arterial ischemia index*, *ankle-brachial index*, or *pedal-brachial index*) is the ratio between ankle systolic pressure and brachial systolic pressure, and is normally equal to or greater than 1. Proximal thigh pressure is normally 20 to 30 mm Hg higher than arm pressure, but pressure measurements at adjacent sites are similar. Normally, venous blood flow fluctuates with respiration, so observing changes in sound wave frequency during respiration helps detect venous occlusive disease. Compression maneuvers can also help detect occlusion of the veins as well as occlusion or stenosis of carotid arteries.

Abnormal images, pressure gradients and altered Doppler signals may indicate the presence of plaque, stenosis, occlusive disease, dissection, aneurysm, carotid body tumor, or arteritis. Confirmation or results may require venography, such as in cases of chronic venous insufficiency and varicose veins.

What needs to be done

• Explain the test to the patient. Check with the vascular laboratory to determine whether special equipment will be used and whether special instructions are necessary.
• Tell the patient that he'll be asked to move his arms to different positions and to perform breathing exercises as measurements are taken. A small ultrasonic probe resembling a microphone is placed at various sites along veins or arteries, and blood pressure is checked at several sites.
• Water-soluble conductive jelly is applied to the tip of the transducer to provide coupling between the skin and the transducer.

Evaluating peripheral arteries

• Peripheral arterial evaluation is always performed bilaterally. The usual test sites in the leg include the common femoral, superficial femoral, popliteal, posterior tibial, and dorsalis pedis arteries; in the arm, the subclavian, brachial, radial, ulnar and, occasionally, palmar arch and digital arteries.
• Instruct the patient to remove all clothing above or below the waist, depending on the test site. After he's placed in the supine position on the examination table or bed, with his arms at his sides, measure his brachial blood pressure and place the transducer at various points along the test arteries.
– Segmental limb blood pressure is obtained to localize arterial occlusive disease. For lower-extremity tests, a blood pressure cuff is wrapped around the calf, pressure readings are obtained, and waveforms are recorded from the dorsalis pedis and posterior tibial arteries. Then the cuff is wrapped around the thigh, and waveforms are recorded at the popliteal artery.
– For upper-extremity tests, a blood pressure cuff is wrapped around the forearm, pressure readings are taken, and waveforms

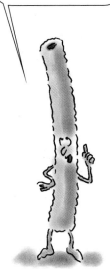

Doppler ultrasonography aids diagnosis of peripheral vascular disease and arterial occlusion, detects abnormal carotid blood flow, and monitors patients after arterial reconstruction and bypass grafts.

are recorded over both the radial and the ulnar arteries. Then the cuff is wrapped around the upper arm, pressure readings are taken, and waveforms are recorded with the transducer over the brachial artery.

• Blood pressure readings and waveform recordings are repeated with the arm in extreme hyperextension and hyperabduction to check for compression factors that may impede arterial blood flow. The upper extremity examination is performed on one arm, with the patient first in a supine position, then sitting. It's repeated on the other arm.

Evaluating peripheral veins

• The usual test sites in the leg are the popliteal, superficial femoral, and common femoral veins and the posterior tibial vein at the ankle; in the arm, the brachial, axillary, subclavian, and jugular veins and, occasionally, the inferior and superior venae cavae.

• Instruct the patient to remove all clothing above or below the waist, depending on the test site. He's placed in the supine position and instructed to breathe normally. The transducer is placed over the appropriate vein, waveforms are recorded, and respiratory modulations noted.

• Proximal limb compression maneuvers are performed and augmentation noted after release of compression, to evaluate venous valve competency. Changes in respiration are monitored. For lower-extremity tests, the patient is asked to perform Valsalva's maneuver, and venous blood flow is recorded. The procedure is repeated for the other arm or leg.

Evaluating extracranial cerebrovascular arteries

• The usual test sites include the supraorbital, common carotid, external carotid, internal carotid, and vertebral arteries.

• The patient is placed in the supine position on the examination table or bed, with a pillow beneath his head for support.

• Brachial blood pressure is then recorded, using the Doppler probe. Next, the transducer is positioned over the test artery, and blood-flow velocity is monitored and recorded. The influence of compression maneuvers on blood-flow velocity is measured, and the procedure is repeated on the opposite side. (See *Detecting thrombi with a Doppler probe*, page 318.)

• After the procedure, remove conductive jelly from the skin.

Now I get it!

Detecting thrombi with a Doppler probe

Typically, the Doppler probe is used to detect venous thrombi. Here's how it works.

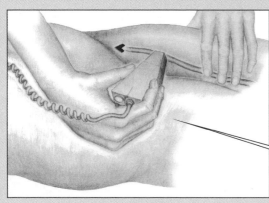

After the transducer is positioned properly, the blood vessel is occluded by compression, as shown here in a normal leg. Water-soluble conductive jelly is applied to the transducer's tip to provide coupling between the skin and the transducer.

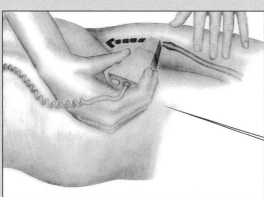

When pressure is released, blood flow resumes. The transducer picks up the sudden augmentation of the flow sound and permits graphic recording of blood blow. If a thrombus is present, compression fails to produce the augmented sound because blood flow, as shown here in the femoral vein, is impaired.

Miscellaneous tests

Breast ultrasound

During breast ultrasound, a transducer is guided over the breast area sending sound waves through the targeted tissue. These sound waves travel at various speeds, depending on the density of the tissue they're passing through. Also called *ultrasound mam-*

mography, this test is useful for differentiating between cystic, solid, and complex breast lesions, in detecting abnormalities in women with very dense breasts, and in fibrocystic breast disease. It may be used in pregnant women discovering a newly palpable mass in the breast, and in women with silicone prosthesis. Although it isn't optimal, it can also provide ultrasound evaluation as an alternative for those who refuse radiographic mammogram or in those who shouldn't be exposed to radiation. However, it isn't an appropriate method for visualizing the presence of microcalcifications.

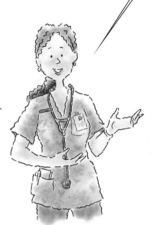

Breast ultrasound helps differentiate between cystic, solid, and complex breast lesions, and helps detect abnormalities in women with very dense breasts, and in fibrocystic breast disease.

What it all means

A normal breast ultrasound shows symmetric patterns in both breasts (this includes the subcutaneous tissue, mammary, and retromammary layers behind the breast).

Abnormal findings may include the presence of cysts, benign solid growths, malignant tumors, metastasis to muscle and lymph nodes, ductal ectasia, or enlarged lymph nodes. (See *Breast ultrasound interference*.)

What needs to be done

- Explain the purpose and procedure of the breast ultrasound. The patient may be shown a videotape explaining the test.
- Tell the patient that she'll be asked to remove clothing above the waistline and may be asked to wear a gown that opens in the front.
- If the breast ultrasound is to be used during a biopsy procedure, a signed informed consent form is required.
- A gel is applied to the exposed breast and a transducer is moved slowly across the breast. Some facilities may use an automated breast scanner whereby the patient must be positioned with the breast immersed in a tank of water. The tank contains transducers that move by remote control, presenting an image of the breast.
- After the test, the breasts are cleaned of gel and dried.

Abdominal ultrasonography

During abdominal ultrasonography, the technician guides a transducer over the area of the patient's body being evaluated. The transducer sends sound waves through the targeted tissue. These sound waves travel at various speeds, depending on the density of the tissue they're passing through.

Stay on the ball

Breast ultrasound interference

If the breast ultrasound is performed on the same day as radiographic mammogram, the patient shouldn't wear any powders, lotions, or other cosmetics to the upper body as it may alter test results.

Tissue densities

After passing through the tissue, sound waves reflect back to the transducer, and are converted into electrical impulses. These impulses are amplified and displayed on a screen. Because tissue densities vary, sound waves pass through them at different speeds. Images displayed on the screen reflect these differences. Cross-sectional images show different shades of gray, which depict various tissue densities. Ultrasound can provide images of many abdominal structures, including the gallbladder and biliary system, liver, spleen, and pancreas. In some patients requiring lower abdominal or pelvic organs (such as ovaries and fallopian tubes) to be assessed, a transvaginal ultrasound using a vaginal probe may be used to provide better visualization of organs.

> Abdominal ultrasound evaluates organ size and structure, differentiates between cysts and solid tumors, and monitors radiation or chemotherapy effects.

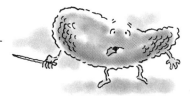

What it all means

A normal abdominal ultrasound shows the normal size, position, and appearance of the liver, gallbladder, bile ducts, pancreas, kidneys, adrenals, and spleen. It also helps visualize the abdominal aorta and inferior vena cava and their major tributaries.

Unwelcome guests

Abdominal ultrasound can detect:
• liver abnormalities, such as cysts, abscesses, tumors, and metastasis, cirrhosis, and variations in portal venous flow
• gallbladder and bile duct abnormalities, including duct dilation or obstruction, gallstones, cholecystitis, and tumors
• pancreas abnormalities, such as pancreatitis, pseudocyst, and cysts and tumors, including adenocarcinoma
• kidney abnormalities, including hydronephrosis, tumors, cysts, calculi, and abscesses
• adrenal abnormalities, such as pheochromocytoma, adrenal hemorrhage, and metastasis
• spleen abnormalities, including splenomegaly, lymph node enlargement, and trauma
• vascular abnormalities, such as abdominal aortic aneurysm, thrombi, and abnormal blood-flow patterns
• other abnormalities including ascites, congenital defects, and hematomas. (See *Abdominal ultrasonography interference.*)

What needs to be done

• Explain the procedure to the patient, and tell him he'll need to put on a hospital gown. Tell him he must remain still during scanning and hold his breath as requested to prevent a distorted image.

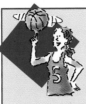

Stay on the ball

Abdominal ultrasonography interference

- Residual contrast media from studies done within the past 24 hours may distort or hinder imaging.
- In a dehydrated patient, body fluid deficiency may prevent ultrasonography from showing the boundaries between organs and tissue structures.
- Obesity interferes with ultrasound transmission, and fatty infiltration of the gland makes distinguishing the pancreas from surrounding tissue difficult.
- Residual barium in the colon or stomach may prevent visualization of the spleen.

- For some testing, the patient may be required to have a full bladder so that lower abdominal organs can be visualized. Check with the ultrasound department for specific testing requirements.

The nose knows

- For a gallbladder and biliary ultrasound, instruct the patient to eat a fat-free meal in the evening and then fast for 8 to 12 hours before the test. This promotes bile accumulation in the gallbladder and enhances ultrasonic visualization. The patient must keep fasting to prevent bile excretion in the gallbladder. Even smelling greasy foods, such as popcorn, can cause the gallbladder to empty.

Fasting before testing

- For ultrasonography of the liver, pancreas, or spleen, the patient must fast for 8 to 12 hours before the test to minimize bowel gas and motility.
- The patient is placed in a supine position.
- The area to be examined is coated with a water-soluble jelly. The transducer then scans the targeted area, projecting the images on the oscilloscope screen. These images are photographed for subsequent examination.
- The patient may be placed in right or left lateral positions for subsequent views and may be repositioned many times to get all necessary scans.
- After the procedure, clean the contact jelly from the skin.
- Tell the patient he may resume his usual diet.

Transcranial Doppler studies

By measuring the velocity of blood flow through cerebral arteries, transcranial Doppler studies provide information about the presence, quality, and changing nature of circulation to an area of the brain. Narrowed blood vessels produce high velocities, indicating possible stenosis or vasospasm. High velocities may also indicate an arteriovenous malformation caused by the accumulated signal from the extra blood flow associated with such lesions.

What it all means

The types of waveforms and velocities obtained indicate whether a pathologic condition exists. Although this test commonly isn't definitive, it provides diagnostic information noninvasively. Typically, high velocities are abnormal and suggest blood flow is too turbulent or the vessel is too narrow. (See *Comparing velocity waveforms*.)

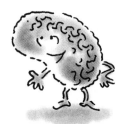

Transcranial Doppler studies measure blood flow in the brain and detect and monitor cerebral vasospasm progression.

Comparing velocity waveforms

A normal transcranial Doppler signal is usually characterized by mean velocities that fall within the normal reported values. Additional information can be gathered by evaluating the shape of the velocity waveform.

Effect of significant proximal vessel obstruction
A delayed systolic upstroke can be seen in a waveform when significant proximal vessel obstruction is present.

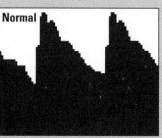
Normal

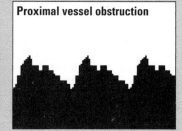
Proximal vessel obstruction

Effect of increased cerebrovascular resistance
Changes in cerebrovascular resistance, as occur with increased intracranial pressure, cause a decrease in diastolic flow.

Normal

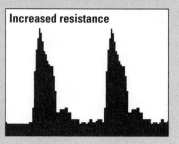
Increased resistance

What needs to be done

• Explain the purpose of the study to the patient or his family.

• The patient reclines in a chair or on a stretcher or bed. A small amount of gel is applied to the transcranial "window," an area where bone is thin enough to allow the Doppler signal to enter and be detected. The most common approaches are temporal, transorbital, and through the foramen magnum.

• The technician directs the signal toward the artery being studied and records the velocities detected. A complete study assesses the middle cerebral arteries, anterior cerebral arteries, ophthalmic arteries, carotid siphon, vertebral arteries, and basilar artery.

• The Doppler signal—measured in millimeters—can be transmitted to varying depths. Waveforms may be printed for later analysis. When the study is complete, wipe the gel away.

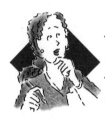

Quick quiz

1. Which statement about M-mode echocardiography is *true?*
   A. A single ultrasound beam strikes the heart using an "ice-pick" view of cardiac structures.
   B. An ultrasound beam sweeps through an arc, producing a fan-shaped view of cardiac structures.
   C. The lateral motion and correct spatial relationships between cardiac structures are recorded.
   D. Retrospective tissues are examined using ultrasound.

Answer: A. In M-mode echocardiography, a single, pencil-like ultrasound beam strikes the heart, producing an "ice-pick," or vertical, view of cardiac structures. This method is especially useful for precise recording of the motion and dimensions of intracardiac structures.

2. When used during echocardiography, amyl nitrate:
   A. has no adverse effects.
   B. is administered by inhalation.
   C. is administered I.V.
   D. is administered orally.

Answer: B. A sweet-smelling gas, amyl nitrate is administered by inhalation during echocardiography.

3.   When teaching a patient about TEE, be sure to mention that:
A.   he doesn't have to restrict his intake before the test.
B.   he doesn't have to remove his dentures before the test.
C.   no complications are associated with the test.
D.   his throat will be sprayed with a topical anesthetic just before the test.

Answer: D. Tell the patient that his throat will be sprayed with a topical anesthetic and that he may gag when the tube is inserted.

4.   Which statement about venous thrombosis is *false*?
A.   It can be detected during Doppler ultrasound.
B.   It can be found during a physical exam.
C.   It causes no change in venous blood-flow velocity in response to Valsalva's maneuver.
D.   It causes a change in venous blood-flow velocity with respirations.

Answer: D. Venous thrombosis is present if venous blood-flow velocity is unchanged by respiration, doesn't increase in response to compression or Valsalva's maneuver, or is absent.

5.   Before an ultrasound of the gallbladder and biliary system, the patient must:
A.   fast for 4 to 6 hours.
B.   eat a high-fat meal.
C.   avoid greasy food odors.
D.   consume only liquids for 3 days before the test.

Answer: C. The odor of greasy foods, such as popcorn, can cause the gallbladder to empty and should be avoided before the test.

Scoring

☆☆☆   If you answered all five questions correctly, yahoo! You're an ultrasonic superstar!

☆☆   If you answered four questions correctly, super! Your comprehension is ultra sound!

☆   If you answered fewer than three questions correctly, don't dunk your Doppler just yet! You'll get the hang of it before long!

Radiography

11

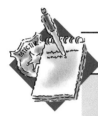

Just the facts

In this chapter, you'll learn:

♦ about radiographic procedures and how they're performed

♦ the patient care associated with these tests

♦ factors that can interfere with these tests

♦ what radiographic results may indicate.

A look at radiography

In radiography, also called *roentgenography*, X-ray beams penetrate bone and tissue and react on specially sensitized film. Soft and bony tissue are evaluated by these short-wave electromagnetic vibrations. X-ray beams travel in straight lines, and as they pass through matter, some of their intensity is absorbed. The denser the matter, the greater the degree of X-ray absorption. Tissue density is displayed in shades of black, white, and gray, much like a negative print of a photograph. Dense structures will appear white; an air-filled area will appear black.

Before radiography, explain the procedure to the patient to ease anxiety. If contrast medium will be used, check the patient's history for hypersensitivity.

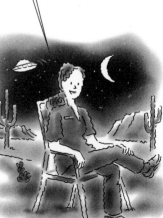

Beam me up! Radiography uses X-ray beams that penetrate bone and tissue.

Neurologic system

Skull radiography

Although skull radiography is of limited value in assessing patients with head injuries, skull X-rays are extremely valuable for studying abnormalities of the skull base and cranial vault, congenital and perinatal anomalies, and systemic diseases that produce bone defects of the skull. Skull X-rays may be done before magnetic resonance imaging (MRI) to detect metal fragments. For more accurate assessment of head injuries as well as of skull and head abnormalities, nonenhanced computed tomography (CT) studies of the head are done.

Skull radiography evaluates the three groups of bones that make up the skull: the calvaria (vault), the mandible (jaw) bone, and the facial bones. The calvaria and the facial bones are closely connected by immovable joints with irregular serrated edges called *sutures*. The skull bones form an anatomic structure so complex that complete skull examination requires several radiologic views of each area.

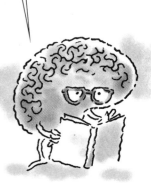

Skull radiography can detect fractures in patients who have suffered head trauma. It also aids diagnosis of pituitary tumors and detects congenital anomalies.

What it all means

A radiologist interprets the X-rays, evaluating the size, shape, thickness, and position of cranial bones as well as the vascular markings, sinuses, and sutures; all should be normal for the patient's age.

Skull radiography can confirm fractures, although basilar fractures may not show on the film if the bone is dense. This test may confirm congenital anomalies and may show erosion, enlargement, or decalcification of the sella turcica caused by increased intracranial pressure (ICP).

Skull X-rays may also show abnormal areas of calcification in such conditions as osteomyelitis (with possible calcification of the skull itself) and chronic subdural hematomas. They can detect neoplasms within the brain that contain calcium. Radiography may also detect other changes in bone structure; for example, those associated with such metabolic disorders as acromegaly or Paget's disease.

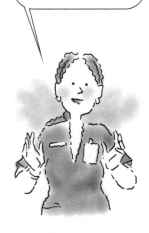

Carefully immobilizing the patient's head during skull radiography can increase his comfort while improving results.

What needs to be done

• Explain the procedure to the patient and tell him he doesn't need to restrict food and fluids before the test. Instruct him to remove glasses, dentures, jewelry, and other metal objects in the radiographic field.

• The patient is placed in the supine position on an X-ray table or seated in a chair and is instructed to keep still while X-rays are taken. A head band, foam pads, or sandbags may be used to immobilize his head and increase comfort. Don't hyperextend or flex the head if cervical injuries are unknown or suspected.

• Routinely, five views are taken: left and right lateral, anteroposterior Towne's, posteroanterior Caldwell's, and axial (or base). Images are developed and checked for quality before the patient leaves the area.

Cerebral angiography

Cerebral angiography allows radiographic examination of the cerebral blood vessels after injection of a contrast medium. Possible injection sites include the femoral, carotid, and brachial arteries. The femoral artery is used most commonly because it allows visualization of four vessels (the carotid and vertebral arteries).

Usually this test is performed on patients with suspected abnormality of the cerebral vasculature; abnormalities may be suggested by intracranial CT, lumbar puncture, MRI, or magnetic resonance angiography.

What it all means

Use of a contrast medium allows visualization of superficial and deep arteries and arterioles as well as superficial and deep veins. The finding of apparently normal (symmetrical) cerebral blood vessels, however, must be correlated with the patient's history and clinical status. (See *Comparing cerebral angiograms*, page 328.)

Suggestive vessels

Changes in the caliber of the vessel's lumina suggests vascular disease possibly resulting from spasms, plaques, fistulas, arteriovenous malformation, or arteriosclerosis. Diminished blood flow to vessels may be related to increased ICP.

Vessel displacement may reflect tumor presence and size, areas of edema, or obstruction of the cerebrospinal fluid (CSF) pathway. Cerebral angiography may also show circulation within a tumor, giving precise information on the tumor's position and nature. Meningeal blood supply originating in the external carotid artery may indicate an extracerebral tumor but usually designates a meningioma. Such a tumor may arise outside the brain substance but still be within the cerebral hemisphere. Treatments may also be administered during the procedure by the interventional radiologist, such as placement of stents or coiling, for abnormalities such as aneurysms, vessel stenosis, or arteriovenous malformations.

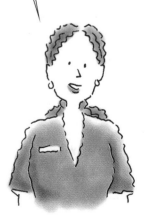

Cerebral angiography helps detect changes in the caliber of cerebral blood vessels.

What needs to be done

• Explain the procedure to the patient. Instruct him to fast for 8 to 10 hours before the test. If ordered, a sedative and an anticholinergic will be given 30 to 45 minutes before the test. Tell the patient that he'll be asked to wear a hospital gown and to remove

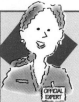

Advice from the experts

Comparing cerebral angiograms

These angiograms show the differences between normal and abnormal cerebral vasculature.

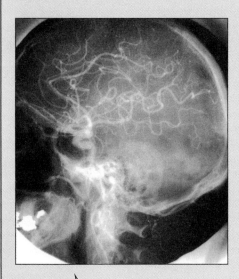

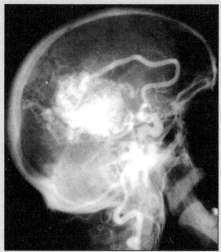

This cerebral angiogram is normal.

This cerebral angiogram shows occluded blood vessels caused by a large arteriovenous malformation.

As in all tests, careful review of the patient history is the key to safe, effective testing. With cerebral angiography, look for iodine hypersensitivity.

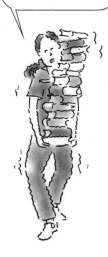

jewelry, dentures, hairpins, and other metal objects in the radiographic field.

• Make sure that pretest blood work results are on the chart to determine bleeding tendency or kidney function.

• The patient may need to discontinue medications such as aspirin or other anticoagulants for 3 days before testing, as ordered.

Historically speaking

• Make sure the patient or responsible family member has signed an informed consent form if required. Check the patient history for hypersensitivity to iodine, iodine-containing substances (such as shellfish), or other contrast media. Also check for contraindications, such as hepatic, renal, or thyroid disease. Mark hypersensitivities on the patient's chart, and notify the practitioner; he may order prophylactic drugs or may cancel the test.

• The patient is placed in the supine position on a radiographic table, and the injection site (femoral, carotid, or brachial artery) is clipped. He's instructed to lie still with his arms at his sides. The skin is cleaned with an antiseptic solution. The local anesthetic is then injected. Sterile technique is used during the procedure.

• The practitioner punctures the artery with the appropriate needle and catheterizes it. If the femoral approach is used, a catheter is threaded up the aortic arch. If the carotid artery is used, the patient hyperextends his neck, and a rolled-up towel or a sandbag is placed under his shoulders. His head is then immobilized with a restraint or tape. If the brachial artery (least common) is used, a blood pressure cuff is placed distal to the puncture site and inflated before injection to prevent the contrast medium from flowing into the forearm and hand.

Contrast medium

• After verifying needle (or catheter) placement by X-ray or fluoroscopy, contrast medium is injected and the patient is observed for a reaction, such as urticaria, flushing, and laryngeal stridor. A first series of lateral and anteroposterior X-rays is taken, developed, and reviewed. Depending on the results of this series, more contrast medium may be injected and another series of X-rays taken. Arterial catheter patency is maintained by continuous or periodic flushing with normal saline solution or heparin solution. Vital and neurologic signs, as well as distal pulses, are monitored throughout the test.

• After obtaining an acceptable series of X-rays, the needle (or catheter) is withdrawn. Firm pressure is applied to the puncture site for 15 minutes.

• The patient is observed for bleeding, distal pulses are checked, and a pressure bandage is applied.

Enforce and observe

• Enforce bed rest for 6 to 8 hours and provide pain medication, as ordered. Monitor vital signs and neurologic status for 24 hours—every hour for the first 4 hours, then every 4 hours.

• Check the puncture site for signs of extravasation, such as redness and swelling. To ease the patient's discomfort and minimize swelling, apply an ice bag to the site. If bleeding occurs, apply firm pressure on the puncture site and inform the practitioner.

Femoral approach

• If the femoral approach was used, keep the affected leg straight for at least 6 hours, and routinely check pulses distal to the site. Check the affected leg's temperature, color, and tactile sensations because thrombosis or hematoma can occlude blood flow. Extravasation can also block blood flow by exerting pressure on the artery.

Carotid artery angle

• If a carotid artery was used as the injection site, watch for dysphagia or respiratory distress, which can result from hematoma or extravasation. Also watch for disorientation and weakness or numbness in the extremities (signs of thrombosis or hematoma) and for arterial spasms, which produce symptoms of transient ischemic attacks. Notify the practitioner if abnormal signs develop.

Brachial route

• If the brachial approach was used, immobilize the arm for at least 6 hours, and routinely check the radial pulse. Place a sign above the patient's bed warning personnel against taking blood pressure readings from the affected arm. Observe the arm and hand, noting any change in color, temperature, or tactile sensations. If they become pale, cool, or numb, notify the practitioner.
• Tell the patient to resume his usual diet.
• For patients who have been receiving aspirin daily, take extra care to compress the puncture site.

Myelography

Myelography combines fluoroscopy and radiography to evaluate the spinal subarachnoid space after injection of a contrast medium. Because the contrast medium is heavier than CSF, it will flow through the subarachnoid space to the dependent area when the patient, lying prone on a fluoroscopic table, is tilted up or down. The fluoroscope allows visualization of the flow of the contrast medium and the outline of the subarachnoid space. X-rays are taken for a permanent record. The radiographic myelogram may be followed by CT imaging for a more thorough analysis of disk spaces of interest and to detect spinal compression.

What it all means

The contrast medium should flow freely through the subarachnoid space, showing no obstruction or structural abnormalities.

The meaning of lesions

This test can identify and localize lesions within or surrounding the spinal cord or subarachnoid space. Common extradural lesions include herniated intervertebral disks and metastatic tumors. Common lesions within the subarachnoid space include neurofibromas and meningiomas; within the spinal cord, ependymomas and astrocytomas. This test may also detect syringo-myelia, a congenital abnormality marked by fluid-filled cavities in the spinal cord and widening of the cord itself. Myelography may also detect arachnoiditis, spinal nerve root injury, and tumors in the posterior fossa of the skull. Test results must be correlated with the patient's history and clinical status.

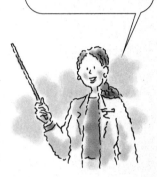

Myelography helps locate a spinal lesion, a ruptured disk, spinal stenosis, or an abscess. It also helps detect arachnoiditis, spinal nerve root injury, and skull tumors.

What needs to be done

• Explain the procedure to the patient. Instruct him to restrict food and fluids for 8 hours before the test.

Consenting adults

• Make sure an informed consent form has been signed. Check the patient's history for hypersensitivity to iodine and iodine-containing substances (such as shellfish), contrast media, and drugs associated with the procedure. Also check for such contraindications as increased ICP or an infection at the puncture site. Notify the radiologist of a history of epilepsy or phenothiazine use. Phenothiazines given with metrizamide during myelography increase the risk of toxicity.

Pretest preliminaries

• Before the test, tell the patient that the head of his bed must be elevated for 6 to 8 hours after the test.
• Instruct the patient to remove jewelry and metal objects in the X-ray field.
• If the puncture is to be performed in the lumbar region, an enema may be ordered.
• A sedative and an anticholinergic, such as atropine sulfate, may be ordered to reduce swallowing during the procedure.

Position and puncture

• The patient may receive a cisternal puncture if lumbar deformity or infection at the puncture site exists. A lumbar puncture is performed. Fluoroscopy verifies proper needle position in the subarachnoid space. Some CSF may be removed for routine laboratory analysis.

Reassure, reposition, and rest

• The patient is then turned to the prone position.
• The contrast medium is injected. If a subarachnoid space obstruction blocks the upward flow of the contrast medium, a cisternal puncture may be performed. The flow of the contrast medium is studied on the fluoroscope, and X-rays are taken.

Now I get it!

Removing contrast media after myelography

Some types of contrast media must be removed after myelography, whereas others are left to be absorbed by the body.

A more mellow medium

Metrizamide is water-soluble and doesn't have to be removed. After it's absorbed into the bloodstream, the kidneys excrete it. However, the patient will need to have his head elevated at least 30 degrees for at least 8 hours because the contrast media can irritate cervical nerve roots and cranial structures.

When removal is a must

Some contrast media, such as Iophendylate, must be removed after the procedure because they aren't water-soluble and won't be excreted. Left in the body, they could cause inflammation or adhesive arachnoiditis. The contrast medium pools in the lumbar region when the patient is in the prone position, facilitating aspiration. If the patient is on his side, (the usual position for lumbar puncture), the dye may be aspirated or allowed to drip from the needle.

Removal of contrast media may cause pain in the buttocks or legs from nerve root irritation. The patient will need to lie flat 8 to 12 hours after receiving oil-based contrast media.

• The contrast medium is withdrawn, if oil-based, and the needle is withdrawn. The puncture site is cleaned and a small dressing is applied. (See *Removing contrast media after myelography.*)
• If a spinal tumor is confirmed, the patient may go directly to the operating room.

Special aftercare

• If the patient received a water-based contrast medium, elevate the head of the bed 30 to 45 degrees for 6 to 8 hours.
• Monitor vital signs, neurologic status, and intake and output. Encourage the patient to drink extra fluids. Notify the practitioner if the patient fails to void within 8 hours after returning to his room.
• If fever, back pain, or signs of meningeal irritation (headache, irritability, or neck stiffness) develop, keep the room quiet and dark, and provide an analgesic or an antipyretic, as ordered.
• The patient may resume his usual diet and activities the day after the test.

> Encourage oral fluids after myelography to help the patient flush out the contrast dye.

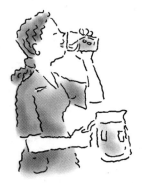

Respiratory system

Chest radiography

In chest radiography (commonly known as *chest X-ray*), X-ray beams penetrate the chest and react on specially sensitized film. Because normal pulmonary tissue is primarily radiolucent, such abnormalities as infiltrates, foreign bodies, fluids, and tumors appear as densities on the film. A chest X-ray is most useful when compared with the patient's previous images because it allows the radiologist to detect changes.

What it all means

For normal and abnormal findings, see *Selected clinical implications of chest X-ray films*, pages 334 and 335. For accurate diagnosis, radiography findings must be correlated with additional radiologic and pulmonary tests as well as with physical assessment findings. Pulmonary hyperinflation with low diaphragm and generalized increased radiolucency may suggest emphysema but may also appear in a healthy person's X-rays.

What needs to be done

- Describe the procedure to the patient.
- Provide a gown without snaps, and ask the patient to remove all jewelry in the radiographic field. Tell him he'll be asked to take a deep breath and hold it momentarily while the film is being taken, to provide a clear view of pulmonary structures.
- For a stationary radiography machine, the patient stands or sits in front of the machine so that films can be taken of the postero-anterior and left lateral views.
- For a portable radiography machine, used at the patient's bedside, help position the patient. Because an upright chest X-ray is preferable, move the patient to the top of the bed if this position can be tolerated. Elevate the head of the bed for maximum upright positioning. Move cardiac monitoring cables, oxygen tubing, I.V. tubing from subclavian lines, pulmonary artery catheter lines, and safety pins as far out of the radiographic field as possible.
- If the patient is intubated, check that no tubes have been dislodged during positioning.
- To avoid exposure to radiation, leave the room or the immediate area while the films are being taken. If you must stay in the area, wear a lead-lined apron.

Chest X-ray helps detect filtrates, foreign bodies, and tumors.

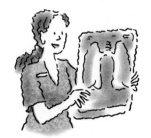

Selected clinical implications of chest X-ray films

Normal anatomic location and appearance	Possible abnormality	Implications
Trachea Visible midline in the anterior mediastinal cavity; translucent tubelike appearance	• Deviation from midline	• Tension pneumothorax, atelectasis, pleural effusion, consolidation, mediastinal nodes or, in children, enlarged thymus
	• Narrowing with hourglass appearance and deviation to one side	• Substernal thyroid or stenosis secondary to trauma
Heart Visible in the anterior left mediastinal cavity; solid appearance due to blood contents; edges may be clear in contrast with surrounding air density of the lung	• Shift	• Atelectasis, pneumothorax
	• Hypertrophy of right heart	• Cor pulmonale, heart failure
	• Cardiac borders obscured by stringy densities ("shaggy heart")	• Cystic fibrosis
Mediastinum (mediastinal shadow) Visible as the space between the lungs; shadowy appearance that widens at the hilum of the lungs	• Deviation to nondiseased side; deviation to diseased side by traction	• Pleural effusion or tumor, fibrosis or collapsed lung
	• Gross widening	• Neoplasms of esophagus, bronchi, lungs, thyroid, thymus, peripheral nerves, lymphoid tissue; aortic aneurysm; mediastinitis; cor pulmonale
Ribs Visible as thoracic cavity encasement	• Break or misalignment	• Fractured sternum or ribs
	• Widening of intercostal spaces	• Emphysema
Spine Visible midline in the posterior chest; straight bony structure	• Spinal curvature	• Scoliosis, kyphosis
	• Break or misalignment	• Fractures
Clavicles Visible in upper thorax; intact and equidistant in properly centered X-ray films	• Break or misalignment	• Fractures

Selected clinical implications of chest X-ray films (continued)

Normal anatomic location and appearance	Possible abnormality	Implications
Hila (lung roots) Visible above the heart, where pulmonary vessels, bronchi, and lymph nodes join the lungs; appear as small, white, bilateral densities	• Shift to one side	• Atelectasis
	• Accentuated shadows	• Pneumothorax, emphysema, pulmonary abscess, tumor, enlarged lymph nodes
Mainstem bronchus Visible; part of the hila with translucent tubelike appearance	• Spherical or oval density	• Bronchogenic cyst
Bronchi Usually not visible	• Visible	• Bronchial pneumonia
Lung fields Usually not visible throughout, except for the blood vessels	• Visible	• Atelectasis
	• Irregular	• Resolving pneumonia, infiltrates, silicosis, fibrosis, metastatic neoplasm
Hemidiaphragm Rounded, visible; right side $3/8''$ to $3/4''$ (1 to 2 cm)	• Elevation of diaphragm (difference in elevation can be measured on inspiration and expiration to detect movement)	• Active tuberculosis, pneumonia, pleurisy, acute bronchitis, active disease of the abdominal viscera, bilateral phrenic nerve involvement, atelectasis
	• Flattening of diaphragm	• Asthma, emphysema
	• Unilateral elevation of either side	• Possible unilateral phrenic nerve paresis
	• Unilateral elevation of left side only	• Perforated ulcer (rare), gas distention of stomach or splenic flexure of colon, free air in abdomen

Fluoroscopy

In fluoroscopy, a continuous stream of X-rays passes through the patient, allowing real-time visualization of the heart, lungs, and diaphragm on a video monitor. It's indicated when visualization of physiologic or pathologic motion of thoracic contents is needed, such as when ruling out paralysis in patients with diaphragmatic elevation or visualizing placement while inserting a central venous catheter.

What it all means

Normal diaphragmatic movement is synchronous and symmetrical. Normal diaphragmatic excursion ranges from $3/4''$ to $1^5/8''$ (2 to 4 cm).

Diminished excursion

Diminished diaphragmatic movement may indicate pulmonary disease. Increased lung translucency (not transparent but permitting light passage) may indicate elasticity loss or bronchiolar obstruction. In elderly people, the lowest part of the trachea may be displaced to the right by an elongated aorta. Diminished or paradoxical diaphragmatic movement may indicate diaphragmatic paralysis, which sometimes occurs after open-heart surgery. However, fluoroscopy may not detect such paralysis if the patient compensates for diminished diaphragm function by forcefully contracting abdominal muscles to aid expiration.

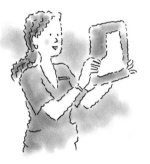

Fluoroscopy can detect bronchiolar obstructions and pulmonary disease. It also aids catheter placement.

What needs to be done

• Describe the procedure to the patient, and explain that this test assesses respiratory structures and their motion. Tell the patient that the test usually takes 5 minutes.
• Instruct the patient to remove all metallic objects, including jewelry, in the X-ray field.
• If necessary, assist with patient positioning. Move cardiac monitoring cables, I.V. tubing from subclavian lines, pulmonary artery catheter lines, and safety pins as far as possible from the X-ray field. During the test, cardiopulmonary motion is observed on a screen.
• If the patient is intubated, check that no tubes have been dislodged during positioning.
• To avoid exposure to radiation, leave the room or the immediate area during the test; if you must stay, wear a lead-lined apron.

Pulmonary angiography

Pulmonary angiography, also known as *pulmonary arteriography*, is the radiographic examination of the pulmonary circulation after injection of a radiopaque contrast agent into the pulmonary artery or one of its branches. This procedure is usually used to confirm symptomatic pulmonary emboli when scans prove nondiagnostic (especially before anticoagulant therapy) or are contraindicated. It also provides accurate preoperative evaluation of patients with congenital heart disease.

Complicating factors

Possible complications include arterial occlusion, myocardial perforation or rupture, ventricular arrhythmias from myocardial irritation, and acute renal failure from hypersensitivity to the contrast agent; bleeding, hematoma formation, or infection may occur at the catheter insertion site.

What it all means

The contrast agent should flow symmetrically and without interruption through the pulmonary circulatory system. Interruption of blood flow may result from emboli, vascular filling defects, or stenosis.

What needs to be done

• Explain the procedure to the patient. Instruct him to fast for 8 hours before the test, or as ordered.

Pretest precautions

• Make sure the patient or a responsible family member has signed the informed consent form. Check his history for hypersensitivity to anesthetics, iodine, seafood, radiographic contrast agents, or anticoagulants, and check for contraindications such as pregnancy. Obtain or check laboratory tests, including prothrombin time, partial thromboplastin time, platelet count, and blood urea nitrogen (BUN) and serum creatinine levels, and notify the radiologist of abnormal results. I.V. hydration may need to be considered, depending on the patient's renal and cardiac status. The radiologist may want to discontinue a heparin infusion 3 to 4 hours before the test.
• Keep emergency equipment available in case of a hypersensitivity reaction to the contrast agent.
• After the patient is placed in a supine position, the local anesthetic is injected and the cardiac monitor is attached to the patient. Blood pressure and pulse oximeter are monitored as per facility protocol. The practitioner makes a puncture at the procedure site and introduces a catheter into the antecubital or femoral vein.

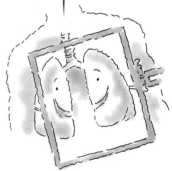

Pulmonary angiography helps detect pulmonary embolism, locate emboli, and evaluate abnormal pulmonary circulation.

Safe passage

• As the catheter passes through the right atrium, right ventricle, and pulmonary artery, the pressures are measured and blood samples are drawn from various regions of the pulmonary circulation.
• Monitor for ventricular arrhythmias caused by myocardial irritation from passage of the catheter through the heart chambers.
• The contrast agent is injected, which circulates through the pulmonary artery and lung capillaries while X-rays are taken.
• Observe for signs and symptoms of hypersensitivity to the contrast agent, such as dyspnea, nausea, vomiting, sweating, increased heart rate, and numbness of extremities.

When it's over

• Have the patient maintain bed rest for about 6 hours.
• Check blood pressure, pulse rate, and the catheter insertion site every 15 minutes for 1 hour, every hour for 4 hours, and then every 4 hours for 16 hours.

Trouble on the way

• Apply pressure over the catheter insertion site for 15 to 20 minutes or until bleeding stops. Observe the site for bleeding and swelling. If they occur, maintain pressure at the insertion site for 10 minutes and notify the practitioner.
• Observe for signs of myocardial perforation or rupture by monitoring vital signs as ordered.
• Be alert for signs of acute renal failure, such as sudden onset of oliguria, nausea, and vomiting. Check BUN and serum creatinine levels.
• Report evidence of a delayed hypersensitivity reaction to the contrast agent or local anesthetic—dyspnea, itching, tachycardia, palpitations, hypotension or hypertension, excitation, and euphoria.
• Measure pulmonary artery pressures. Right ventricular end-diastolic pressure is usually less than or equal to 20 mm Hg, and pulmonary artery systolic pressure is usually less than or equal to 70 mm Hg. Pressures greater than this increase the risk of mortality associated with this procedure.

Back to normal

• Advise the patient of any activity restrictions, and tell him he may resume his usual diet.
• Encourage the patient to drink fluids, or give him I.V. fluids to help flush the contrast agent from his body.

Gastrointestinal system

Barium swallow

Barium swallow, also known as *esophagography*, is the radiographic or fluoroscopic examination of the pharynx and the fluoroscopic examination of the esophagus after ingestion of thick and thin mixtures of barium sulfate. This test, most commonly performed as part of the upper GI series, is indicated for patients with a history of dysphagia and regurgitation. Further testing is usually required for a definitive diagnosis. Cholangiography and the barium enema test, if ordered, may precede the barium swallow because ingested barium may obscure anatomic details on the X-rays.

What it all means

After the barium is swallowed, it pours over the base of the tongue into the pharynx. A peristaltic wave propels it through the entire length of the esophagus in about 2 seconds. When the peristaltic wave reaches the base of the esophagus, the cardiac sphincter opens, allowing the barium to enter the stomach. After passage of the barium, the cardiac sphincter closes. Normally, it evenly fills and distends the lumen of the pharynx and esophagus, and the mucosa appears smooth and regular.

Inside view

Barium swallow may reveal reflux, hiatal hernia, diverticula, or presence of varices. Although strictures, tumors, polyps, ulcers, and motility disorders, such as pharyngeal muscular disorders, esophageal spasms, and achalasia (cardiospasm), may be detected, a definitive diagnosis requires endoscopic biopsy or, for motility disorders, manometric studies. (See *GI motility study*, page 340.)

What needs to be done

• Explain to the patient that this test evaluates the function of the pharynx and esophagus. Instruct the patient to fast after midnight before the test. If the patient is an infant, delay feeding to ensure complete digestion of barium.
• Tell the patient he'll first receive a barium mixture to drink during the examination. Inform him that he'll be placed in various positions on a tilting X-ray table and that X-rays will be taken.

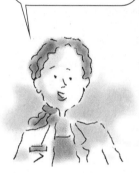

A barium swallow diagnoses hiatal hernia, diverticula, and varices. It also helps detect strictures, ulcers, tumors, polyps, and motility disorders.

Now I get it!

GI motility study

When intestinal disease is strongly suspected, the GI motility study may follow the upper GI and small-bowel series. This study, which evaluates intestinal motility and the integrity of the mucosal lining, records barium passage through the lower digestive tract.

Riding the time line

About 6 hours after barium ingestion, the head of the barium column is usually in the hepatic flexure and the tail is in the terminal ileum. The barium completely opacifies the large intestine by 24 hours after ingestion.

Because the amount of barium passing through the large intestine isn't sufficient to fully extend the lumen, spot films taken 24, 48, or 72 hours after barium ingestion prove inferior to the barium enema. However, when spot films suggest intestinal abnormalities, the barium enema and colonoscopy can provide more specific, confirming diagnostic information.

- If gastric reflux is suspected, withhold antacids, histamine-2 (H_2) blockers, and proton pump inhibitors, as ordered. Just before the procedure, instruct the patient to put on a hospital gown without snap closures and to remove jewelry, dentures, hairpins, and other radiopaque objects from the X-ray field.
- Check the patient history for contraindications to the barium swallow, such as intestinal obstruction and pregnancy. Radiation may have teratogenic effects.
- The patient is placed in an upright position behind the fluoroscopic screen and undergoes examination of his heart, lungs, and abdomen. He's then instructed to take one swallow of the thick barium mixture, after which the pharyngeal action is recorded. The patient is then told to take several swallows of the thin barium mixture. The passage of the barium is examined fluoroscopically, and spot films of the esophageal region are taken.

Location, location, location

- Esophageal strictures and obstruction of the esophageal lumen by the lower esophageal ring are best detected when the patient is upright.
- The patient is then secured to the X-ray table and is rotated to the Trendelenburg position to evaluate esophageal peristalsis or to demonstrate hiatal hernia and gastric reflux. Again, he's instructed to take several swallows of barium while the esophagus is examined fluoroscopically, and spot films of significant findings are taken when indicated.

• After the table is rotated to a horizontal position, the patient is told to take several swallows of barium so that the esophagogastric junction and peristalsis can be evaluated. The passage of barium is then fluoroscopically observed, and spot films of significant findings are taken with the patient in supine and prone positions.

• During fluoroscopic examination of the esophagus, the cardia and fundus of the patient's stomach are also carefully studied because neoplasms in these areas may invade the esophagus and cause obstruction.

• The patient may resume his usual diet, as ordered, after all images are completed. Check with radiology to see if additional images or repeat fluoroscopic evaluation are required before resuming diet.

• Instruct the patient to drink plenty of fluids, unless contraindicated, and administer a cathartic, if ordered, to help eliminate the barium. (See *After barium swallow*.)

• Check the patient for abdominal distention and absent bowel sounds, which are associated with constipation and may suggest barium impaction.

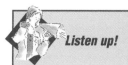

Listen up!

After barium swallow

After your patient undergoes barium swallow, inform him that his stools will be chalky and light-colored for 24 to 72 hours. Explain that barium retained in the intestine may harden, causing obstruction. Tell him to notify the practitioner if he hasn't had a bowel movement in 2 to 3 days.

Upper GI and small-bowel series

The upper GI and small-bowel series test involves the fluoroscopic examination of the esophagus, stomach, and small intestine after the patient ingests barium, a contrast agent. As the barium passes through the digestive tract, fluoroscopy shows peristalsis and the mucosal contours of the respective organs, and spot films record significant findings. This test is indicated for patients who have upper GI symptoms (difficulty swallowing, regurgitation, burning or gnawing epigastric pain), signs of small-bowel disease (diarrhea, weight loss), and signs of GI bleeding (hematemesis, melena).

Before and after

Although this test can detect various mucosal abnormalities, many patients need a biopsy afterward to rule out cancer or to distinguish specific inflammatory diseases. Endoscopy, barium enema, and routine X-rays should always precede this test because retained barium interferes with visualization.

What it all means

After the barium suspension is swallowed, it's propelled by a peristaltic wave through the cardiac sphincter to enter the stomach. Then the cardiac sphincter closes and barium enters the stomach's outlining folds, called *rugae*. When the stomach is complete-

The upper GI and small-bowel series help detect hiatal hernia, diverticula, varices, and motility disorders. They also aid in diagnosis of strictures, ulcers, tumors, and malabsorption syndrome.

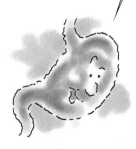

ly filled with barium, its outline appears smooth and regular without evidence of flattened, rigid areas that suggest lesions.

Looping through the duodenum

After barium enters the stomach, it quickly empties into the duodenal bulb. Circular folds become apparent as barium enters the duodenal loop. These folds deepen and become more numerous in the jejunum. Barium temporarily lodges between these folds, producing a speckled pattern on the X-ray film. As barium enters the ileum, the circular folds become less prominent and, except for their broadness, resemble those in the duodenum. The film also shows that the diameter of the small intestine tapers gradually from the duodenum to the ileum.

Experiencing the esophagus

Radiographic studies of the esophagus may reveal strictures, tumors, hiatal hernia, diverticula, varices, and ulcers (particularly in the distal esophagus). Benign strictures usually dilate the esophagus, whereas malignant ones cause erosive changes in the mucosa. Tumors produce filling defects in the column of barium, but only malignant ones change the mucosal contour. Nevertheless, a biopsy is necessary for a definitive diagnosis of esophageal strictures and tumors.

Erratic behavior

Motility disorders such as esophageal spasm are usually difficult to detect because spasms are erratic and transient. Achalasia is strongly suggested when the distal esophagus appears to narrow. Gastric reflux appears as a backflow of barium from the stomach into the esophagus.

Searching the stomach

Radiographic studies of the stomach may reveal tumors and ulcers. Malignant tumors, usually adenocarcinomas, appear as filling defects and usually disrupt peristalsis. Benign tumors, such as adenomatous polyps and leiomyomas, appear as outpouchings of the gastric mucosa and generally don't affect peristalsis. Ulcers occur most commonly in the stomach and duodenum, particularly in the duodenal bulb. Benign ulcers usually show evidence of partial or complete healing and are characterized by radiating folds extending to the edge of the ulcer crater. Malignant ulcers usually have radiating folds that extend beyond the ulcer crater to the edge of the mass. However, only a biopsy provides a definitive diagnosis of tumors and ulcers.

Radiographic studies of the small intestine may reveal regional enteritis, malabsorption syndrome, and tumors.

What needs to be done

• Explain the procedure to the patient. Instruct him to maintain a low-residue diet, as ordered, for 2 or 3 days before the test and then to fast and avoid smoking after midnight before the test.
• Tell him he must drink the barium to help visualize the stomach and small intestines.

What to withhold

• As ordered, withhold most oral medications after midnight and anticholinergics and opioids for 24 hours because these drugs affect small-intestine motility. Antacids, H_2-receptor antagonists, and proton pump inhibitors are also sometimes withheld for several hours if gastric reflux is suspected.

A lovely gown...but no accessories

• Just before the procedure, instruct the patient to put on a hospital gown without snap closures and to remove jewelry, dentures, hairpins, and other objects that might obscure anatomic detail.
• After the patient is secured in a supine position on the X-ray table, the table is tilted until the patient is erect, and the heart, lungs, and abdomen are examined fluoroscopically.
• Then the patient is instructed to take several swallows of the barium suspension. During fluoroscopic examination, images are taken from lateral angles and from right and left posteroanterior angles.

Palpation station

• When barium enters the stomach, the patient's abdomen is palpated or compressed to ensure adequate coating of the gastric mucosa with barium. To perform a double-contrast examination, the patient may be asked to swallow a substance that produces carbon dioxide gas. As he does so, air is introduced into the stomach to allow detailed examination of the gastric rugae, and images are taken. As the patient ingests the remaining barium suspension, filling of the stomach and emptying into the duodenum are observed fluoroscopically and images are obtained as indicated.

Nearing the end

• Barium passage into the remainder of the small intestine is observed fluoroscopically, and images are taken at lengthy intervals until the barium reaches the ileocecal valve and the region around it (this can be at 30- to 60-minute intervals). If small intestine abnormalities are detected, the area is palpated and compressed to help clarify the defect, and images are taken. When the barium enters the cecum, the examination ends.

Finishing up

- Make sure additional X-rays haven't been ordered before allowing the patient food, fluids, and oral medications (if applicable).
- Tell the patient to drink plenty of fluids (unless contraindicated) to help eliminate the barium.
- Administer a cathartic or enema to the patient as ordered. Tell him his stools will be light-colored for 24 to 72 hours. Record and describe any stools that he passes in the hospital. Because barium retention in the intestine may cause obstruction or fecal impaction, notify the practitioner if the patient doesn't pass barium within 2 to 3 days.
- Tell the patient to report abdominal fullness or pain or a delay in return to brown stools.

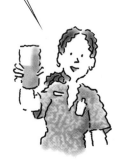

Banish the barium! Have the patient drink fluids galore to flush it out.

Barium enema

Barium enema, also known as a *lower GI examination*, is the radiographic examination of the large intestine after rectal instillation of barium (single-contrast technique) or barium and air (double-contrast technique). This test is indicated for patients with a history of altered bowel habits, lower abdominal pain, or passage of blood, mucus, or pus in the stools. It may also be performed after colostomy or ileostomy; in such patients, barium (or barium and air) may be instilled through the stoma.

What to be wary of

Possible complications of barium enema include perforation of the colon, water intoxication, barium granulomas and, in rare cases, intraperitoneal and extraperitoneal extravasation of barium and barium embolism.

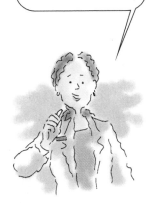

Barium enema aids diagnosis of colorectal cancer and inflammatory disease and detects polyps, diverticula, and structural changes in the large intestine.

What it all means

In a single-contrast test, the intestine is uniformly filled with barium, and colonic haustral markings are clearly apparent. The intestinal walls collapse as the barium is expelled, and the mucosa has a regular, feathery appearance.

In the double-contrast test, the intestine is uniformly distended with air, with a thin layer of barium providing excellent detail of the mucosal pattern. As the patient is assisted to various positions, the barium collects on the dependent walls of the intestine by force of gravity.

Abnormal findings

Barium enema may reveal adenocarcinoma. However, endoscopic biopsy may be necessary to confirm the diagnosis.

Barium enema demonstrates and defines the extent of inflammatory diseases, such as diverticulitis, ulcerative colitis, and granulomatous colitis. This test may also reveal polyps; structural changes in the intestine, such as intussusception, telescoping of the bowel, sigmoid volvulus (360-degree turn or greater), and sigmoid torsion (a turn of up to 180 degrees); gastroenteritis; irritable colon; vascular injury caused by arterial occlusion; and selected cases of acute appendicitis. (See *Barium enema interference.*)

What needs to be done

• Explain the procedure to the patient.

Bowel prep

• Instruct the patient to restrict dairy products and to follow a liquid diet for 24 hours before the test. Tell the patient to drink five 8-oz (237-ml) glasses of water or clear liquids for 12 to 24 hours before the test to ensure adequate hydration. Withhold breakfast before the procedure; if the test is scheduled for late afternoon or is delayed, clear liquids may be allowed. Administer a bowel preparation supplied by the radiography department (A GoLYTELY preparation isn't recommended because it leaves the bowel too wet and the barium won't coat the walls of the bowel.) An enema or repeat enemas may be ordered until return is clear.

Proceed with caution

• Although various diets, laxatives, and enemas may be used, remember that certain conditions, such as ulcerative colitis and active GI bleeding, may prohibit the use of laxatives and enemas, so check the patient history for any of these conditions. Also check for such contraindications as tachycardia, fulminant ulcerative colitis associated with systemic toxicity and megacolon, toxic megacolon, or suspected perforation and pregnancy.
• After the patient is in a supine position on a tilting X-ray table, scout films of the abdomen are taken. The patient is assisted to Sims' position. A well-lubricated rectal tube is inserted through the anus. If the patient can't retain the tube, a rectal tube with a retaining balloon may be inserted. The barium is then administered slowly, and the filling process is monitored fluoroscopically. To aid filling, the table may be tilted or the patient assisted to various positions.
• Patients with colostomy or ileostomy are typically imaged with a water-based iodinated contrast medium instead of barium, because of the risk of peritoneal leakage. In most cases the contrast medium will be administered both through the stoma and through the rectum.

Stay on the ball

Barium enema interference

Performing a barium swallow within a few days of a barium enema may impair the quality of radiographic films.

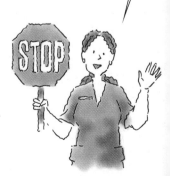

Don't give laxatives or enemas to a patient with ulcerative colitis or active GI bleeding.

• As the flow of barium is observed, spot images are taken of significant findings. When the intestine is filled with barium, overhead films of the abdomen are taken, and the rectal tube is withdrawn. The patient is escorted to the toilet or given a bedpan and told to expel as much barium as possible. After evacuation, an additional overhead film is taken to record the mucosal pattern of the intestine and evaluate the efficiency of colonic emptying.

Double-contrast time

• A double-contrast barium enema may be performed separately with a thicker contrast medium. When the double-contrast technique is performed separately, a colloidal barium suspension is instilled, filling the patient's intestine to either the splenic flexure or the middle of the transverse colon. The suspension is then aspirated, and air is forcefully injected into the intestine.
• The patient is then assisted to erect, prone, supine, and lateral decubitus positions in sequence. Barium filling is monitored fluoroscopically, and spot images are taken of significant findings. After the required films are taken, the patient is escorted to the toilet or provided with a bedpan.

Rest and fluids

• Make sure further studies haven't been ordered before allowing the patient food and fluids. Encourage extra fluid intake as ordered to prevent dehydration and help eliminate the barium.
• Encourage rest because this test and the bowel preparation that precedes it exhaust most patients.
• Because barium retention after this test can cause intestinal obstruction or fecal impaction, administer a mild cathartic or an enema as ordered. Tell the patient his stools will be light-colored for 24 to 72 hours. Record and describe any stools that the patient passes in the hospital. Notify the practitioner if the patient doesn't have a bowel movement within 2 to 3 days.

Endoscopic retrograde cholangiopancreatography

Endoscopic retrograde cholangiopancreatography (ERCP) is the radiographic examination of the pancreatic ducts and hepatobiliary tree after injection of a contrast medium into the duodenal papilla. It's indicated in patients with confirmed or suspected pancreatic disease or with obstructive jaundice of unknown etiology. Complications may include cholangitis and pancreatitis.

What it all means

The duodenal papilla appears as a small, red, or sometimes pale erosion extending into the lumen. Its orifice is commonly bordered by a fringe of white mucosa, and a longitudinal fold running perpendicular to the deep circular folds of the duodenum helps mark its location. Although the pancreatic and hepatobiliary ducts usually unite in the ampulla of Vater and empty through the duodenal papilla, separate orifices are sometimes present. The contrast agent uniformly fills the pancreatic duct, the hepatobiliary tree, and the gallbladder.

Abnormal findings

Examination of the hepatobiliary tree may reveal calculi, strictures, or irregular deviations that suggest biliary cirrhosis, primary sclerosing cholangitis, or cancer of the bile ducts. Examination of the pancreatic ducts may show calculi, strictures, and irregular deviations that may indicate pancreatic cysts and pseudocysts, pancreatic tumor, cancer of the head of the pancreas, chronic pancreatitis, pancreatic fibrosis, carcinoma of the duodenal papilla, or papillary stenosis.

> ERCP assesses obstructive jaundice; diagnoses cancer of the duodenal papilla, pancreas, and biliary ducts; and locates calculi and stenosis in the hepatobiliary tree and pancreatic ducts.

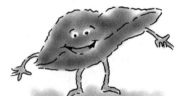

What needs to be done

• Explain to the patient that this procedure permits examination of the liver, gallbladder, and pancreas through X-rays taken after injection of a contrast medium. Instruct him to fast for 4 hours before the test.
• Just before the test, tell the patient to remove all metal and other radiopaque objects and constricting undergarments and to void to ease the discomfort of urine retention after the test.

Contraindication and consent

• Make sure the patient or responsible family member has signed an informed consent form. Check the patient history for such contraindications as pregnancy (because of the risk of fetal harm secondary to radiation exposure), infectious disease, pancreatic pseudocysts, stricture or obstruction of the esophagus or duodenum, or acute pancreatitis, cholangitis, or cardiorespiratory disease. Check for allergies to contrast media or medications.
• Obtain baseline vital signs just before the procedure and attach the patient to continuous electrocardiogram monitoring and pulse oximetry.
• An I.V. infusion is started with 150 ml of normal saline solution. First, the local anesthetic is administered as ordered; this usually takes effect in about 10 minutes. If a spray is used, ask the patient to hold his breath while his mouth and throat are sprayed. Then place him in a left lateral position and give him an emesis basin and tissues. Encourage him to let saliva drain from the side of his mouth. Then insert the mouth guard.

• While the patient remains in the left lateral position, diazepam or midazolam is administered I.V.; an opioid analgesic is also administered this way, if needed. When ptosis or dysarthria develops, the patient's head is bent forward, and he's asked to open his mouth. The practitioner inserts his left index finger into the patient's mouth and guides the tip of the endoscope. As the endoscope passes through the posterior pharynx, have the patient slowly extend his head to assist the advance of the scope.

• When the scope is advanced well into the esophagus, the patient's chin is moved toward the table or a continuous suction catheter is placed in his mouth to allow drainage of saliva. The practitioner advances the endoscope through the remainder of the esophagus and into the stomach. When the pylorus is located, a small amount of air is insufflated and the tip of the endoscope is angled upward and passed into the duodenum.

Descending to the duodenum

• After the endoscope is rotated clockwise to enter the descending duodenum, the patient is assisted into the prone position. An anticholinergic or glucagon I.V. is administered. Air is insufflated, and the endoscope is manipulated until the duodenal papilla is located. Then the cannula, filled with contrast medium, is passed through the biopsy channel of the endoscope and into the ampulla of Vater. The pancreas is visualized first.

Getting it on film

• The cannula is repositioned, and the hepatobiliary tree is visualized by injection of contrast medium. After each injection, rapid-sequence X-rays are taken and reviewed. When the required images have been obtained, the cannula is removed. Before the endoscope is withdrawn, a tissue specimen may be obtained or fluid aspirated for examination.

Postprocedure care

• Observe the patient closely for signs of cholangitis, pancreatitis, and perforation, such as abdominal pain, bleeding, and fever.

• Tell the patient that he may experience a feeling of fullness, some cramping, and passage of flatus several hours after the test.

• Continue to watch for signs of respiratory depression, apnea, hypotension, excessive diaphoresis, bradycardia, and laryngospasm. Be sure to have available emergency resuscitation equipment and a benzodiazepine antagonist such as flumazenil, or an opioid antagonist such as naloxone.

• Check vital signs every 15 minutes for 1 hour, every 30 minutes for the next 2 hours, every hour for the next 4 hours, then every 4 hours thereafter, as indicated.

• Withhold food and fluids until the gag reflex returns. Test the gag reflex by touching the back of the throat with a tongue blade. When the gag reflex returns, allow fluids and a light meal.
• Discontinue or maintain the I.V. infusion as ordered.
• Check for signs of urine retention. Notify the practitioner if the patient hasn't voided within 8 hours.
• If this test is performed on an outpatient basis, make sure that transportation is available. Patients who have undergone anesthesia or sedation shouldn't operate an automobile for at least 12 hours postprocedure. Alcohol should be avoided for 24 hours.

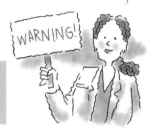

Thumbs down on food and fluids until the patient's gag reflex returns.

Genitourinary and reproductive systems

Kidney-ureter-bladder radiography

Usually the first step in diagnostic testing of the urinary system, kidney-ureter-bladder (KUB) radiography surveys the abdomen to determine the position of the kidneys, ureters, and bladder and to detect gross abnormalities. This test, also known as a *scout film* or *flat plate* of the abdomen, doesn't require intact renal function and may aid differential diagnosis of urologic and GI diseases, which commonly produce similar signs and symptoms. However, KUB radiography has many limitations and nearly always must be followed by more elaborate tests, such as excretory urography or renal CT. KUB radiography shouldn't follow recent instillation of barium, which obscures the urinary system.

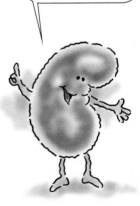

Check me out! KUB helps evaluate my size, structure, and position. It's used to screen for abnormalities, such as calcifications, soft-tissue masses, and malformations.

What it all means

The shadows of the kidneys appear bilaterally, the right slightly lower than the left. Both kidneys should be approximately the same size. The ureters are visible only when an abnormality such as calcification is present. Visualization of the bladder depends on the density of its muscular wall and on the amount of urine in it. Generally, the bladder's shadow can be seen but not as clearly as the kidneys' shadows.

KUB abnormality

Bilateral renal enlargement may result from polycystic kidney disease, multiple myeloma, lymphoma, amyloidosis, hydronephrosis, or compensatory renal hypertrophy. A tumor, a cyst, or hydronephrosis may cause unilateral enlargement. Abnormally small kidneys may suggest end-stage glomerulonephritis or bilateral atrophic pyelonephritis. An apparent decrease in the size of one kidney suggests possible congenital hypoplasia, atrophic pyelonephritis, or ischemia. Renal displacement may be caused by a retroperitoneal tumor such as an adrenal tumor.

Congenital anomalies

Congenital anomalies, such as abnormal location or absence of a kidney, may be suggested by renal axes that parallel the vertebral column, especially if the inferior poles of the kidneys can't be clearly distinguished. A lobulated edge or border may indicate polycystic kidney disease or patchy atrophic pyelonephritis.

Opaque bodies may reflect calculi or vascular calcification caused by aneurysm or atheroma; they may also suggest cystic tumors, fecaliths, foreign bodies, or abnormal fluid collection. (See *KUB interference.*)

What needs to be done

• Explain to the patient that the test shows the position of the urinary system organs and helps detect abnormalities in them. Explain that the test takes only a few minutes.
• Place the patient on an adjustable X-ray table in the supine position and in correct body alignment. Tell him to extend his arms overhead, and then check for symmetrical positioning of the iliac crests. If the patient can't extend his arms or stand, he may lie on his left side with his right arm up. A single X-ray is taken.
• The male patient should have gonadal shielding to prevent irradiation of the testes. The female patient's ovaries can't be shielded because they're too close to the kidneys, ureters, and bladder.

Excretory urography

The cornerstone of a urologic workup, excretory urography allows visualization of the renal parenchyma, calyces, and pelvis as well as the ureters, bladder and, in some cases, the urethra after I.V. administration of a contrast medium. This test is also known as *intravenous pyelography* (*I.V. pyelography* or *IVP*). In some facilities, a nonenhanced CT scan of the urinary tract is commonly performed instead of this test if urinary tract stones are suspect.

What it all means

The kidneys, ureters, and bladder show no gross evidence of soft- or hard-tissue lesions. Prompt visualization of the contrast medium in the kidneys demonstrates bilateral renal parenchyma and pelvicaliceal systems of normal conformity. The ureters and bladder should be outlined, and the postvoiding should show no mucosal abnormalities and little residual urine.

System abnormalities

Excretory urography can demonstrate many urinary system abnormalities, including renal and ureteral calculi; abnormal size, shape, or structure of the kidneys, ureters, or bladder; supernumerary or absent kidney; polycystic kidney disease associated with renal hypertrophy; redundant pelvis or ureter; space-occupying lesions; pyelonephritis; renal tuberculosis; hydronephrosis; and renovascular hypertension. (See *Excretory urography interference* and *Abnormal excretory urogram*, page 352.)

> Excretory urography evaluates the structure and excretory function of the kidneys, ureters, and bladder.

What needs to be done

• Explain the procedure to the patient. After ensuring he's well hydrated, instruct him to fast for 8 hours before the test.
• Make sure the patient or responsible family member has signed an informed consent form. Check the patient history for hypersensitivity to iodine, iodine-containing foods, or contrast media containing iodine. Mark any sensitivities on the chart, and notify the practitioner. Premedication with corticosteroids may be indicated for patients with severe asthma or a history of sensitivity to the contrast medium.
• The patient is placed in the supine position on the table. A KUB X-ray is performed to detect gross abnormalities of the urinary system. If no such abnormalities are found, the contrast medium is injected, and the patient is observed for signs and symptoms of hypersensitivity. The first X-ray, visualizing the renal parenchyma, is obtained about 1 minute after the injection. This may be supplemented by CT if small, space-occupying masses—such as cysts or tumors—are suspected. Films are then exposed at regular intervals—usually 5, 10, and 15 or 20 minutes after the injection.

On to the inflated bladders

• Ureteral compression may be performed through a compression device positioned before the KUB scout image so bladder placement is verified. Two inflated rubber bladders are placed on the abdomen on both sides of the midline, and secured by a fastener. The inflated bladders occlude the ureters and promote retention of the contrast medium by the upper urinary tract. (Ureteral compression is contraindicated in ureteral calculi, aortic aneurysm,

Stay on the ball

Excretory urography interference

The following factors may cause poor-quality film:
• end-stage renal disease
• fecal matter or gas in the colon
• recent barium enema or GI or gallbladder series.

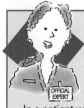

Advice from the experts

Abnormal excretory urogram

In a patient with suspected renal hypertension, an excretory urogram taken 8 minutes after injection of a contrast medium shows normal filling of the right kidney but delayed filling of the left kidney and ureter (see below).

This impaired excretion of the contrast material commonly results from narrowing of the renal artery feeding the subject kidney. Constriction hinders blood flow to the glomerulus and leads to increased renal absorption of water and decreased urine output. Demonstration of delayed filling can distinguish unilateral renal hypertension from essential hypertension.

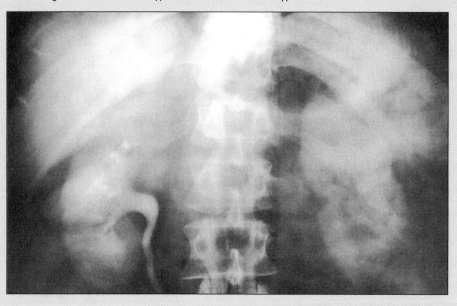

pregnancy, or recent abdominal trauma or surgical procedure.) After the 10-minute image is exposed, ureteral compression is released. As the contrast flows into the lower urinary tract, images are taken of the lower ureters and bladder.

• At the end of the procedure, the patient voids, and another image is taken to visualize residual bladder contents or mucosal abnormalities of the bladder or urethra.

Aftercare

• After the procedure, monitor vital signs and observe for delayed reactions to the contrast medium.
• Continue I.V. fluids or provide oral fluids to increase hydration.

Renal angiography

Renal angiography permits radiographic examination of the renal blood vessels and parenchyma after arterial injection of a contrast medium. As the contrast agent goes through the renal blood vessels, rapid-sequence X-rays show the vessels during three phases of filling: arterial, nephrographic, and venous. This procedure usually follows standard bolus aortography, which shows individual variations in number, size, and condition of the main renal arteries; aberrant vessels; and the relationship of the renal arteries to the aorta.

What it all means

Renal arteriographs show normal formation of the vascular tree and renal parenchyma.

Abnormal findings

Renal tumors usually show hypervascularity; renal cysts typically appear as clearly delineated masses. Renal artery stenosis caused by arteriosclerosis produces a noticeable constriction in the blood vessel; this is a crucial finding in confirming renal hypertension.

In renal infarction, blood vessels may appear to be absent or cut off and the normal tissue replaced by scar tissue. Another typical finding is the appearance of triangular areas of infarcted tissue near the periphery of the affected kidney. The kidney itself may appear shrunken because of tissue scarring.

Renal angiography may also...

Renal angiography may also detect renal artery aneurysms (saccular or fusiform), severe or chronic pyelonephritis, renal abscesses, or inflammatory masses. When angiography is used to evaluate renal trauma, it may detect intrarenal hematoma, parenchymal laceration, shattered kidney, and areas of infarction; it may also be useful in evaluating donors and recipients before and after kidney transplantation. (See *Renal angiography interference*.)

What needs to be done

• Explain the procedure to the patient. Instruct him to fast for 8 hours before the test and to drink extra fluids the day before the test and after the test to maintain adequate hydration (or he may have an I.V. line started, if needed). Tell him that he may receive a laxative or an enema the evening before the test.
• Before the test, instruct the patient to put on a hospital gown and to remove all metallic objects that may interfere with test results.

> Renal angiography assesses renal vessels before surgery and helps determine the cause of renal hypertension. It's also used to evaluate chronic renal disease, assess renal masses and trauma, and detect complications after a kidney transplant.

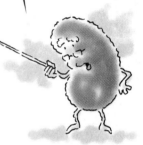

Stay on the ball

Renal angiography interference

The following factors may interfere with the quality of X-rays and their interpretation:
• patient movement during the test
• recent contrast studies such as a barium enema
• presence of feces or gas in the GI tract.

- Check the patient's history for hypersensitivity to iodine-based contrast media or iodine-containing foods such as shellfish.
- Make sure the patient or a responsible family member has signed an informed consent form. Administer medication, if ordered (usually an opioid analgesic and a sedative). Record baseline vital signs. Ensure that recent laboratory test results (BUN, serum creatinine, bleeding studies) are documented on the patient's chart. Verify adequate renal functioning and adequate clotting ability. Evaluate peripheral pulse sites, and mark them for easy access in postprocedure assessment.
- The patient is placed in the supine position, and a peripheral I.V. infusion is started. The skin over the arterial puncture site is cleaned with antiseptic solution, and a local anesthetic is injected.
- The femoral artery is punctured and, with the aid of fluoroscopy, cannulated. (If a femoral pulse is absent or the artery is otherwise inaccessible, another approach may be used.) After passing the flexible guide wire through the artery, the cannula is withdrawn, leaving several inches of wire in the lumen.

Here comes the catheter

- Next, a catheter is passed over the wire and advanced up the femoroiliac vessels to the aorta. The guide wire is removed, and the catheter is flushed with heparin flush solution to prevent clotting in the catheter tip. At this juncture, the contrast medium is injected and screening aortograms are taken before proceeding. On completion of the aortographic study, a renal catheter is exchanged for the former one.
- To determine the position of the renal arteries and to ensure that the tip of the catheter is in the lumen, a test bolus of contrast dye is injected immediately. This prevents subintimal injection or arterial spasm that may mimic a renal artery lesion. If the patient has no adverse reaction, 20 to 25 ml of contrast dye is injected just below the origin of the renal arteries so that it doesn't reach the mesenteric vessels first, obscuring the renal arteries. After this injection, a series of rapid-sequence films of the filling of the renal vascular tree is exposed.
- If further selective studies are needed, the catheter remains in place while the films are examined. If the films are satisfactory, the catheter is removed and a sterile dressing is firmly applied to the puncture site for 15 minutes. Before the patient returns to his room, the puncture site is observed for hematoma.

Wait and watch

- Keep the patient flat in bed; keep the leg on the affected side straight for at least 6 hours or as ordered.
- Check vital signs every 15 minutes for 1 hour, every 30 minutes for 2 hours, and then every hour until they stabilize. Monitor

popliteal and dorsalis pedis pulses for adequate perfusion at least every hour for 4 hours. Note the color and temperature of the involved extremity, and compare them with those of the uninvolved extremity. Watch for pain or paresthesia in the involved limb.

• Watch for bleeding or hematomas at the injection site. Keep the pressure dressing in place, and check for bleeding when you check all vital signs. If bleeding occurs, notify the practitioner promptly and apply direct pressure or a weighted sandbag to the site.

• Apply cold compresses to the puncture site to lessen edema and pain.

• Provide extra fluids (2,000 to 3,000 ml in the 24-hour period after the test) to prevent nephrotoxicity from the contrast medium.

Mammography

Mammography, using film-screen or digital method, is a radiographic technique used to detect breast cysts or tumors, especially those not palpable on physical examination. Biopsy of suspicious areas may be required to confirm malignancy. Although 90% to 95% of malignant breast tumors can be detected by mammography, this test produces many false-positive results. Mammography may follow such screening procedures as ultrasonography. (See *Using ultrasound to detect breast cancer*, and *Understanding ductal lavage*, page 356.)

The American College of Radiologists and the American Cancer Society have established separate guidelines for the use and

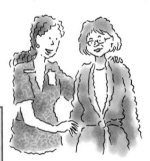

Mammography is used for breast cancer screening and to monitor breast cancer patients who have been treated with breast-conserving surgery and radiation.

Now I get it!

Using ultrasound to detect breast cancer

Ultrasonography—especially useful for diagnosing tumors less than ¼″ (0.6 cm) in diameter—also helps distinguish cysts from solid tumors in dense breast tissue. As in other ultrasound techniques, a transducer is used to focus a beam of high-frequency sound waves through the patient's skin and into the breast. The sound waves bounce back to the transducer as an echo that varies in strength with density of the underlying tissues. A computer processes these echoes and displays the resulting image on a screen for interpretation.

Ultrasound can show all breast areas, including the difficult area close to the chest wall, which is hard to study with X-rays. When used as an adjunct to mammography, ultrasound increases diagnostic accuracy. When used alone, it's more accurate than mammography in examining the denser breast tissue of young patients.

Now I get it!

Understanding ductal lavage

Ductal lavage is a procedure that can identify cancerous and precancerous cells in the milk ducts of the breast. The technique uses a nonsurgical approach to identify abnormal cells—possibly before they become cancerous.

In step one of this two-step procedure, a breast pump applies gentle suction to the patient's nipple. This may cause a drop of fluid to appear at the duct opening. Fluid is more likely to appear at the opening of a duct with abnormal cells than a duct with normal cells.

Under pressure

If ductal fluid is present, ductal lavage progresses to step two. After an anesthetic is applied to the nipple, a flexible catheter is inserted about $1/2''$ into the nipple's duct opening. Then saline solution is infused through the catheter into the duct and aspirated back out. Cells collected in the aspirated fluid are analyzed.

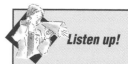

Listen up!

Mammography screening advice

Tell your patient that the American Cancer Society recommends that all healthy women have a screening mammogram annually after age 40. Women at high risk should receive magnetic resonance imaging and a mammogram yearly. Breast self-examinations may be done monthly; clinical examinations yearly, as recommended.

potential risks of mammography. (See *Mammography screening advice.*) Both groups agree that despite low radiation levels, the test is contraindicated during pregnancy.

MRI is becoming a more popular method of breast imaging; it tends to be highly sensitive but not very specific, leading to biopsies of many benign lesions.

What it all means

A normal mammogram reveals normal ducts, glandular tissue, and fat architecture. No abnormal masses or calcifications should appear.

Benign or malignant?

Well-outlined, regular, and clear spots suggest benign cysts; irregular, poorly outlined, and opaque areas suggest a malignant tumor. Malignant tumors are generally solitary and unilateral, whereas benign cysts tend to occur bilaterally. Findings that suggest cancer require further tests, such as biopsy, for confirmation. (See *Mammography interference.*)

What needs to be done

• Assess the patient's understanding of the test, answer her questions, and correct any misconceptions. Assure her that the test may be uncomfortable, but not painful. Tell the patient not to use underarm deodorant or powder the day of her examination to avoid having confusing shadows on the film. If she has breast implants, tell her to inform the staff when she schedules the mammogram so that a technologist familiar with imaging breast implants is on duty.

• Inform her that although the test takes only about 15 minutes, she may be asked to wait while the images are checked to make sure they're readable. Advise her that the test has a high rate of false-positive results. Give her a gown that opens in the front and ask her to remove all jewelry and clothing above the waist.

• The patient is asked to rest one of her breasts on a table above an X-ray cassette. The technologist places the compression device on the breast and tells the patient to hold her breath.

• An X-ray is taken of the craniocaudal view. The machine is rotated, the breast is compressed again, and an X-ray of the lateral view is taken. The procedure is repeated on the other breast. After the films are developed, they're checked to make sure they're readable.

Stay on the ball

Mammography interference

• Highly glandular breasts (common before age 30), previous breast surgery, and active lactation can impair readability of films.

• Breast implants may prevent detection of masses.

Skeletal system

Bone densitometry

Bone densitometry assesses bone mass quantitatively. This noninvasive technique, also known as *dual energy X-ray absorptiometry* or *DEXA scan*, uses an X-ray tube to measure bone mineral density, but exposes the patient to only minimal radiation. The images detected are computer-analyzed to determine bone mineral status. The computer calculates the size and thickness of the bone as well as its volumetric density to determine its potential resistance to mechanical stress. It may be performed in the radiology department of a hospital, a practitioner's office, or a clinic.

The test is useful in identifying the risk of osteoporosis, as well as evaluating clinical response to therapy for reducing the rate of bone loss. The value and reliability of bone densitometry as a predictor of fractures remain under investigation. Also, large-scale studies are being conducted to establish an "at-risk" level of bone density to help predict fractures.

Bone densitometry assesses bone mass quantitatively, and is useful in identifying the risk of osteoporosis, as well as evaluating clinical response to therapy for reducing the rate of bone loss.

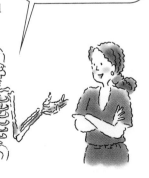

What it all means

Computer-analyzed results of the bone densitometry scan are within normal limits for the patient's age, sex,

Now I get it!

Bone densitometry

These illustrations show the difference between normal bone and a bone with osteoporosis. The osteoporotic bone has much less density, making it less resistant to trauma.

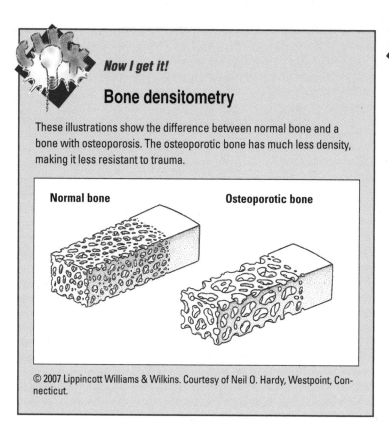

Normal bone   **Osteoporotic bone**

© 2007 Lippincott Williams & Wilkins. Courtesy of Neil O. Hardy, Westpoint, Connecticut.

Stay on the ball

Bone densitometry interference

Osteoarthritis, fractures, the size of the region being scanned, and the fat tissue distribution all influence the accuracy of test results.

and height. (*See Bone densitometry.*) The patient's rate of bone loss can be trended over time. A T-score above –1 is normal, while a T-score between –1 and –2.5 may suggest osteopenia, and a T-score at or below –2.5 may suggest osteoporosis. (*See Bone densitometry interference.*)

What needs to be done

• Reassure the patient that the bone densitometry test is painless and that the exposure to radiation is minimal.
• Check the patient's history to determine if contraindications to testing are present. This test is contraindicated during pregnancy.
• Instruct the patient to remove all metallic objects from the area to be scanned.
• The patient is positioned on a table under the scanning device, with the radiation source below and the detector above. The detector measures the bone's radiation absorption and produces a digital readout.

Vertebral radiography

Vertebral radiography visualizes all or part of the vertebral column. A commonly performed test, it's used to evaluate the vertebrae for deformities, fractures, dislocations, tumors, and other abnormalities. Bone films determine bone density, texture, erosion, and changes in bone relationships. X-rays of the cortex of the bone reveal the presence of any widening, narrowing, and signs of irregularity. Joint X-rays can reveal the presence of fluid, spur formation, narrowing, and changes in the joint structure.

The type and extent of vertebral radiography depends on the patient's clinical condition. For example, a patient with lower back pain requires study of only the lumbar and sacral segments. Some purposes for which this test may be performed include detecting vertebral degeneration, infection, and congenital disorders; detecting disorders of the intervertebral disks; and determining the vertebral effects of arthritic and metabolic disorders.

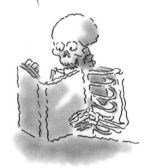

Vertebral radiography is used to evaluate the vertebrae for deformities, fractures, dislocations, tumors, and other abnormalities.

What it all means

Normal vertebrae show no fractures, subluxations, dislocations, curvatures, or other abnormalities. Specific positions and spacing of the vertebrae vary with the patient's age. In the lateral view, adult vertebrae are aligned to form four alternately concave and convex curves. The cervical and lumbar curves are convex anteriorly; the thoracic and sacral curves are concave anteriorly. Although the structure of the coccyx varies, it usually points forward and downward. Neonatal vertebrae form only one curve, which is concave anteriorly.

Vertebrae variations

The vertebral X-ray readily shows spondylolisthesis, fractures, subluxations, dislocations, wedging, and such deformities as kyphosis, scoliosis, and lordosis.

To confirm other disorders, spinal structures and their spatial relationships on the X-ray must be examined, and the patient's history and clinical status must be considered. These disorders include congenital abnormalities, such as torticollis (wryneck), absence of sacral or lumbar vertebrae, hemivertebrae, and Klippel-Feil syndrome; degenerative processes, such as hypertrophic spurs, osteoarthritis, and narrowed disk spaces; tuberculosis (Pott's disease); benign or malignant intraspinal tumors; ruptured disk and cervical disk syndrome; and systemic disorders, such as rheumatoid arthritis, Charcot's disease, ankylosing spondylitis, osteoporosis, and Paget's disease.

Depending on radiographic results, definitive diagnosis may also require additional tests, such as myelography or CT scanning.

What needs to be done

• Explain to the patient that vertebral radiography permits examination of the spine through the use of X-rays.
• Inform the patient that he need not restrict food and fluids.
• Advise the patient that he'll be placed in various positions for the X-ray films. Tell the patient that although some positions may cause slight discomfort, his cooperation is needed to ensure accurate results.
• Stress to the patient that he must keep still, and hold his breath during the procedure.
• Initially, the patient is placed in a supine position on the X-ray table for an anteroposterior view.
• The patient may be repositioned for lateral or right and left oblique views; specific positioning depends on the vertebral segment or adjacent structure of interest.
• Analgesics or local heat applications may relieve pain.
• Check the patient's history for contraindications to the test. Vertebral radiography is contraindicated during the first trimester of pregnancy, unless the benefits outweigh the risk of fetal radiation exposure.
• Exercise extreme caution when handling a trauma patient with suspected spinal injuries, particularly of the cervical area. He should be filmed while on the stretcher to avoid further injury during transfer to the X-ray table.

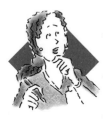

Quick quiz

1. After any angiographic procedures, pressure should be held on the puncture site for a minimum of:
    A.   1 minute.
    B.   5 minutes.
    C.   10 minutes.
    D.   15 minutes.

Answer: D. Pressure should be applied to the puncture site for a minimum of 15 minutes to reduce complications from bleeding.

2. Perforation is a complication associated with ERCP. Signs and symptoms suggesting that perforation has occurred include:

    A.   shortness of breath, abdominal pain, and fever.

    B.   abdominal pain, bleeding, and fever.

    C.   cramping, hypertension, and fever.

    D.   rash, itching, and blotchy skin.

Answer: B. Signs and symptoms of perforation include abdominal pain, bleeding, and fever.

3. When the contrast medium is injected during excretory urography, the patient may experience:

    A.   shortness of breath.

    B.   metallic taste.

    C.   headache.

    D.   fever.

Answer: B. When the contrast medium is injected, the patient may experience a transient burning sensation and a metallic taste.

4. After renal angiography, nursing responsibilities include:

    A.   keeping your patient flat in bed, with the affected side straight for at least 24 hours.

    B.   comparing the color and temperature of the involved and uninvolved extremities.

    C.   applying warm compresses to the puncture site to lessen edema and pain.

    D.   ambulating the patient as soon as possible to avoid complications.

Answer: B. After renal angiography, you should compare the color and temperature of the involved and uninvolved extremities to watch for adequate perfusion.

5. A dual energy X-ray absorptiometry (DEXA) scan is useful in identifying the risk of:

    A.   pneumonia.

    B.   cholecystitis.

    C.   osteoporosis

    D.   spondylolisthesis.

Answer: C. A DEXA scan is useful in identifying the risk of osteoporosis as well as evaluating clinical rseponse to therapy for reducing the rate of bone loss.

6. The American Cancer Society recommends that all healthy women over age 40 hav a screening mammogram every:
    A.   6 months.
    B.   year.
    C.   2 years.
    D.   3 years.

Answer: B. All healthy women over age 40 should have a screening mammogram annually.

Scoring

☆☆☆   If you answered all six questions correctly, you nailed it! X-ray marks the spot!

☆☆   If you answered four or five questions correctly, stellar! Your knowledge of radiography rules!

☆   If you answered fewer than four questions correctly, hang tight! You're bound to catch the radiography ride next time it comes around!

Computed tomography and magnetic resonance imaging

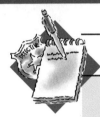

Just the facts

In this chapter, you'll learn:

♦ about computed tomography and magnetic resonance imaging and how they're performed

♦ the patient care associated with each procedure

♦ factors that can interfere with test results

♦ what test results may indicate.

A look at CT and MRI

Computed tomography (CT) records detailed internal images of a predetermined plane of body tissue to produce thin, cross-sectional images. Multiple X-rays pass through this body area and are measured, while detectors measure differences in tissue densities. A computer processes and reconstructs this data as a two-dimensional image on a video monitor. Because CT images avoid superimposition of structures, this technique permits practitioners to make fine distinctions among various tissues and organs.

Before the procedure, explain the test to the patient to ease his anxiety. Make sure the patient or a responsible family member has signed an informed consent form, if required. If the patient is restless or apprehensive, notify the practitioner, who may order a sedative. Tell the patient he'll need to remove all metal objects and jewelry before the test.

After a procedure involving a contrast medium, observe the patient for evidence of an allergic reaction (itching, increased or decreased blood pressure, diaphoresis, tachycardia, and urticaria).

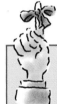

Memory jogger

To remember the signs and symptoms of a hypersensitivity reaction to contrast media, think of the mnemonic **PURR**.

Pruritus

Urticaria

Rash

Respiratory distress

A message about a medium

If the patient will receive a contrast medium (which accentuates tissue density differences), check his chart for hypersensitivity to shellfish, iodine, or radiographic contrast agents. Then start an I.V. saline lock. Tell him he may experience warmth, facial flushing, and a metallic taste when the contrast medium is injected.

Of magnets and spinning atoms

Magnetic resonance imaging (MRI) relies on the atom's magnetic properties. The MRI scanner uses a powerful magnetic field and radiofrequency (RF) energy to produce images based on hydrogen content of body tissues. Exposed to an external magnetic field, positively charged electrons align uniformly. RF energy directed at the atoms knocks them out of magnetic alignment and causes them to precess, or spin. When the RF pulse stops, the atoms realign themselves with the magnetic field, emitting RF energy as a tissue-specific signal based on the relative density of nuclei and the realignment time. A computer processes these signals and displays information as a high-resolution video image.

Before an MRI, explain the procedure to the patient to ease his anxiety. Tell him that although MRI is painless, he may feel uncomfortable while remaining still inside a small space. Tell him he'll be positioned on a narrow bed, which slides into a large cylinder housing MRI magnets. Mention that the scanner will make clicking, whirring, and thumping noises as it moves inside its housing to obtain different images; note that he may receive earplugs.

Ask if claustrophobia might be an issue; if so, the patient may not be able to tolerate the procedure or might need sedation. Although open scanners have been developed for patients with ex-

Memory jogger

The simple mnemonic **SIC** will help you remember what allergies to ask the patient about before a CT scan or MRI that requires a contrast medium.

Shellfish

Iodine

Contrast media (prior sensitive reaction)

Now I get it!

Open MRI: A better choice for claustrophobes

With an open magnetic resonance imaging (MRI) unit, the patient isn't completely enclosed in a tunnel. This is ideal for patients with claustrophobia. Open MRI units are low-field units (0.2 to 0.5 Tesla), whereas closed MRI units are typically high-field units (1 to 1.5 or greater Tesla).

But not ideal

Image quality is almost always better in a high-field unit because of field strength, gradient speed and strength, surface coils, and software. Also, accurate diagnosis may be difficult unless the interpreting radiologist has experience reading low-field units.

treme claustrophobia or morbid obesity, tests using such machines take longer. (See *Open MRI: A better choice for claustrophobes.*)

Reassure the patient that he'll be able to communicate with the technician at all times and that the procedure will be stopped if he feels claustrophobic.

Check your metal at the door

Immediately before the test, instruct the patient to remove all metal objects. (See *MRI and metals don't mix.*)

At the scanner room door, the patient is checked one last time for metal objects. Discontinue I.V. infusion pumps, feeding tubes with metal tips, pulmonary artery catheters, and similar devices before the test.

Computed tomography

CT of the intracranium

CT of the intracranium is a CT of the head or brain, and provides a series of images that represent cross-sectional images of various brain layers. This technique can reconstruct cross-sectional, horizontal, sagittal, and coronal plane images.

What it all means

The density of tissue determines the amount of radiation that passes through it. Tissue densities appear as black, white, or shades of gray on the CT image.

White, gray, or black

Bone, the densest tissue, appears white; brain matter appears in shades of gray; ventricular and subarachnoid cerebrospinal fluid (CSF)—the least dense—appears black. Structures are evaluated according to their density, size, shape, and position.

CT scans may indicate intracranial tumor, hematoma, cerebral atrophy, infarction, edema, or congenital anomalies such as hydrocephalus.

MRI and metals don't mix

Before your patient undergoes magnetic resonance imaging (MRI), make sure he doesn't have a pacemaker or a surgically implanted joint, pin, clip, valve, or pump containing metal. Such objects could be attracted to the strong MRI magnet. Also ask whether he has ever worked with metals or has metal in his eyes. (Some facilities may have a checklist that covers all pertinent questions regarding metals, clips, pins, pacemakers, and other devices.) If he does have such a device, he won't be able to undergo the test.

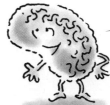

Check me out! A CT scan of the intracranium helps diagnose lesions and abnormalities and helps monitor the effects of cancer treatment.

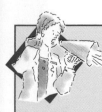

Teaching about CT scans

Cover the following points if your patient will undergo a computerized tomography (CT) scan:
• Tell the patient he'll have to lie still during the procedure.
• Inform him that he'll be placed in a supine position on an X-ray table and that the table will be advanced into the opening of the scanner.
• Explain that the scanner will revolve around him and make clicking noises as it takes the films.
• Tell him that after the first film series, he'll receive an I.V. injection, if a contrast medium is necessary.
• Warn him that he may experience a feeling of warmth during the injection and experience a salty, metallic taste in his mouth, which will last about 2 minutes.
• Instruct him to notify you immediately if he experiences nausea, vomiting, dizziness, headache, hives, or itching.

What needs to be done

• Explain the procedure to the patient and make sure that an informed consent was obtained. Tell him he need not restrict food or fluids. (See *Teaching about CT scans.*)
• The patient is placed in a supine position on an X-ray table, with his head immobilized by straps, if required. The head of the table is moved into the scanner, which rotates around the patient's head, taking X-rays at 1-degree intervals in a 180-degree arc.
• When this series of X-rays is complete, a contrast medium is administered, if ordered. Usually, 50 to 100 ml of the contrast medium are injected by I.V. infusion or by I.V. drip over 1 to 2 minutes.
• After injection of the contrast medium, another series of scans is taken.
• No specific posttest care is necessary if the test was performed without contrast enhancement. If a contrast agent was used, watch for residual adverse reactions after the test.

CT of the biliary tract and liver

In CT of the biliary tract and liver, multiple X-rays pass through the upper abdomen and are measured while detectors record differences in tissue attenuation. A computer reconstructs this data as a two-dimensional image on a monitor. CT scanning distinguishes the biliary tract and the liver if the ducts are large. Use of an I.V. contrast medium can further emphasize differences in tissue density.

What it all means

Normally, the liver has a uniform density that's slightly greater than that of the pancreas, kidneys, and spleen. Areas of slightly lower density, representing hepatic vessels, may interrupt this uniform appearance. The portal vein is usually visible; the hepatic artery usually isn't. I.V. contrast medium enhances both vessels and the main portion of the liver, and they become dense.

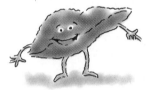

A CT of the biliary tract and liver can be used to detect abscesses, cysts, and hematomas, and it also helps distinguish between obstructive and nonobstructive jaundice.

Obstruction detective

A CT scan of the biliary tract and liver can detect small lesions, hepatic abscesses and cysts, and hepatic hematoma. Dilation of the biliary ducts indicates obstructive jaundice. If the biliary ducts aren't dilated, then nonobstructive jaundice is present. Use of an I.V. contrast medium helps detect biliary dilation, especially when the ducts are only slightly dilated. CT scans can usually identify the cause of obstruction, such as calculi or pancreatic carcinoma.

What needs to be done

• Explain the procedure to the patient and make sure that an informed consent form was signed. Tell him he'll be given a contrast medium to drink and should fast until after the examination. If contrast won't be used, fasting isn't necessary.
• Give the patient the oral contrast agent supplied by the radiology department.

Photo op

• The patient is placed in a supine position on an X-ray table and then positioned in the opening of the scanner. A series of X-rays is taken and recorded on magnetic tape.
• When the first series of films is completed, I.V. contrast enhancement may be ordered. After the contrast medium is injected, a second series of films is taken.
• Observe for a delayed allergic reaction to the contrast dye. (See *Biliary tract and liver CT scan interference*.)

CT of the pancreas

In CT of the pancreas, multiple X-rays penetrate the upper abdomen, while a detector records differences in tissue density, which are then displayed as an image on a monitor. A series of cross-sectional views can provide a detailed look at the pancreas. CT scanning accurately distinguishes the pancreas and surrounding organs and vessels if enough fat is present between the structures. Use of an I.V. or oral contrast medium can further accentuate differences in tissue density.

Stay on the ball

Biliary tract and liver CT scan interference

• An oral or I.V. contrast medium excreted in the bile in previous diagnostic studies can interfere with detection of biliary dilation.
• Barium studies performed within 4 days before a computed tomography (CT) scan may obscure the image.

What it all means

The pancreas generally lies obliquely across the upper abdomen and its parenchyma shows a uniform density (particularly if an I.V. contrast medium is used). The gland normally thickens from tail to head and generally has a smooth surface. An oral contrast medium opacifies the adjacent stomach and duodenum and helps outline the pancreas, particularly in people with little peripancreatic fat, such as children and very thin adults.

Because the tissue density of pancreatic cancer resembles that of normal pancreatic tissue, changes in pancreas size and shape help demonstrate pancreatitis, carcinoma, and pseudocysts. Use of an I.V. contrast medium helps detect metastasis by highlighting the pancreatic and hepatic tissues.

What needs to be done

• Explain the procedure to the patient and ensure that an informed consent was obtained. Inform him that he may be given a contrast medium I.V. or orally to aid pancreas visualization. Instruct him to fast after administration of the oral contrast medium. Describe possible adverse effects of the contrast agent, and tell him to report these.
• Check the patient history for recent barium studies. Give him the oral contrast agent as ordered.
• The patient is placed in the supine position on an X-ray table, and the table is positioned in the opening of the scanner.
• A series of transverse X-rays is taken and recorded on magnetic tape. After the first series of films is completed, I.V. contrast enhancement may be ordered.
• After the I.V. contrast medium is administered, another series of films is taken. (See *Pancreatic CT scan interference.*)
• Observe for delayed allergic reaction to the contrast dye, if used.

> **Stay on the ball**
>
> ## Pancreatic CT scan interference
>
> Barium retained in the GI tract from an earlier test may obscure visualization.

> CT of the pancreas is used to detect pancreatic cancer, pseudocysts, and pancreatitis distress.

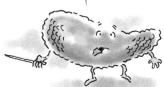

CT of the spine

CT scans of the spine provide detailed images in the cross-sectional, longitudinal, sagittal, and lateral planes. Multiple X-ray beams from a computerized body scanner are directed at the spine from different angles; they pass through the body and strike radiation detectors, producing electrical impulses. A computer converts these impulses into digital information, which appears as a three-dimensional image on a monitor.

What it all means

In the CT image, spinal tissue appears black, white, or gray, depending on its density. Vertebrae, the densest tissues, are white; soft tissues appear in shades of gray; CSF is black.

A dense crowd

By highlighting areas of altered density and depicting structural malformation, CT scanning can reveal spinal lesions and abnormalities. It's particularly useful in detecting and localizing tumors, which appear as masses of varying density. Measuring this density and noting the configuration and location relative to the spinal cord can identify the type of tumor. For example, a neurinoma (schwannoma) appears as a spherical mass dorsal to the cord; a darker, wider mass lying more laterally or ventrally to the cord may be a meningioma.

CT scanning also reveals degenerative processes and structural changes in detail as well as paraspinal cysts, vascular malformations, and congenital spinal malformations.

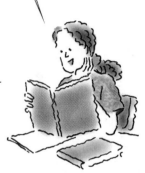

You learn something new every day! It says here that CT of the spine helps diagnose spinal lesions and abnormalities and helps monitor the effects of surgery and treatment.

What needs to be done

- Explain the procedure to the patient and ensure that an informed consent form was signed. Tell the patient that he doesn't need to restrict food or fluids.
- For a patient with significant back pain, administer analgesics before the scan, if ordered, so he can lie still comfortably.
- The patient is placed in the supine position on an X-ray table and is told to lie still. The table is then slid into the circular opening of the body CT scanner. The scanner revolves around the patient, taking X-rays at preselected intervals.
- After the first set of scans, the patient is removed from the scanner and a contrast medium is administered. Then he's moved back into the scanner, and another series of scans is taken.
- Observe the patient for any residual effects if a contrast medium was used (headache, nausea, vomiting).

CT of bone

CT scanning of bone provides a series of tomograms, translated by a computer and displayed on a monitor, that represent cross-sectional images of various bone layers. This technique can reconstruct cross-sectional, horizontal, sagittal, and coronal plane images.

What it all means

The scan should reveal no disease in the bones or joints. Because of its ability to display cross-sectional anatomy, CT scanning can obtain images of the shoulder, spine, hip, and pelvis. It can reveal primary bone and soft-tissue tumors as well as skeletal metastasis. It can also reveal joint abnormalities that other methods can't detect.

What needs to be done

• Explain the procedure to the patient and make sure that an informed consent was obtained. Tell him he doesn't need to restrict food or fluids.
• If the patient has significant pain, give analgesics, as ordered, so the patient can lie still comfortably during the scan.
• The patient is placed in a supine position on an X-ray table and told to lie as still as possible. The table is then moved into the circular opening of the CT scanner. The scanner revolves around the patient, taking scans at preselected intervals.
• After the first set of scans is taken, the patient is removed from the scanner and a contrast medium is administered, if ordered.

Pete and repeat

• After the injection, the patient is moved back into the scanner and another series of scans is taken.
• Urge the patient to drink lots of fluids to help eliminate the contrast agent.
• Monitor for any adverse effects of the contrast media.

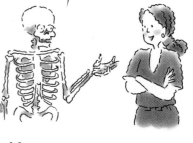

Bone CT detects and assesses the extent of primary bone tumors, skeletal metastasis, soft-tissue tumors, ligament or tendon injuries, and fractures.

CT of the thorax

Thoracic CT scanning provides cross-sectional views of the chest by passing an X-ray beam from a computerized scanner through the body at different levels. CT scanning may be done with or without an injected contrast agent, which is used primarily to highlight blood vessels and to allow greater visualization.

What it all means

Black and white areas on a thoracic CT scan refer, respectively, to air and bone densities. Shades of gray correspond to fluid, fat, and soft-tissue densities.

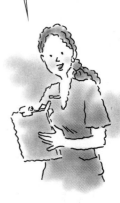

CT of the thorax helps locate tumors, plan radiation treatment, and evaluate lymph nodes, aortic aneurysms, and lung disease severity.

Abnormal thoracic CT scan findings include tumors, nodules, cysts, aortic aneurysms, enlarged lymph nodes, pleural effusions, and accumulations of blood, fluid, or fat.

What needs to be done

- Explain the procedure to the patient and make sure that an informed consent form was signed. If contrast enhancement will be used, he may need to fast for 4 hours before the test.
- After the patient is placed in a supine position on the X-ray table and while the contrast agent is being injected, the machine scans the patient at different levels.
- Encourage fluid intake if a contrast agent was used and monitor for adverse effects.

CT of the heart and calcium scoring

A cardiac scoring CT is a series of tomograms, translated by a computer and displayed on an oscilloscope screen, usually using a contrast medium. This provides layers of cross-sectional images of the heart and reconstructs cross-sectional, horizontal, sagittal, and coronal-plane images. This test is used to diagnose coronary artery calcium content, as well as to screen for coronary artery calcium content in high-risk patients and patients with chest pain of unknown origin (See *CT of the heart and calcium scoring test interference.*)

The test isn't recommended during pregnancy because of potential risk to the fetus.

What it all means

A score of 100 or less is normal and indicates that the risk of significant coronary artery disease (CAD) is minimal, and it's unlikely that the patient has a narrowing of the arteries.

Watch that score

A score between 101 and 400 indicates a significant amount of calcified plaque in the arteries. This score indicates an increased risk of myocardial infarction in the future, and further testing is suggested. A score greater than 400 signifies extensive calcification and that the patient may have a critical narrowing of the arteries due to plaque. Further assessment is required immediately.

What needs to be done

- Make sure the patient has signed an informed consent form.

> A cardiac-scoring CT helps diagnose coronary artery calcium content, and screens for coronary artery calcium content in high-risk patients and patients with chest pain of unknown origin.

Stay on the ball

CT of the heart and calcium scoring test interference

- The presence of coronary stents may alter the quality of the picture.

- Note and report allergies.
- Tell the patient that he doesn't need to restrict food or fluid. Also tell him that he may be asked to hold his breath at times during the test.
- Caution that the patient will hear clacking sounds as the head of the table moves into the scanner, which rotates around the patient.
- The patient is assisted into the supine position on an X-ray table and asked to lie as still as possible to ensure accurate results.
- The table slides into the circular opening of the CT scanner, and the scanner revolves around the patient, taking X-rays at preselected intervals.
- After the test, have the patient resume his usual diet and medications unless otherwise ordered.

CT of the kidney

Renal CT scanning provides an image of the kidneys from a series of tomograms, which are translated by a computer and displayed on a special screen. The image reflects the amount of radiation absorbed by renal tissue and permits identification of masses and other lesions. An I.V. contrast medium may be injected to highlight tissue density and help differentiate renal masses.

What it all means

Normal renal tissue is slightly denser than the liver but less dense than bone, which appears white on a CT scan. The collecting system usually exhibits low (black) density, unless a contrast medium is used to enhance it to a higher (whiter) density. Kidney position is evaluated according to the surrounding structures; kidney size and shape are determined by counting cuts between the superior and inferior poles and following the kidney's contour.

Demonstrating densities

Renal masses appear as areas of different density from normal tissue, possibly altering the kidneys' shape or projecting beyond their margins. Renal cysts, for example, appear as smooth, sharply defined masses, with thin walls and a lower density than normal tissue. Such tumors as renal cell carcinoma usually have thick walls and nonuniform density. (See *Abnormal renal CT scan.*)

When a contrast medium is used, solid tumors show a higher density than renal cysts but a lower density than normal tissue. Tumors with hemorrhage, calcification, or necrosis show higher densities. Vascular tumors are more clearly defined with contrast enhancement. Adrenal tumors are confined masses that are usually detached from the kidneys and other retroperitoneal organs.

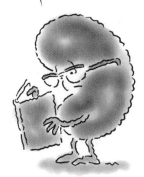

How revealing! A renal CT scan can show all my secrets: renal tumor, obstruction, calculi, polycystic kidney disease, congenital anomalies, and abnormal fluid accumulation.

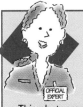

Advice from the experts

Abnormal renal CT scan

This photograph of a renal computed tomography (CT) scan reveals a renal adenocarcinoma that has displaced and distorted the right kidney and that now exceeds the kidney in size. The left kidney appears normal, the spine is sharp and white in the center of the photograph, and the stomach is equally clear at the top.

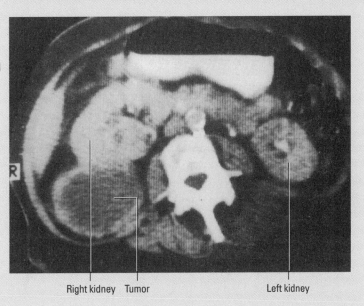

Right kidney   Tumor   Left kidney

Renal CT scans may also identify obstructions, calculi, polycystic kidney disease, congenital anomalies, and abnormal fluid accumulation around the kidneys, such as from hematomas, lymphoceles, and abscesses.

What needs to be done

- Explain the procedure to the patient and make sure that an informed consent form was signed. If a contrast medium will be used, he may need to fast for 4 hours before the test.
- The patient is placed in the supine position on the scanning table and is secured with straps. The table is moved into the scanner, and the patient is instructed to lie still. The scanner rotates around the patient, taking multiple images at different angles.
- When one series of tomograms is complete, an I.V. contrast medium may be administered. Another series of tomograms is then taken.

Magnetic resonance imaging

MRI of bone and soft tissue

A noninvasive technique, MRI produces clear, sensitive tomographic images of bone and soft tissue. It provides superior contrast of body tissues and allows imaging of multiple planes in regions that can't be easily visualized with X-rays or CT scans.

Magnetic resonance images are easily generated from the proton of the hydrogen atom. Each water molecule has two hydrogen atoms, but the distribution of water molecules varies with the specific body tissue. For example, bone is considered "dry" because it contains little hydrogen. Consequently, bone produces a weak signal and can't be visualized. Normal bone marrow has the brightest signal and can be seen well.

What it all means

MRI should reveal no disease in bone, muscles, and joints. It's an excellent method for visualizing disease of the spinal canal and cord and for identifying primary and metastatic bone tumors. MRI is also useful in providing anatomic delineation of muscles, ligaments, and bones. The images show superior contrast of body tissues and sharply define healthy, benign, and malignant tissues.

What needs to be done

• First, make sure the scanner can accommodate the patient's weight and abdominal girth. Explain to the patient that this test assesses bone and soft tissue. Explain that a contrast medium may be used. Make sure that an informed consent was obtained.
• The patient is placed on a narrow, padded table that moves into the scanner tunnel. Fans continuously circulate air in the tunnel, and an intercom is used to maintain verbal contact with the technician. The patient must remain still.
• While the patient lies within the strong magnetic field, the area to be studied is stimulated with RF waves. The MRI computer measures resulting energy changes at these body sections and uses them to generate images. The images resemble two-dimensional slices through the tissues, bone, or organs.
• Provide comfort measures and pain medication, as needed, because of prolonged positioning in the scanner.
• If the patient is unstable, make sure all equipment is compatible with MRI imaging. If necessary, monitor his oxygen saturation, cardiac rhythm, and respiratory status during the test.

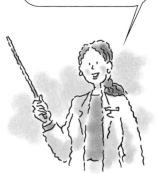

MRI of bone and soft tissue helps evaluate tumors and identify changes in the bone marrow cavity. It also helps identify spinal disorders.

MRI of the breast

MRI of the breast produces detailed analysis of complex breast lesions. It can help identify early breast cancer not detected through other means, especially in those with dense breast tissue, in those who have implants or scar tissue, and those at high risk. MRI of the breast isn't a replacement for mammography or ultrasound imaging but is considered a supplemental tool for detecting and staging breast cancer as well as other abnormalities. It may also be used to screen women younger than 40 and in women at high risk for breast cancer.

What it all means

MRI normally should reveal no disease in breast tissue. The MRI can help determine the integrity of breast implants, distinguish between scar tissue and recurrent tumors, assess multiple tumor locations, and check the progress of chemotherapy. Before surgery, the MRI can identify sites of tumors within the breast, or those that have spread into the chest wall.

Without contrast material, an MRI of the breast can show breast tissue density, cysts, enlarged ducts, hematomas, or leaking or ruptured breast implants. An MRI can help determine whether an abnormality looks benign or malignant (cancerous). The size and location of any abnormality can be determined, as well as the presence of enlarged lymph nodes.

What needs to be done

• First, make sure the scanner can accommodate the patient's weight and abdominal girth. Explain to the patient that this test assesses breast tissue. Explain that a contrast medium may be used. Make sure that an informed consent was obtained.
• The patient is placed on a narrow, padded table that moves into the scanner tunnel. Fans continuously circulate air in the tunnel, and an intercom is used to maintain verbal contact with the technician. The patient must remain still.
• While the patient lies within the strong magnetic field, the area to be studied is stimulated with RF waves. The MRI computer measures resulting energy changes at these body sections and uses them to generate images. The images resemble two-dimensional slices through the tissues, bone, or organs.

MRI of the breast is a supplemental tool that can help identify early breast cancer not detected through other means. It isn't a replacement for mammography or ultrasound imaging.

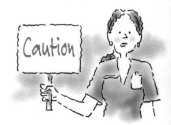

Caution

MRI of the cardiovascular system

A great asset in diagnosing cardiac disorders, MRI can see through bone and delineate fluid-filled soft tissue in great detail as well as produce images of organs and vessels in motion. For this noninvasive procedure, the patient is placed in a magnetic field and cross-sectional images of the anatomy are viewed in multiple planes and recorded for a permanent record.

What it all means

MRI should reveal no anatomic or structural dysfunction in cardiovascular tissue.

MRI can detect cardiomyopathy and pericardial disease as well as atrial or ventricular septal defects and other congenital defects. The test also can be used to identify paracardiac or intracardiac masses and evaluate the extent of pericardial or vascular disease.

What needs to be done

• Explain the procedure to the patient and make sure that an informed consent was obtained.
• The patient is placed in a supine position on a padded, nonmetallic bed, which slides to the desired position inside the scanner. RF energy is directed at the patient's chest. The resulting images appear on a monitor and are recorded on film or magnetic tape. During the procedure, the patient must remain still.
• Monitor the sedated patient's hemodynamic, cardiac, respiratory, and mental status until the sedative effects have worn off.
• If the patient is unstable, make sure that all equipment is compatible with MRI imaging. If necessary, monitor the patient's oxygen saturation, cardiac rhythm, and respiratory status during the test.

Cardiac MRI helps detect congenital heart disease, valvular heart disease, and vascular anomalies such as thoracic aneurysm. It also helps detect cardiac tumors and structural anomalies.

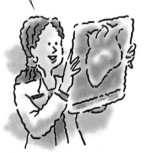

MRI of the neurologic system

Like CT, MRI produces cross-sectional images of the brain and spine in multiple planes. The greatest advantage of an MRI is its ability to "see through" bone and to delineate fluid-filled soft tissue. The magnetic fields and RF energy used for MRI are imperceptible to the patient; no harmful effects have been documented.

What it all means

MRI can show details of the normal central nervous system anatomy in any plane, without interference from bone. Brain and spinal cord structures should appear distinct and sharply defined.

MRI of the neurologic system helps identify intracranial lesions and diagnose spinal lesions and soft-tissue abnormalities.

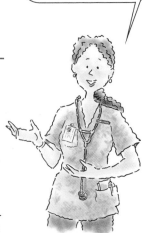

Represents dense tissues

Because the MRI signal represents the proton density (water content) of tissue, MRI shows structural changes resulting from disorders that increase tissue water content, such as cerebral edema, demyelinating disease, and pontine and cerebellar tumors.

What needs to be done

• Explain the procedure to the patient. Tell him it takes up to 90 minutes and that a radioactive contrast dye may be used.

• The patient is placed in the supine position on a narrow bed, which moves to the desired position inside the scanner. RF energy is directed at his head or spine; the resulting images are displayed on a monitor and recorded on film or magnetic tape. The patient must remain still during the procedure.

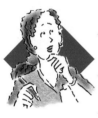

Quick quiz

1. Before CT involving a contrast medium, you should ask the patient whether he's allergic to:

    A.   shellfish.

    B.   nuts.

    C.   penicillin.

    D.   caffeine.

Answer: A. Before CT, you should question the patient about allergies to shellfish, iodine, and contrast media.

2. Hypersensitivity reactions to an I.V. contrast medium, such as respiratory distress, urticaria, and rash, usually develop within:

    A.   10 minutes.

    B.   30 minutes.

    C.   60 minutes.

    D.   90 minutes.

Answer: B. Hypersensitivity reactions usually develop within 30 minutes of contrast medium injection.

3. A nurse is caring for a comatose patient with a head injury who requires mechanical ventilation. Which test is most appropriate for evaluating this patient's brain tissues?

    A.   Skull X-rays

    B.   MRI of the neurologic system

    C.   CT of the intracranium

    D.   Reflex testing

Answer: C. Although MRI has surpassed CT scanning in diagnosing neurologic disorders, CT can be performed when the patient is on a ventilator, whereas MRI can't.

4.   A patient has a score of 450 when a CT of the heart and calcium scoring test is performed. This indicates:
    A.   a normal test with minimal risk of CAD.
    B.   the patient doesn't have narrowing of the arteries.
    C.   significant amount of calcified plaque.
    D.   extensive calcification needing further assessment.

Answer: D. A score greater than 400 signifies extensive calcification and that the patient may have a critical narrowing of the arteries due to plaque.

5.   A CT of the biliary tract and liver will be performed without contrast. Dietary instructions for the patient include:
    A.   that fasting isn't necessary.
    B.   not eating or drinking anything for 8 hours before the test.
    C.   not eating or drinking anything for 24 hours before the test.
    D.   fasting after midnight before the test.

Answer: A. If contrast won't be used for the scan, fasting isn't necessary.

Scoring

☆☆☆ If you answered all five questions correctly, fantastic! Congratulations on a magnetic and resounding success!

☆☆ If you answered four questions correctly, super! You've done a good job of computing tomographies!

☆ If you answered fewer than four questions correctly, don't let it affect your self-image! You'll get the hang of it in no time!

Nuclear medicine scans

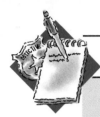

Just the facts

In this chapter, you'll learn:

♦ about nuclear medicine scans and how they're performed

♦ the patient care associated with each procedure

♦ factors that can interfere with test results

♦ what test results may indicate.

A look at nuclear medicine scans

In nuclear medicine scans, a radiopharmaceutical agent is inhaled or injected. A specialized camera detects the amount and changing distribution of the agent in the area or organ, and feeds the information into a computer. The computer then processes the data and produces two-dimensional images for immediate visualization, which are analyzed to diagnose certain conditions.

Explain the procedure to the patient in easily understood terms. Make sure he or a responsible family member has signed an informed consent form, if necessary.

A lung perfusion scan helps assess arterial perfusion. It's also useful for detecting pulmonary emboli and evaluating lung function before resection.

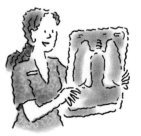

Lung perfusion scan

A lung perfusion scan produces a visual image of pulmonary blood flow after I.V. injection of a radiopharmaceutical, either human serum albumin microspheres or macroaggregated albumin bonded to technetium. This test is useful for confirming pulmonary vascular obstruction such as pulmonary or septic emboli. When performed in addition to a lung ventilation scan, this scan assesses ventilation-perfusion ratios.

Stay on the ball

Lung perfusion scan interference

• Scheduling the patient for more than one radionuclide test per day (especially if different trace substances are used) can inhibit diffusion of the radioactive substance in the second test.
• I.V. injection of the radiopharmaceutical while the patient is sitting can produce abnormal images because many particles settle to the lung bases.
• Such conditions as chronic obstructive pulmonary disease, vasculitis, pulmonary edema, tumor, sickle cell disease, and parasitic disease may cause poor imaging.

What it all means

Hot spots (areas of high radioactive substance uptake) indicate normal blood perfusion. A normal lung shows a uniform uptake pattern. Cold spots (areas of low radioactive substance uptake) indicate poor perfusion, suggesting an embolism; however, a ventilation scan is necessary to confirm the diagnosis. Decreased regional blood flow that occurs without vessel obstruction may indicate pneumonitis.

What needs to be done

• Explain the procedure to the patient and ensure that an informed consent has been signed, if required.

Smile...you're on candid camera!

• Inform the patient that a radiopharmaceutical will be injected into a vein in his arm.
• With the patient in a supine position and taking moderately deep breaths, the radiopharmaceutical is injected slowly over 5 to 10 seconds.
• After uptake of the radiopharmaceutical, the camera takes a series of single stationary images of the various views of the chest. Images projected on a special screen show the distribution of radioactive particles. (See *Lung perfusion scan interference*.)

Lung ventilation scan

A lung ventilation scan—a nuclear scan performed after inhalation of air mixed with radioactive gas—delineates areas of the lung ventilated during respiration. During the scan, the distribution of the gas is recorded in three phases: during the buildup of

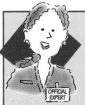

Advice from the experts

Comparing normal and abnormal ventilation scans

The normal ventilation scan on the left, taken 30 minutes to 1 hour after the wash-out phase, shows equal gas distribution. The abnormal scan on the right, taken 1½ to 2 hours after the start of the wash-out phase, shows unequal gas distribution, represented by the area of poor wash-out on both the left and right sides.

Normal scan

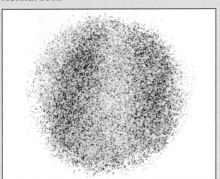

Abnormal scan

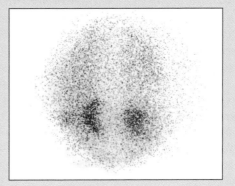

radioactive gas (wash-in phase), after the patient rebreathes from a bag and the radioactivity reaches a steady level (equilibrium phase), and after removal of the radioactive gas from the lungs (wash-out phase). (See *Comparing normal and abnormal ventilation scans.*)

What it all means

Gas should be equally distributed in both lungs, and wash-in and wash-out phases should be normal.

It's a gas, gas, gas

Unequal gas distribution in both lungs indicates poor ventilation or airway obstruction in areas with low radioactivity. When compared with a lung perfusion scan, in vascular obstructions such as pulmonary embolism, perfusion to the embolized area is decreased, but ventilation to this area is maintained; in parenchymal diseases such as pneumonia, both ventilation and perfusion are abnormal within the areas of consolidation.

Hmmmm...it says here that a lung ventilation scan can help diagnose pulmonary emboli, atelectasis, obstructing tumors, and chronic obstructive pulmonary disease.

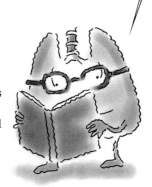

What needs to be done

• Explain the procedure to the patient and tell him he doesn't need to restrict food and fluids. Ensure that an informed consent form has been signed.
• Instruct the patient to remove all metal objects in the scanning field. Tell him that he'll be asked to hold his breath for a short time after inhaling gas and to remain still while a machine scans his chest. Explain that the mask is tight-fitting; monitor for panic attacks during the procedure.
• After the patient inhales air mixed with a small amount of radioactive gas through a mask, its distribution in the lungs is monitored on a nuclear scanner. The patient's chest is scanned as the gas is exhaled.

Radioactive iodine uptake test

The radioactive iodine uptake (RAIU) test evaluates thyroid function by measuring the amount of orally ingested radioactive isotopes of iodine, ^{123}I or ^{131}I, that accumulate in the thyroid gland after a period of time (1 or 2, 6, and 24 hours). An external single-counting probe measures the radioactivity in the thyroid as a percentage of the original dose, thus indicating the gland's ability to trap and retain iodine.

What it all means

After 2 hours, 4% to 12% of the radioactive iodine should have accumulated in the thyroid; after 6 hours, 5% to 20%; after 24 hours, 8% to 29%. The remaining radioactive iodine is excreted in the urine.

Comprehending percentages

Local variations in the normal range of iodine uptake may stem from regional differences in dietary iodine intake or procedural differences among individual laboratories.

Below-normal percentages of iodine uptake may indicate hypothyroidism, subacute thyroiditis, or iodine overload. Above-normal percentages may indicate hyperthyroidism, early Hashimoto's disease, hypoalbuminemia, ingestion of lithium, or iodine-deficient goiter. However, in hyperthyroidism, the rate of turnover may be so rapid that the 24-hour measurement appears falsely normal.

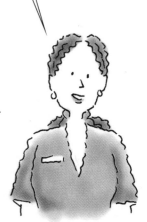

RAIU testing evaluates thyroid function and, when used with other tests, helps distinguish between primary and secondary thyroid disorders.

Stay on the ball

RAIU test interference

Thyroid hormones, thyroid hormone antagonists, salicylates, penicillins, antihistamines, anticoagulants, corticosteroids, and phenylbutazone may cause decreased iodine uptake.

What needs to be done

• Explain the procedure to the patient. Instruct him to fast from midnight before the test.
• Check the patient history for past or present iodine exposure, which may interfere with test results. If the patient previously had radiologic tests using contrast media or nuclear medicine procedures or if he's currently receiving iodine preparations or thyroid medications, note this on the request.
• At 2, 6, and 24 hours after an oral dose of radioactive iodine is administered, the patient's thyroid is scanned by placing the anterior portion of the patient's neck in front of an external single counting probe. The amount of radioactivity that the probe detects is compared with the amount in the original dose to determine the percentage of radioactive iodine retained by the thyroid.
• As ordered, instruct the patient to resume his usual diet. (See *RAIU test interference*.)

Radionuclide thyroid imaging

Radionuclide thyroid imaging allows visualization of the thyroid gland by a gamma camera after administration of a radioisotope—usually iodine ^{123}I, ^{131}I, or technetium-99m (^{99m}Tc) pertechnetate. This test is usually performed concurrently with measurement of serum triiodothyronine (T_3) levels, serum thyroxine levels, and thyroid uptake tests.

What it all means

Radionuclide thyroid imaging should reveal a thyroid gland that's about 2″ (5.1 cm) long and 1″ (2.5 cm) wide, with a uniform uptake of the radioisotope and without nodules. The gland should be butterfly-shaped, with the isthmus located at the midline. Occasionally, a third lobe called the *pyramidal lobe* may be present; this is a normal variant.

> Radionuclide thyroid imaging assesses thyroid size, structure, and position and helps evaluate thyroid function.

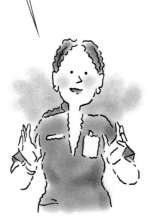

Where's the hot spot?

During radionuclide thyroid imaging, hyperfunctioning nodules (areas of excessive iodine uptake) appear as black regions called *hot spots*. The presence of hot spots requires a follow-up T_3 thyroid suppression test to determine whether the hyperfunctioning areas are autonomous.

Hey, cool!

Hypofunctioning nodules (areas of little or no iodine uptake) appear as white or light gray regions called *cold spots*. If a cold spot appears, thyroid ultrasonography may be performed later to rule out cysts; in addition, fine-needle aspiration and biopsy of such nodules may be performed to rule out a malignant tumor.

What needs to be done

• Explain the procedure to the patient and ensure that an informed consent form has been signed. If he's scheduled to receive an oral dose of ^{123}I or ^{131}I, instruct him to fast after midnight the night before the test.
• Check the patient history for tests within the past 60 days that used radiographic contrast media. Note such tests or the use of drugs that may interfere with iodine uptake on the X-ray request. (See *Getting ready for radionuclide thyroid imaging*.)
• The test is performed 24 hours after oral administration of ^{123}I or ^{131}I or 20 to 30 minutes after I.V. injection of ^{99m}Tc pertechnetate. The patient receiving an oral radioisotope should fast for another 2 hours after administration. Just before the test, tell the pa-

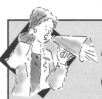

Listen up!

Getting ready for radionuclide thyroid imaging

If your patient will undergo radionuclide thyroid imaging, cover the following points to help prepare him for the test.
• Instruct him to stop taking thyroid hormones, thyroid hormone antagonists, iodine preparations (Lugol's solution, some multivitamins, and cough syrups) 2 to 3 weeks before the test as ordered. Phenothiazines, corticosteroids, salicylates, anticoagulants, and antihistamines should be stopped 1 week before the test as ordered.
• Tell him to avoid iodized salt, iodinated salt substitutes, and seafood for 14 to 21 days.
• Instruct him to discontinue liothyronine, propylthiouracil, and methimazole 3 days before the test and to discontinue thyroxine 10 days before the test as ordered.

tient to remove his dentures and any jewelry that could interfere with visualization of the thyroid.

• The patient's thyroid gland is palpated. Then with the patient in a supine position and his neck extended, the gamma camera is placed over the anterior portion of his neck. The radioactive substance within the thyroid gland projects an image of the gland on a display screen and X-ray film. Three views of the thyroid are obtained: one straight-on anterior view and two bilateral oblique views. (See *Thyroid imaging interference*.)

Cardiac blood pool imaging

Cardiac blood pool imaging evaluates regional and global ventricular performance after I.V. injection of human serum albumin or red blood cells (RBCs) tagged with the isotope ^{99m}Tc pertechnetate. In first-pass imaging, a scintillation camera records the radioactivity emitted by the isotope in its first pass through the left ventricle. Higher counts of radioactivity occur during diastole because there's more blood in the ventricle; lower counts occur during systole as the blood is ejected. The portion of isotope ejected during each heartbeat can then be calculated to determine the ejection fraction; the presence and size of intracardiac shunts can also be determined.

Signals, camera, action!

Gated cardiac blood pool imaging, performed after first-pass imaging or as a separate test, has several forms; however, most forms use signals from an electrocardiogram (ECG) to trigger the scintillation camera. In two-frame gated imaging, the camera records left ventricular end-systole and end-diastole for 500 to 1,000 cardiac cycles; superimposition of these gated images allows assessment of left ventricular contraction to find areas of hypokinesia or akinesia.

In multiple-gated acquisition (MUGA) scanning, the camera records 14 to 64 points of a single cardiac cycle, yielding sequential images that can be studied like motion picture films to evaluate regional wall motion and determine the ejection fraction and other indices of cardiac function. In the stress MUGA test, the same test is performed at rest and after exercise to detect changes in ejection fraction and cardiac output. In the nitroglycerin MUGA test, the scintillation camera records points in the cardiac cycle after sublingual nitroglycerin administration to assess its effect on ventricular function.

Blood pool imaging is more accurate and involves less risk to the patient than left ventriculography in assessing cardiac function. Cardiac blood pool imaging is contraindicated during pregnancy.

Cardiac blood pool imaging evaluates regional and global ventricular performance after I.V. injection of human serum albumin or RBCs tagged with the isotope ^{99m}Tc.

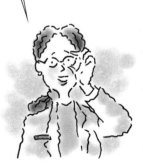

What it all means

Normally, the left ventricle contracts symmetrically, and the isotope appears evenly distributed in the scans. Normal ejection fraction is 55% to 65%.

Abnormal results

Coronary artery disease (CAD) shows asymmetrical blood distribution to the myocardium, which produces segmental abnormalities of ventricular wall motion. Abnormalities may also result from preexisting conditions such as myocarditis.

Cardiomyopathy shows globally reduced ejection fractions. In a left-to-right shunt, the recirculating radioisotope prolongs the downslope of the curve of scintigraphic data. Early arrival of activity in the left ventricle or aorta signifies a right-to-left shunt.

What needs to be done

• Explain the test and tell the patient that he doesn't need to restrict food and fluids.
• Explain to the patient that he'll receive an I.V. injection of a radioactive tracer and that a detector positioned above his chest will record the circulation of this tracer through the heart. Reassure the patient that the tracer poses no radiation hazard and rarely produces adverse effects.

The sound of silence

• Instruct the patient to remain silent and motionless during imaging, unless otherwise instructed.
• Make sure that the patient or a responsible family member has signed an informed consent form.
• The patient is placed in a supine position beneath the detector of a scintillation camera, and 15 to 20 millicuries of albumin or RBCs tagged with ^{99m}Tc pertechnetate are injected intravenously.
• For the next minute, the scintillation camera records the first pass of the isotope through the heart so that the aortic and mitral valves can be located.
• Then, using an ECG, the camera is gated for selected 60-msec intervals, representing end-systole and end-diastole, and 500 to 1,000 cardiac cycles are recorded on X-ray or Polaroid film.

Position change

• To observe septal and posterior wall motion, the patient may be assisted to a modified left anterior oblique position or to a right anterior oblique position and given 0.4 mg of nitroglycerin sublingually. The scintillation camera then records additional gated images to evaluate abnormal contraction in the left ventricle.

- The patient may be asked to exercise as the scintillation camera records gated images.
- If the patient is elderly or physically compromised, assist him to a sitting position and make sure he isn't dizzy. Then help him get off the examination table.

Thallium imaging

Thallium imaging (also called *cardiac nuclear imaging, cold spot myocardial imaging,* or *myocardial perfusion scan*) evaluates blood flow after I.V. injection of the radioisotope thallium-201 or Cardiolyte. Areas with poor blood flow and ischemic cells fail to take up the isotope and thus appear as cold spots on a scan.

What it all means

Thallium imaging should show normal distribution of the isotope throughout the left ventricle and no defects (cold spots). The results may be normal if the patient has narrowed coronary arteries but adequate collateral circulation.

Persistent defects indicate myocardial infarction (MI); transient defects (those that disappear after a 3- to 6-hour rest) indicate ischemia caused by CAD. After coronary artery bypass surgery, improved regional perfusion suggests patency of the graft. Increased perfusion after ingestion of antianginal drugs can show that the drugs relieve ischemia. Improved perfusion after balloon angioplasty suggests increased coronary flow.

What needs to be done

- The procedure varies with the type of imaging. Make sure that an informed consent form has been signed.
- Explain to the patient that this test helps determine whether any areas of the heart muscle aren't receiving an adequate supply of blood. (See *Teaching about thallium imaging,* page 388.)

Stressin' out

- For stress imaging, instruct the patient to restrict alcohol, tobacco, and nonprescription medications for 24 hours and to have nothing by mouth after midnight the night before the test. Tell him that initial testing takes 45 to 90 minutes and that additional scans may be required.
- Tell the patient he'll receive a radioactive tracer I.V. and that multiple images of his heart will be scanned.
- For stress imaging, instruct the patient to wear walking shoes during the treadmill exercise and to report fatigue, pain, or shortness of breath immediately.

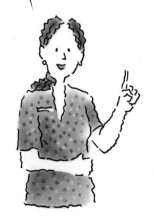

Thallium imaging assesses the location and extent of an MI. It also evaluates graft patency and the effectiveness of antianginal therapy or balloon angioplasty.

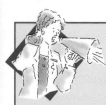

Listen up!

Teaching about thallium imaging

Explain to the patient that the thallium-imaging test can be performed either in a resting state or after stress.

Resting imaging can detect acute myocardial infarction (MI) within the first few hours of symptoms but doesn't distinguish an old from a new infarct. Stress imaging is performed after the patient exercises on a treadmill to the point of angina or rate-limiting fatigue. It can assess known or suspected coronary artery disease and evaluate the effectiveness of antianginal therapy or balloon angioplasty. It's also used to determine graft patency after coronary artery bypass surgery. Complications of stress testing include arrhythmias, angina pectoris, and MI.

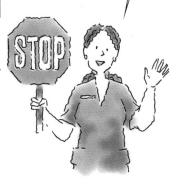

Thallium imaging is contraindicated in pregnancy, impaired neuromuscular function, acute MI or myocarditis, aortic stenosis, acute infection, unstable metabolic conditions, digoxin toxicity, and recent pulmonary infarction.

Stress imaging

- The patient, wired with electrodes, walks on a treadmill at a regulated pace that's gradually increased while his ECG, blood pressure, and heart rate are monitored. When the patient reaches peak stress, the examiner injects thallium into the antecubital vein, or infuses Cardiolyte. The patient exercises an additional 45 to 60 seconds to permit circulation and uptake of the isotope and then lies on his back under the camera. If the patient is asymptomatic, the precordial leads are removed. Scanning begins after 10 minutes, with the patient in anterior, left anterior oblique, and left lateral positions. Additional scans may be taken after the patient rests and occasionally after 24 hours. Taking a scan after the patient rests is helpful in differentiating between an ischemic area and an infarcted or scarred area of the myocardium.
- Monitor the patient carefully during the testing. Stop stress imaging at once if the patient develops chest pain, dyspnea, fatigue, syncope, hypotension, ischemic ECG changes, significant arrhythmias, or critical signs (pale, clammy skin, confusion, or staggering).

Resting imaging

- Within the first few hours of MI symptoms, the patient receives an injection of thallium I.V. or Cardiolyte. Scanning begins after 10 minutes, with the patient positioned as described previously.
- If further scanning is required, have the patient rest, and restrict foods and beverages other than water. (See *Thallium scan interference.*)

Stay on the ball

Thallium scan interference

• Cold spots may result from sarcoidosis, myocardial fibrosis, cardiac contusion, attenuation caused by soft tissue and artifacts (for example, diaphragm, implants, breast, electrodes), apical cleft, or coronary spasm.
• Absence of cold spots in a patient with coronary artery disease may result from an insignificant obstruction, inadequate stress, delayed imaging, single-vessel disease (particularly the right or left circumflex coronary arteries), or collateral circulation.

Persantine-thallium imaging

Persantine-thallium imaging is an alternative method of assessing coronary vessel function for the patient who can't tolerate exercise or stress ECG. Dipyridamole (Persantine) infusion simulates the effects of exercise by increasing blood flow to the collateral circulation and away from the coronary arteries, thereby inducing ischemia. Thallium infusion allows the examiner to evaluate the cardiac vessels' response. The heart is scanned immediately after the thallium infusion and again 2 to 4 hours later. Diseased vessels can't deliver thallium to the heart, and thallium lingers in diseased areas of the myocardium. It's used to identify exercise- or stress-induced arrhythmias as well as the presence and degree of cardiac ischemia.

What it all means

Imaging should reveal characteristic distribution of the isotope throughout the left ventricle and no visible defects.

A different depression

The presence of ST-segment depression, angina, and arrhythmias strongly suggests CAD. Persistent ST-segment depression generally indicates an MI. In contrast, transient ST-segment depression indicates ischemia from CAD.

Cold spots usually indicate CAD, but may result from sarcoidosis, myocardial fibrosis, cardiac contusion, attenuation due to soft tissue (for example, breast and diaphragm), apical cleft, and coronary spasm. The absence of cold spots in the presence of CAD may result from insignificant obstruction, single-vessel disease, or

> Persantine-thallium imaging is an alternative method of assessing coronary vessel function for the patient who can't tolerate exercise or stress ECG.

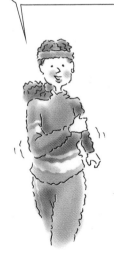

collateral circulation. (See *Persantine-thallium imaging interference.*)

What needs to be done

• Tell the patient that a 5- to 10-minute baseline ECG will precede Persantine-thallium imaging.
• Explain to the patient that he'll need to restrict food and fluids before the test. Tell him to avoid caffeine and other stimulants (which may cause arrhythmias).
• Instruct the patient to continue to take all his regular medications, with the possible exception of beta-adrenergic blockers, as prescribed.
• Explain to the patient that an I.V. line infuses the medications for the study. Inform the patient that he may experience mild nausea, headache, dizziness, or flushing after Persantine administration. Reassure him that these adverse reactions are usually temporary and rarely need treatment.
• Make sure that the patient or a responsible family member has signed an informed consent form.

Take a load off

• The patient reclines or sits while a resting ECG is performed. Then Persantine is given either orally or I.V. over 4 minutes. Blood pressure, pulse rate, and cardiac rhythm are monitored continuously.
• After Persantine administration, the patient is asked to get up and walk. After it takes effect, thallium is injected.
• The patient is placed in a supine position for about 40 minutes while the scan is performed. Then the scan is reviewed. If necessary, a second scan is performed.
• If the patient must return for further scanning, tell him to rest and to restrict food and fluids in the interim.
• Monitor the patient for arrhythmias, angina, ST-segment depression, or bronchospasm. Make sure resuscitation equipment is readily available. Monitor for more common adverse reactions such as nausea, headache, flushing, dizziness, and epigastric pain.

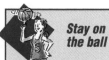

Stay on the ball

Persantine-thallium imaging interference

Failure to observe pretest restrictions may result in altered results. Artifacts, such as implants and electrodes may cause possible false-positive results. Absence of cold spots with coronary artery disease may occur, indicating a possible delay in imaging.

Bone scan

A bone scan permits imaging of the skeleton by a scanning camera after I.V. injection of a radioactive tracer compound. The tracer of choice, technetium diphosphonate, collects in bone tissue in increased concentrations at sites of abnormal metabolism. When scanned, these sites appear as hot spots that are commonly detectable months before radiography can reveal a lesion.

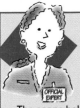

Advice from the experts

Comparing normal and abnormal bone scans

The scans below compare a normal bone scan with an abnormal scan.

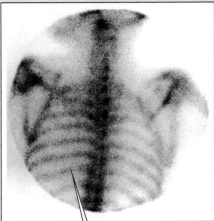

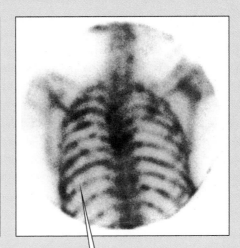

This scan is normal because the isotope is distributed evenly throughout the skeletal tissue.

This scan is abnormal because the isotope has accumulated in multiple areas of metastasis in the ribs and spine.

A bone scan can detect bone cancer, bone trauma associated with pathologic fractures, and infection. It also helps stage cancer and monitor degenerative bone disorders.

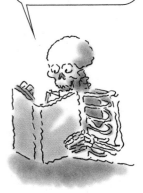

What it all means

The tracer concentrates on bone tissue at sites of new bone formation or increased metabolism. The epiphyses of growing bone are normal sites of high concentration. (See *Comparing normal and abnormal bone scans.*)

Although a bone scan demonstrates hot spots that identify sites of bone formation, it doesn't distinguish between normal and abnormal bone formation. However, scan results can identify all types of bone cancer, infection, fracture, and other disorders if viewed in light of the patient's medical and surgical history, radiographic findings, and laboratory test results.

What needs to be done

• Explain the procedure to the patient and make sure that an informed consent was obtained. In the interval between tracer injection and actual scanning (about 1 to 3 hours), advise him to drink lots of fluids.

• Instruct the patient to void immediately before the procedure (otherwise, a urinary catheter may be inserted to empty the bladder). Position the patient on the scanner table.

• As the scanner head moves over the patient's body, it detects low-level radiation emitted by the skeleton and translates this into a film or paper chart, or both, to produce two-dimensional pictures of the area scanned. The patient may have to be repositioned several times during the test to obtain adequate views.

• Check the injection site for redness and swelling.

• Don't schedule other radionuclide tests for this patient for the next 24 to 48 hours.

Hydration station

• Instruct the patient to drink lots of fluids and to empty his bladder frequently for the next 24 to 48 hours.

• Provide analgesics, as needed, for pain resulting from positioning on the scanning table. (See *Bone scan interference*.)

> **Stay on the ball**
>
> ## Bone scan interference
>
> A distended bladder may obscure pelvic detail.

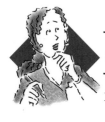

Quick quiz

1. A lung perfusion scan is useful for detecting:
  A. obstructing tumors.
  B. chronic obstructive pulmonary disease.
  C. pulmonary emboli.
  D. congenital heart defects.

Answer: C. A lung perfusion scan helps assess arterial perfusion of the lungs. Therefore, it's useful for detecting pulmonary emboli.

2. What dietary instructions should you give the patient who will be undergoing RAIU testing?
  A. Resume a light diet 2 hours after taking the oral dose of ^{123}I or ^{131}I.
  B. Fast after midnight before the test.
  C. No dietary restrictions are necessary before the test.
  D. Remain on clear liquids 3 days before the test.

Answer: A. As ordered, instruct the patient to resume a light diet 2 hours after taking the oral dose of ^{123}I or ^{131}I. After the complete study, he can resume his normal diet.

3. In most patients who have had an MI, hot spots on a technetium scan disappear after:
  A. 1 hour.
  B. 12 hours.
  C. 72 hours.
  D. 1 week.

Answer: D. Typically, hot spots disappear 1 week after MI. In some patients, they persist for several months if necrosis continues in the infarction area.

4. A patient needs further radionuclide tests following a bone scan. How soon after the bone scan should you schedule the tests?
  A. Immediately after
  B. At least 6 hours after
  C. At least 12 hours after
  D. At least 24 hours after

Answer: D. You shouldn't schedule other radionuclide tests for the patient receiving a bone scan until at least 24 hours after the scan, as it may interfere with testing results.

5. A patient has had a lung perfusion scan and asks what hot spots on the scan indicate. Which of the following is a correct statement?
  A. Hot spots indicate normal blood perfusion.
  B. Hot spots indicate increased areas of blood perfusion.
  C. Hot spots indicate decreased areas of blood perfusion.
  D. Hot spots indicate the need for further testing.

Answer: A. Hot spots (areas of high radioactive substance uptake) indicate normal blood perfusion. A normal lung shows a uniform uptake pattern.

Scoring

☆☆☆ If you answered all five questions correctly, outstanding! You're a nuclear power plant!

☆☆ If you answered four questions correctly, not bad! You know how to tell fact from fission!

☆ If you answered fewer than four questions correctly, don't worry! You just need to build on the nucleus of knowledge you already have!

Monitoring, catheterization, and miscellaneous tests

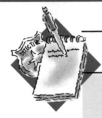

Just the facts

In this chapter, you'll learn:

♦ about monitoring, catheterization, and miscellaneous tests and how they're performed
♦ the patient care associated with each procedure
♦ factors that can interfere with test results
♦ what test results may indicate.

A look at monitoring, catheterization, and miscellaneous tests

Monitoring, catheterization, and miscellaneous tests help diagnose various disorders, evaluate the effectiveness of treatment, and identify complications. Before the patient undergoes testing, explain the procedure in terms he can easily understand. Make sure an informed consent form has been signed, if necessary. These tests may cause anxiety, so be sure to provide emotional support.

Monitoring tests

External fetal monitoring

In external fetal monitoring, a noninvasive test, an electronic transducer and a cardiotachymeter amplify and record the fetal heart rate (FHR) while a pressure-sensitive transducer—the tokodynamometer—simultaneously records uterine contractions. This procedure records the baseline FHR (average FHR over two contraction cycles or 10 minutes), periodic fluctuations in the baseline FHR, and beat-to-beat heart rate variability.

What it all means

Normally, FHR baseline ranges from 120 to 160 beats/minute, with 5 to 25 beats/minute variability.

Low fetal heart rate

Bradycardia—an FHR of less than 120 beats/minute—may indicate fetal heart block, malposition, or hypoxia. Fetal bradycardia may also be drug-induced.

Rapid fetal heart rate

Tachycardia—an FHR of more than 160 beats/minute—may result from vagolytic drugs; maternal fever, tachycardia, or hyperthyroidism; early fetal hypoxia; or fetal infection or arrhythmia.

Less fluctuation

Decreased variability—FHR fluctuation of less than 5 beats/minute—may stem from fetal cardiac arrhythmia or heart block, vagolytic drugs, fetal hypoxia, central nervous system (CNS) malformation, or infection. FHR accelerations may result from early hypoxia. They may precede or follow variable decelerations and may indicate a breech position.

Nonstressful situation

During an antepartum nonstress test, the fetus is considered healthy and should remain so for another week if two fetal movements associated with FHR acceleration of more than 15 beats/minute from baseline occur within 20 minutes. Nonstress testing is also done for postdate fetal well-being. A normal healthy fetus usually has three FHR rises in 10 to 15 minutes, but a fetus may sleep up to 45 minutes at a time. A positive nonstress test result (fewer than two FHR accelerations of more than 15 seconds each, with a heart rate acceleration over 15 beats/minute) indicates an exaggerated risk of perinatal morbidity and mortality and usually necessitates a contraction stress test (CST) or biophysical profile test. The fetus is assessed by watching fetal movements, muscle tone, fetal breathing, and amniotic fluid index.

External fetal monitoring helps measure FHR and uterine contractions. It also evaluates fetal health during stressful and nonstressful situations.

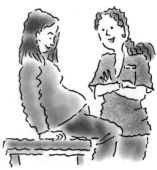

What needs to be done

• Explain the procedure to the patient. If monitoring will be performed antepartum, instruct her to eat a meal just before the test to increase fetal activity, which decreases the test time. If the patient is still smoking, advise her to abstain for 2 hours before testing because smoking decreases fetal activity.

• Place the patient in the semi-Fowler or left lateral position with her abdomen exposed. Cover the ultrasonic transducer with ultrasound transmission gel. After palpating the abdomen to identify the fetal chest area, locate the most distinct fetal heart sounds and secure the ultrasound transducer over this area with the elastic band, stockinette, or abdominal strap. Check the recordings to ensure an adequate printout, and verify the fetal monitor's alarm boundaries.

Chasin' the baseline

• If the patient is undergoing antepartum monitoring with a nonstress test, tell her to hold the pressure transducer in her hand and push it each time she feels the fetus move. Within a 20-minute period, monitor the baseline FHR until you record two fetal movements of more than 15 seconds each and cause heart rate accelerations of more than 15 beats/minute from the baseline. If you can't obtain two FHR accelerations, wait 30 minutes, shake the patient's abdomen to stimulate the fetus, and repeat the test.

Contraction action

• If the patient is undergoing intrapartum monitoring, secure the pressure transducer with an elastic band, stockinette, or abdominal strap over the area of greatest uterine electrical activity during contractions (usually the fundus). Adjust the machine to record 0 to 10 mm Hg pressure between palpable contractions. Review the tracing frequently. Record maternal movement, drug administration, and procedures performed directly on the tracing so tracing changes can be evaluated in view of these activities. Report abnormalities immediately. (See *External fetal monitoring interference.*)

• As labor progresses, reposition the pressure transducer as needed so it remains on the fundal portion of the uterus. You may also need to reposition the ultrasonic transducer as fetal position changes.

Stay on the ball

External fetal monitoring interference

• Maternal obesity or excessive maternal or fetal activity may inhibit recording of uterine contractions or fetal heart rate (FHR).
• Drugs that affect the sympathetic and parasympathetic nervous systems may depress FHR.

Internal fetal monitoring

For internal fetal monitoring, an invasive procedure, an electrode attached directly to the fetal scalp measures the FHR—especially its beat-to-beat variability—and a fluid-filled catheter placed in the uterine cavity measures the frequency and pressure of uterine contractions. This procedure is performed exclusively during labor, after the membranes have ruptured and the cervix has dilated 3 cm, with the fetal head lower than the –2 station.

Maternal risks (perforated uterus or intrauterine infection) and fetal risk (scalp abscess or hematoma) are minimal.

What it all means

Normally, FHR ranges from 120 to 160 beats/minute with a variability of 5 to 25 beats/minute from FHR baseline.

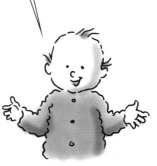

A valuable tool for evaluating intrapartal fetal health, internal fetal monitoring helps assess FHR and the frequency and pressure of uterine contractions.

Slowin' down

Bradycardia—an FHR below 120 beats/minute—may indicate fetal heart block, malposition, hypoxia, or maternal ingestion of certain drugs, such as propranolol or opioid analgesics.

Speedin' up

Tachycardia—an FHR above 160 beats/minute—may result from maternal use of vagolytic drugs, early fetal hypoxia, fetal infection or arrhythmia, prematurity, or maternal fever, tachycardia, or hyperthyroidism.

Even-keeled

Decreased variability—fluctuation of fewer than 5 beats/minute from FHR baseline—may result from maternal use of vagolytic drugs, fetal cardiac arrhythmia or heart block, or fetal hypoxia, CNS malformation, or infection.

Slowin' down early

Early decelerations (FHR slowing at contraction onset, with recovery to baseline not greater than 15 seconds after completion of the uterine contraction) are related to fetal head compression and usually mean the fetus is healthy.

Slowin' down late

Late decelerations (FHR slowing, with onset after the contraction starts, a lag time greater than 20 seconds, and a recovery time greater than 15 seconds) may indicate uteroplacental insufficiency, fetal hypoxia, or acidosis.

What needs to be done

• Prepare for two separate procedures: electrode insertion for FHR monitoring and probe insertion for monitoring contractions.
• Explain the procedure to the patient.

Picking up the FHR

• Place the patient in the dorsal lithotomy position, and prepare her perineal area for a vaginal examination. After the vaginal examination, the fetal scalp is palpated and an area not over a fontanel is identified. Then the plastic guide tube surrounding the small corkscrew-type electrode is introduced into the cervix, pressed firmly against the fetal scalp, and rotated 180 degrees clockwise to insert the electrode into the scalp. After the electrode wire is tugged slightly to make sure it's attached properly, the tube is withdrawn, leaving the electrode in place.

• Next, a leg plate with a conduction medium is strapped to the mother's thigh. Electrode wires are attached to the leg plate, and a cable from the leg plate is plugged into the fetal monitor. To check proper placement of the scalp electrode, the monitor is turned on and the electrocardiogram (ECG) button is pressed; an FHR signal indicates proper electrode attachment. (See *Understanding internal fetal monitoring*, page 400.)

Converting contractions

• *To measure uterine contractions:* Before inserting the uterine catheter, fill it with sterile normal saline solution to prevent air emboli. Ask the patient to breathe deeply through her mouth and relax her abdominal muscles. After the vagina has been examined and the fetal presenting part has been palpated, the fluid-filled catheter and catheter guide are inserted $3/8''$ to $3/4''$ (1 to 2 cm) into the cervix, usually between the fetal head and the posterior cervix. The catheter is then gently inserted into the uterus until the black mark on the catheter is flush with the vulva. (The catheter guide should *never* be passed deeply into the uterus.) Next, the guide is removed and the catheter is connected to a transducer that converts the intrauterine pressure, as measured by fluid in the catheter, to an electrical signal. To standardize pressure readings, the transducer is exposed to air (it should measure zero pressure). The system is then closed to the air, and intrauterine pressure readings are checked.

• After removal of the fetal scalp electrode, apply antiseptic or antibiotic solution to the attachment site and watch for signs of fetal scalp abscess or maternal intrauterine infection. (See *Internal fetal monitoring interference*.)

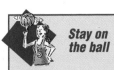

Stay on the ball

Internal fetal monitoring interference

Drugs that affect the parasympathetic and sympathetic nervous systems may influence fetal heart rate.

Now I get it!

Understanding internal fetal monitoring

In internal fetal monitoring, an electrode is attached to the fetal scalp. The resultant fetal electro-cardiograms (FECGs) are transmitted to an amplifier. A cardiotachometer then measures the interval between FECGs and plots a continuous fetal heart rate (FHR) graph, which is displayed on a two-channel oscilloscope screen. Intrauterine catheters attached to a transducer in the leg plate measure the frequency and pressure of uterine contractions, which are plotted below the FHR graph.

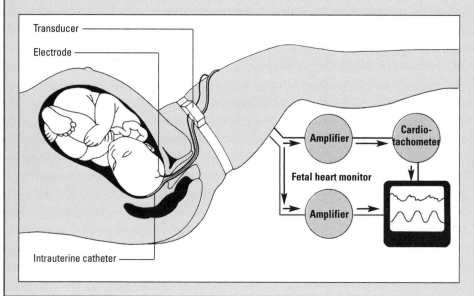

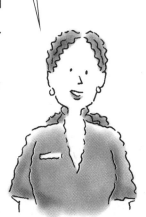

The CST helps evaluate the fetus's hypoxia risk and ability to withstand uterine contractions. It also helps assess whether the placenta can supply sufficient oxygen to the fetus.

Contraction stress test

The CST, also known as the *oxytocin challenge test,* measures the fetus's ability to withstand decreased oxygen supply and the stress of contractions induced before actual labor begins. Oxytocin is infused to stimulate uterine contractions while the FHR is assessed to evaluate the placenta's ability to provide sufficient oxygen to the fetus.

What it all means

Three contractions occur in a 10 minute period with no slowing (or late decelerations) of FHR in response to contractions. A negative result occurs when FHR is within normal range (120 to 160 beats/minute), indicating that the fetus can tolerate the stress of labor.

Asphyxia indicator

Late decelerations of the FHR occur in response to the contractions, indicating a problem that requires further testing or delivery.

What needs to be done

• Explain the procedure to the patient. Inform her that food and fluids may be restricted before the test, as ordered. If the patient smokes, tell her not to smoke for 2 hours before the test.
• Have the patient empty her bladder.
• Assist the patient into a semi-Fowler, side-lying position, and drape her for privacy.
• Monitor the patient's blood pressure before and every 10 minutes during the procedure.
• Place the fetal monitor on the patient's abdomen to monitor FHR and the tokodynamometer on the lower abdomen to monitor contractions. A baseline recording is made, and then the FHR is monitored and recorded continuously.
• If the patient isn't having contractions, ask her to stimulate one of her nipples for a brief time, until contractions begin. In some cases oxytocin is given I.V. to stimulate contractions.
• An I.V. line is inserted, and diluted I.V. oxytocin is administered via I.V. pump as ordered, increasing until the patient experiences three contractions within 10 minutes, each lasting longer than 45 seconds). The FHR and contractions are monitored and recorded, and the infusion is discontinued to determine the FHR response to the contractions.
• Encourage the patient to use deep-breathing and relaxation skills while the oxytocin is administered and she feels the contractions.
• Continue to monitor FHR for 30 minutes as uterine movements return to normal.
• If premature labor begins, note the frequency, strength, and length of contractions and prepare for labor or cesarean delivery.

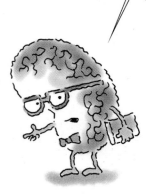

EEG diagnoses epilepsy and intracranial lesions and confirms brain death.

Electroencephalography

In EEG, electrodes attached to standard areas of the patient's scalp record a portion of the brain's electrical activity. These electrical impulses are transmitted to an electroencephalograph, which magnifies them 1 million times and records them as brain waves on moving strips of paper.

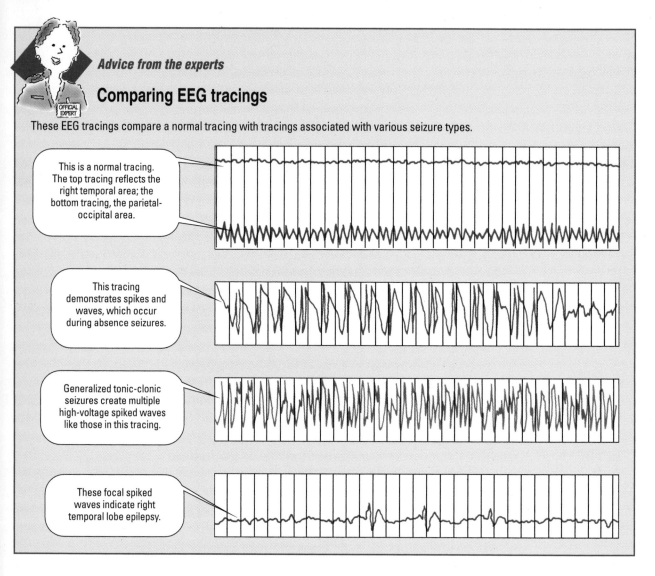

Advice from the experts

Comparing EEG tracings

These EEG tracings compare a normal tracing with tracings associated with various seizure types.

This is a normal tracing. The top tracing reflects the right temporal area; the bottom tracing, the parietal-occipital area.

This tracing demonstrates spikes and waves, which occur during absence seizures.

Generalized tonic-clonic seizures create multiple high-voltage spiked waves like those in this tracing.

These focal spiked waves indicate right temporal lobe epilepsy.

What it all means

EEG records a portion of the brain's electrical activity as waves; some are irregular, whereas others demonstrate common patterns. Among the basic waveforms are the alpha, beta, theta, and delta rhythms. (See *Comparing EEG tracings*.)

Usually, a strip of the recording is evaluated, with special focus on basic waveforms, symmetry of cerebral activity, transient discharges, and response to stimulation. A specific diagnosis depends on the patient's clinical status.

Now I get it!

Wrap your brain around EEG techniques

During an EEG, your patient may be asked to perform certain stress-producing activities so brain wave patterns can be documented. For example, he may be asked to hyperventilate (breathe deeply and rapidly for 3 minutes) to produce brain wave patterns typical of seizure disorders or other abnormalities. This technique is commonly used to detect absence seizures.

Light the way
Photic stimulation, another EEG technique, tests central cerebral activity in response to bright light, accentuating abnormal activity in the absence of myoclonic seizures. In this procedure, a strobe light in front of the patient flashes 1 to 20 times per second. Recordings are made with the patient's eyes opened and closed.

Losing consciousness

EEG may reveal epilepsy, absence seizures, generalized tonic-clonic seizures, temporal lobe epilepsy, focal seizures, intracranial lesions (such as tumors or abscesses), or vascular lesions (such as cerebral infarcts and intracranial hemorrhages). Generally, any condition that causes a diminishing level of consciousness alters the EEG pattern in proportion to the degree of consciousness lost.

What needs to be done

• Explain the procedure to the patient. Tell him to restrict caffeine intake before the test. Smoking is prohibited for at least 8 hours before the test.
• Thoroughly wash and dry the patient's hair to remove hair sprays, creams, or oils. Check his medication history for drugs that may interfere with test results.
• If a sleep EEG is ordered, keep the patient awake the night before the test and, as ordered for some patients, administer a sedative (such as chloral hydrate) to help him sleep during the test.
• The patient is positioned comfortably, and electrodes are attached to his scalp. Before the recording procedure begins, the patient is instructed to close his eyes, relax, and remain still. During the recording, the patient is carefully observed through a window in an adjoining room. Blinking, swallowing, talking, or other movements that may cause artifacts are noted. The recording may be stopped periodically to let the patient reposition himself and get comfortable. (See *Wrap your brain around EEG techniques*.)

• Observe the patient for seizures, and provide a safe environment.
• If the test is done to confirm brain death in a comatose patient, provide emotional support for the family. (See *EEG interference*.)

Electromyography

Electromyography (EMG) is the recording of electrical activity of selected skeletal muscle groups at rest and during voluntary contraction. In this test, a needle electrode is inserted percutaneously into a muscle. The muscle's electrical discharge (or motor unit potential) is then measured and displayed on an oscilloscope screen.

What it all means

At rest, a normal muscle exhibits minimal electrical activity. During voluntary contraction, however, electrical activity increases markedly. A sustained contraction or one of increasing strength produces a rapid "train" of motor unit potentials that can be heard as a crescendo of sounds, similar to the sound of an outboard motor, over the audio amplifier.

Catching a wave

Closely spaced waveforms indicate a high frequency; widely spaced waveforms signify a low frequency. In primary muscle disease, such as muscular dystrophies, motor unit potentials are short (low amplitude), with frequent, irregular discharges. In such disorders as amyotrophic lateral sclerosis and peripheral nerve disorders, motor unit potentials are isolated and irregular but show increased amplitude and duration. In myasthenia gravis, motor unit potentials may be normal initially but diminish in amplitude progressively with continuing contractions. The interpreter distinguishes waveforms that indicate a muscle disorder from those indicating denervation.

What needs to be done

• Explain the procedure to the patient. In some cases, the practitioner may restrict cigarettes, coffee, tea, and cola for 2 to 3 hours before the test.
• Check his history for medications that may interfere with test results.

That's some signal!

• The patient lies on a stretcher or bed or sits on a chair, depending on the muscles to be tested. The arm or leg is positioned so the muscle to be tested is at rest. The skin is cleaned with alcohol,

EMG is used to diagnose neuromuscular disorders and spinal nerve disorders.

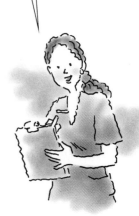

the needle electrodes are quickly inserted into the selected muscle, and a metal plate is placed under the patient to serve as a reference electrode. The muscle's resulting electrical signal (motor unit potential), recorded during rest and contraction, is amplified 1 million times and displayed on an oscilloscope screen or computer screen. Recorder leadwires are usually attached to an audioamplifier so voltage fluctuations within the muscle can be heard.

• If the patient experiences residual pain, apply warm compresses and administer analgesics, as ordered. (See *EMG interference.*)

Stay on the ball

EMG interference

Drugs that affect myoneural junctions, such as cholinergics, anticholinergics, and skeletal muscle relaxants, interfere with electromyography (EMG) results.

Electrocardiography

ECG, the most commonly used test for evaluating cardiac status, graphically records the electric current (electrical potential) generated by the heart. This current radiates from the heart in all directions and, on reaching the skin, is measured by electrodes connected to an amplifier and strip chart recorder. The standard resting ECG uses five electrodes to measure the electrical potential from 12 different leads: the standard limb leads (I, II, III), the augmented limb leads (aV_F, aV_L, and aV_R), and the precordial, or chest, leads (V_1 through V_6).

ECG tracings usually consist of three identifiable waveforms: the P wave, the QRS complex, and the T wave. The P wave depicts atrial depolarization; the QRS complex, ventricular depolarization; and the T wave, ventricular repolarization.

Computerized ECG machines use small electrode tabs that peel off a sheet and adhere to the patient's skin. The entire ECG tracing is displayed on a screen so abnormalities can be corrected before printing; then it's printed on one sheet of paper. Electrode tabs can remain on the patient's chest, arms, and legs to provide continuous lead placement for serial ECG studies.

What it all means

The lead II waveform, known as the *rhythm strip*, depicts the heart's rhythm more clearly than any other waveform. (See *Normal ECG waveforms*, page 406.)

In lead II, the normal P wave doesn't exceed 2.5 mm (0.25 mV) in height or last longer than 0.12 second. The PR interval, which includes the P wave and PR segment, persists for 0.12 to 0.20 second for cardiac rates over 60 beats/minute. The QT interval varies with the cardiac rate and lasts 0.40 to 0.52 second for rates above 60; R wave voltage in the V_1 through V_6 leads doesn't exceed 27 mm. The total QRS interval lasts 0.06 to 0.1 second.

ECG helps identify primary conduction abnormalities, cardiac arrhythmias, cardiac hypertrophy, pericarditis, electrolyte imbalance, myocardial ischemia, and myocardial infarction site and extent. It also helps evaluate the effectiveness of cardiac drugs.

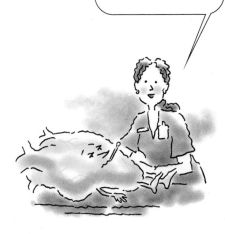

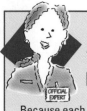

Advice from the experts

Normal ECG waveforms

Because each lead takes a different view of heart activity, it generates its own characteristic tracing. The tracings shown here are representative of each of the 12 leads. Leads aVR, V_1, V_2, V_3, and V_4 usually show strong negative deflections. Negative deflections indicate that the current is moving away from the positive electrode; positive deflections, that the current is moving toward the positive electrode.

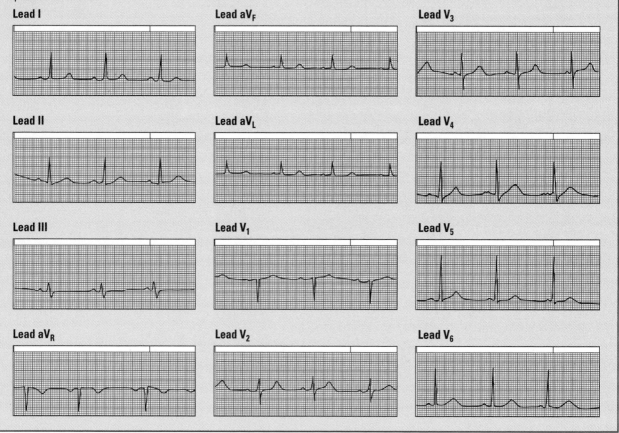

Lead I

Lead aV$_F$

Lead V$_3$

Lead II

Lead aV$_L$

Lead V$_4$

Lead III

Lead V$_1$

Lead V$_5$

Lead aV$_R$

Lead V$_2$

Lead V$_6$

The lowdown on levels

An abnormal ECG may show myocardial infarction (MI), right or left ventricular hypertrophy, arrhythmias, right or left bundle-branch block, ischemia, conduction defects or pericarditis, electrolyte abnormalities such as hypokalemia, or the effects of cardioactive drugs. Sometimes, an ECG reveals abnormal waveforms only during episodes of angina or during exercise.

Standard 12-lead ECG

In a standard 12-lead electrocardiogram (ECG), ten electrodes (four limb, six chest) record the heart's electrical potential from 12 different views, or leads. Lead I connects the left and right arms. Lead II connects the left leg and right arm. Lead III connects the left leg and left arm.

Mind your limbs and Vs

Unipolar augmented limb leads (aV_F, aV_L, and aV_R), which use the same electrode placement as standard limb leads, measure electrical potential between one augmented limb lead and the electrical midpoint of the remaining two leads (determined electronically by the ECG machine). Both standard and augmented leads measure electrical potential while viewing the heart from the front, in a vertical plane.

All walled off

The six unipolar chest leads (V_1 through V_6) shown here depict the electrical potential from a horizontal plane that helps locate disorders in the heart's lateral, anterior, and posterior walls. The ECG machine averages the electrical potentials of all three limb lead electrodes. Recordings made with the V connection show electrical potential variations that occur under the chest electrode as its position changes.

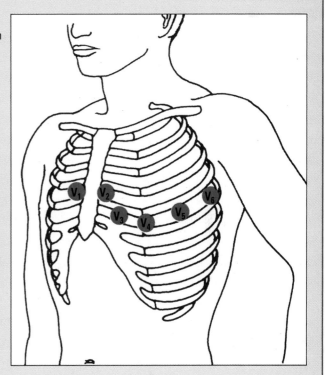

What needs to be done

• Explain the procedure to the patient and ask that the patient remain still and not talk during the test.

• Place the patient in the supine or semi-Fowler position. Expose his chest, both ankles, and both wrists for electrode placement. Drape the female patient's chest until chest leads are applied.

• Place electrodes on the inner aspect of the wrists, the medial aspect of the lower legs, and on the chest. (For the proper chest positions, see *Standard 12-lead ECG*.) Then connect the leadwires after all electrodes are in place.

• Press the START button and input any required information. The machine will produce a printout showing all 12 leads simultaneously.

• If the wave peaks beyond the top edge of the recording grid, adjust the machine to bring the wave inside the boundaries.

Setting the pace

- If the patient has a pacemaker, the ECG may be performed with or without a magnet. Indicate on the request and the patient's record that a pacemaker is present and whether a magnet is used. Many pacemakers function only when the heart rate falls below a preset level; a magnet makes the pacemaker fire regularly, which permits evaluation of pacemaker performance.

Finishing up

- When the machine finishes the tracing, remove the electrodes and reposition the patient's gown and bed covers.
- Label each ECG strip with the patient's name and room number (if applicable), date and time of the procedure, and the practitioner's name. Some equipment models require this input into a computer before initiation of testing; follow manufacturer recommendations. Note whether the ECG was performed during or on resolution of a chest pain episode.

Exercise electrocardiography

Exercise ECG, commonly known as a *stress test*, evaluates heart action during physical stress—when oxygen demand increases—and thus provides important diagnostic information that can't be obtained from a resting ECG alone.

In this test, ECG and blood pressure readings are taken while the patient walks on a treadmill or pedals a stationary bicycle, and his response to a constant or an increasing workload is observed. Unless complications develop, the test continues until the patient reaches the target heart rate, determined by an established protocol (usually 85% of maximum predicted heart rate for the patient's age and gender) or experiences chest pain or fatigue.

What it all means

In a normal exercise ECG, the P, QRS, and T waves and the ST segment change slightly; a slight ST-segment depression occurs in some patients, especially women. The heart rate rises in direct proportion to the workload and metabolic oxygen demand; systolic blood pressure also rises as workload increases. The normal patient attains endurance levels appropriate for his age and the exercise protocol.

Hypotension resulting from exercise, ST-segment depression of 3 mm or more, downsloping ST segments, and ischemic ST segments appearing within the first 3 minutes of exercise and lasting 8 minutes into the posttest recovery period may indicate multivessel or left coronary artery disease (CAD). ST-segment elevation

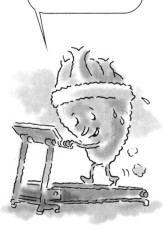

Exercise ECG helps screen for asymptomatic CAD, set limitations for an exercise program, and evaluate myocardial perfusion.

may indicate dyskinetic left ventricular wall motion or severe transmural ischemia. This test's value in predicting CAD varies with the patient's history and gender.

What needs to be done

• Explain the procedure to the patient. Tell him not to eat, smoke, or drink alcoholic or caffeinated beverages for 3 hours before the test. Instruct him to continue his drug regimen unless the practitioner directs otherwise. Instruct the patient to inform the practitioner or technician if he has taken an erectile dysfunction drug within the past 24 hours.
• Tell the patient to wear comfortable clothing for the procedure.
• The electrode sites are thoroughly cleaned and prepared.
• Electrodes are placed for 12-lead ECG monitoring. The leadwire cable is placed over the patient's shoulder, and the leadwire box is placed on his chest. The cable is secured and the leadwires are connected to the chest electrodes.
• The monitor is started, and a stable baseline tracing is obtained. A blood pressure reading is taken, and the patient is auscultated for S_3 or S_4 gallops and crackles.

Steppin' up

• For the treadmill test, the treadmill is turned on to a slow speed, and the patient is shown how to step onto it and use the support railings to maintain balance but not to support weight. He's instructed to step onto the treadmill, and is kept on a slow speed until he gets used to walking on it. Exercise intensity is increased every 3 minutes by slightly increasing the treadmill speed while raising the incline 3%.

Biking to nowhere

• For the bicycle test, the patient is instructed to sit on the bicycle, not to grip the handlebars tightly, and to pedal until he reaches the desired speed, as shown on the speedometer.

Combo-test

• In both tests, a monitor is observed continuously for changes in the heart's electrical activity. The rhythm strip is checked at preset intervals for arrhythmias, premature ventricular contractions (PVCs), ST-segment changes, and T-wave changes. The test level and the amount of time it took to reach that level are marked on each strip. Blood pressure is monitored, and systolic changes are noted. Common responses to maximal exercise are dizziness, light-headedness, leg fatigue, dyspnea, diaphoresis, and a slightly ataxic gait.

When to stop an exercise ECG

You should stop an exercise electrocardiogram (ECG) test immediately if:
• the ECG shows three consecutive premature ventricular contractions (PVCs) or a significant increase in ectopy
• the patient's systolic blood pressure falls below the resting level
• the patient's heart rate falls 10 beats/minute or more below the resting level
• the patient becomes exhausted or complains of significant shortness of breath.

Other dicey situations

Depending on the patient's condition, the test may be stopped in the following situations:
• the ECG shows bundle-branch block, ST-segment depression exceeding 1.5 mm, persistent ST-segment alteration, or frequent or complicated PVCs
• blood pressure fails to rise above resting level
• systolic pressure exceeds 220 mm Hg
• the patient experiences angina.

• If symptoms become severe, the test is stopped. Usually, testing stops when the patient reaches the target heart rate. As the treadmill speed slows, he may be instructed to keep walking for several minutes to prevent nausea or dizziness. (See *When to stop an exercise ECG.*)
• Assist the patient to a chair, and continue monitoring heart rate and blood pressure for 10 to 15 minutes or until the ECG returns to baseline.
• Auscultate for S_3 or S_4 gallops. In many patients, an S_4 gallop develops after exercise from increased blood flow volume and turbulence. However, an S_3 gallop, indicating transient left ventricular dysfunction, is more significant than an S_4 gallop.
• Remove the electrodes, and clean the electrode sites. (See *Exercise ECG interference.*)

Holter monitoring

Holter monitoring, also called *ambulatory ECG* or *dynamic monitoring*, is the continuous recording of heart activity as the patient follows his normal routine, usually for 24 hours, or about 100,000 cardiac cycles. The patient wears a small cassette tape recorder connected to chest electrodes and keeps a diary of activities and associated symptoms. At the end of the recording period, the tape is analyzed and a report is printed, permitting correlation of cardiac irregularities, such as arrhythmias and ST-segment changes, with the patient's activities.

(Text continues on page 411.)

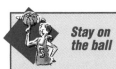

Stay on the ball

Exercise ECG interference

• Use of beta-adrenergic blockers may make test results hard to interpret.
• Use of cardiac glycosides may cause false-positive results.
• Conditions that cause left ventricular hypertrophy may interfere with ischemia testing.

Echocardiography

An echocardiograph uses ultra-high-frequency waves to help examine the size, shape, and motion of the heart's structures. Here's how it works.

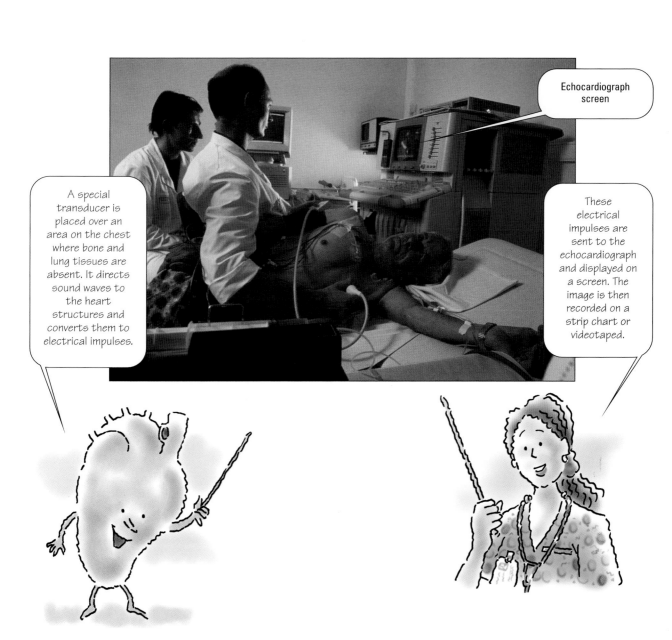

Echocardiograph screen

A special transducer is placed over an area on the chest where bone and lung tissues are absent. It directs sound waves to the heart structures and converts them to electrical impulses.

These electrical impulses are sent to the echocardiograph and displayed on a screen. The image is then recorded on a strip chart or videotaped.

Intracranial computed tomography

Intracranial computed tomography provides a series of tomograms, or radiographs, of a selected layer of the body (in this case, the brain). These tomograms, which are translated by a computer and displayed on a screen, represent cross-sectional images of various layers (or slices) of the brain. Intracranial tumors and other brain lesions may be identified.

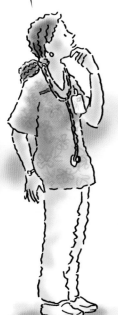

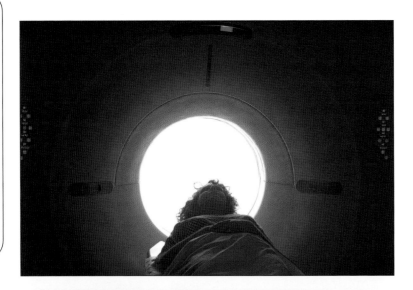

The patient is placed in a supine position on an X-ray table with her head immobilized. The head of the table moves into the scanner, which rotates around the patient's head, taking radiographs at 1-degree intervals in a 180-degree arc.

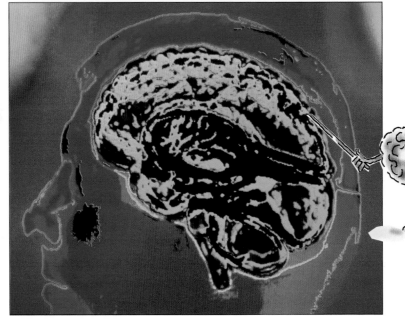

This image shows a normal brain. Whew!

The density of tissue determines the amount of radiation that passes through it. Areas of altered density or displaced vasculature or other structures may indicate a tumor, an infarction, or a hematoma. Let's take a look at a few abnormal intracranial computed tomography scans.

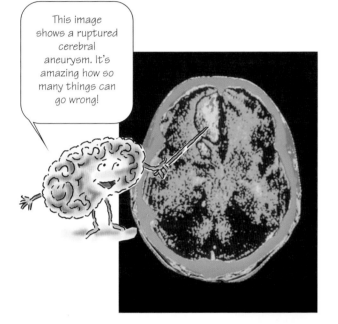

This image shows a ruptured cerebral aneurysm. It's amazing how so many things can go wrong!

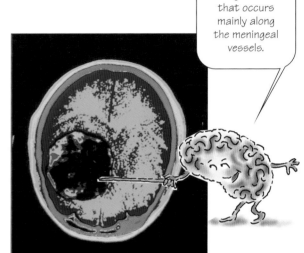

Here we see a calcified meningioma, a benign tumor that occurs mainly along the meningeal vessels.

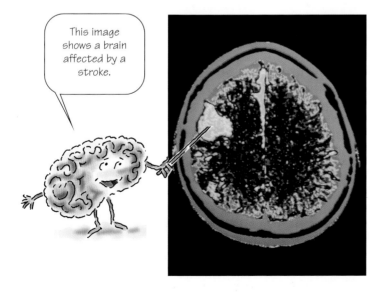

This image shows a brain affected by a stroke.

Endoscopic ultrasound

Endoscopic ultrasound combines ultrasonography with endoscopy to visualize the GI tract. An ultrasound probe, incorporated at the end of an endoscope, allows ultrasonic imaging in addition to typical endoscopy.

Images can be transmitted onto a screen for better visualization.

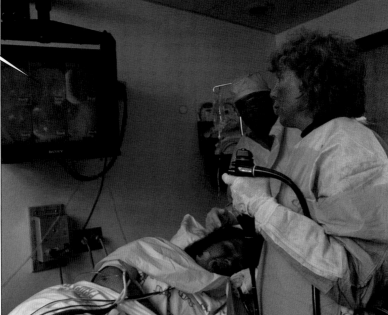

The practitioner passes the endoscope through the esophagus. When examination of the esophagus and the cardiac sphincter is complete, she advances it into the stomach.

After examining the stomach lining, the practitioner advances the endoscope into the duodenum. She examines the duodenum and then slowly withdraws the endoscope.

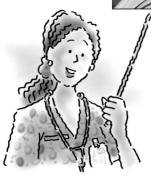

What it all means

When evaluated along with the patient's diary, a normal ECG pattern shows no significant arrhythmias or ST-segment changes. Heart rate changes normally occur during various activities.

Cardiac abnormalities detected by Holter monitoring include PVCs, conduction defects, tachyarrhythmias, bradyarrhythmias, and bradycardia-tachycardia syndrome.

What needs to be done

- Explain the procedure to the patient.
- Show him how to position the recorder when he lies down. Tell him to continue his routine activities during the monitoring period. Instruct him to keep a log of these activities as well as emotional upsets, physical symptoms, and drug use; show the patient a sample diary. Demonstrate how to mark the tape at the symptom onset, if applicable. (If a patient-activated monitor is being used, show him how to press the EVENT button to activate the monitor when he experiences unusual sensations.)

Magnetic attraction

- Instruct the patient to wear loose-fitting clothing with front-buttoning tops during monitoring and not to tamper with the monitor. Provide bathing instructions. Instruct him to avoid magnets, metal detectors, high-voltage areas, and electric blankets. Show him how to check the recorder to make sure it's working properly. Tell him to notify you if an electrode comes off.
- Clean the electrode sites with an alcohol pad and gently abrade them until they redden. Apply the electrodes to the correct sites, and press the sides and bottom of each electrode firmly. Then press the center of the electrode lightly to promote good contact between the jelly and the patient's skin. Attach the electrode cable securely to the monitor, and position the monitor (and case) as the patient will wear it; then attach the leadwires to the electrodes.
- Install a new or fully charged battery in the recorder, insert the tape, and turn on the recorder. Test the electrode attachment circuit by connecting the recorder to a standard ECG machine. (See *Holter monitoring interference.*)
- If the patient won't be returning to the facility immediately after the monitoring period, show him how to remove and store the equipment. Remind him to bring the diary when he returns.

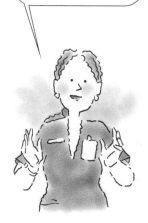

It's versatile! Holter monitoring can help detect cardiac arrhythmias, evaluate chest pain, and monitor the effectiveness of therapy.

Stay on the ball

Holter monitoring interference

Physiologic variation in arrhythmia frequency and severity may cause an arrhythmia to be missed during 24-hour Holter monitoring.

Catheterization tests

Cardiac catheterization

Simply stated, cardiac catheterization is the passing of a catheter into the right or left side or both sides of the heart. This procedure can determine blood pressure and blood flow in the heart's chambers, permit blood sample collection, and record films of the ventricles (contrast ventriculography) and arteries (coronary arteriography or angiography).

What it all means

Cardiac catheterization should reveal no abnormalities of heart chamber size or configuration, wall motion or thickness, or direction of blood flow or valve motion. Coronary arteries should have a smooth and regular outline. (For more information on normal findings, see *Maximum normal cardiac pressures*.)

Common abnormalities and defects that can be confirmed by cardiac catheterization include CAD, myocardial incompetence, valvular heart disease, and septal defects.

What needs to be done

• Explain the procedure to the patient. Tell him to restrict food and fluids for at least 6 hours before the test. Inform him that the test takes 1 to 2 hours. Tell him that he may receive a mild sedative but will remain conscious during the procedure.
• Have the patient void just before the procedure.
• Check the patient history for hypersensitivity to shellfish, iodine, or contrast media used in other diagnostic tests. Discontinue any anticoagulant therapy as ordered.

Supine is fine

• The patient is placed in the supine position. ECG leads are applied, and an I.V. line is started. After the local anesthetic is injected at the catheterization site, a small incision or percutaneous puncture is made into the artery or vein, depending on where studies will be performed, and the catheter is passed through the sheath into the vessel. The catheter is guided to the cardiac chambers or coronary arteries using fluoroscopy. When the catheter is in place, the contrast medium is injected through it to visualize

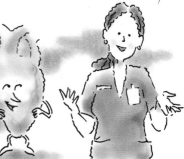

Cardiac catheterization evaluates valvular insufficiency or stenosis, septal defects, congenital anomalies, myocardial function and blood supply, and cardiac wall motion.

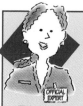

Advice from the experts

Maximum normal cardiac pressures

This chart shows the upper limits of normal pressure in the cardiac chambers and great vessels of recumbent (lying down) adults.

Chamber or vessel	Pressure
Right atrium	6 mm Hg (mean)
Right ventricle	30/6 mm Hg*
Pulmonary artery	30/12 mm Hg* (mean, 18)
Left atrium	12 mm Hg (mean)
Left ventricle	140/12 mm Hg*
Ascending aorta	140/90 mm Hg* (mean, 105)
Pulmonary artery wedge	Almost identical to left atrial mean pressure (±1 to 2 mm Hg)

Peak systolic and end-diastolic

the cardiac vessels and structures. Vital signs are monitored frequently.

• After the procedure, the catheter is removed and direct pressure is applied to the incision site for 30 minutes; a dressing is applied when hemostasis occurs.

• Monitor vital signs every 15 minutes for 2 hours, every 30 minutes for the next 2 hours, and then every hour for 2 hours. If no hematoma or other problems arise, check every 4 hours. If signs are unstable, check every 5 minutes and notify the doctor.

• Observe the insertion site for a hematoma or blood loss, and reinforce the pressure dressing, as needed.

• Check the patient's color, skin temperature, and peripheral pulse below the puncture site. The brachial approach carries a higher incidence of vasospasm (characterized by cool fingers and hand and weak pulses on the affected side); this usually resolves within 24 hours.

• Enforce bed rest for 8 hours. If the femoral route was used for catheter insertion, keep the patient's leg extended for 6 to 8 hours; if the antecubital fossa route was used, keep the arm extended for at least 3 hours.

- Resume medications withheld before the test as ordered. Administer analgesics as ordered.
- Obtain a posttest ECG to check for possible myocardial damage. (See *Cardiac catheterization interference*.)

Pulmonary artery catheterization

Pulmonary artery (PA) catheterization (also known as *Swan-Ganz catheterization*) uses a balloon-tipped, flow-directed catheter to provide intermittent occlusion of the pulmonary artery. (See *A primer on PA catheters*.)

When the catheter is in place, this procedure permits measurement of both pulmonary artery pressure (PAP), and pulmonary artery wedge pressure (PAWP).

The PAWP reading accurately reflects left atrial pressure and left ventricular end-diastolic pressure, although the catheter itself never enters the left side of the heart.

What it all means

Normal pressures are:
- *right atrial pressure:* 1 to 6 mm Hg
- *systolic right ventricular pressure:* 20 to 30 mm Hg

Now I get it!

A primer on PA catheters

The flexible pulmonary artery (PA) catheter used in PA catheterization comes in two-lumen, three-lumen, and four-lumen (thermodilution) models and in various lengths.

Can you make do with two?
In the two-lumen catheter, one lumen contains the balloon, 1 mm behind the catheter tip. The other lumen, which opens at the tip, measures pressure in front of the balloon. The two-lumen catheter measures pulmonary artery pressure and pulmonary artery wedge pressure and can be used to sample mixed venous blood and to infuse I.V. solutions.

Three gives you CVP
The three-lumen catheter has an additional proximal lumen that opens 12" (30.5 cm) behind the tip. When the tip is in the main pulmonary artery, the proximal lumen lies in the right atrium, permitting fluid administration or monitoring of right atrial pressure (central venous pressure [CVP]).

Four means a thermistor
The four-lumen type includes a transistorized thermistor for monitoring blood temperature and allows cardiac output measurement. A four-lumen catheter with thermodilution and pacer port mode is used to allow pacing, if necessary. The introducer part of the system may also be used to infuse large amounts of fluids.

- *end-diastolic right ventricular pressure:* less than 5 mm Hg
- *systolic PAP:* 20 to 30 mm Hg
- *diastolic PAP:* 10 to 15 mm Hg
- *mean PAP:* less than 20 mm Hg
- *PAWP:* 6 to 12 mm Hg
- *left atrial pressure:* about 10 mm Hg.

High, low, and in between

An abnormally high right atrial pressure can indicate pulmonary disease, right-sided heart failure, fluid overload, cardiac tamponade, tricuspid stenosis and insufficiency, or pulmonary hypertension.

Elevated right ventricular pressure can result from pulmonary hypertension, pulmonary valvular stenosis, right-sided heart failure, pericardial effusion, constrictive pericarditis, chronic heart failure, or ventricular septal defects.

An abnormally high PAP is characteristic of increased pulmonary blood flow, as in a left-to-right shunt secondary to atrial or ventricular septal defect; increased pulmonary arteriolar resistance, as in pulmonary hypertension or mitral stenosis; chronic obstructive pulmonary disease; pulmonary edema or embolus; and left-sided heart failure from any cause.

PA systolic pressure is the same as right ventricular systolic pressure. PA diastolic pressure is the same as left atrial pressure, except in patients with severe pulmonary disease causing pulmonary hypertension; in such patients, catheterization is still important diagnostically.

Elevated PAWP can result from left-sided heart failure, mitral stenosis and insufficiency, cardiac tamponade, or cardiac insufficiency; depressed PAWP, from hypovolemia.

What needs to be done

- Explain the procedure to the patient.
- Set up the equipment according to the manufacturer's directions and the facility's procedure. Place the patient in the supine position, and position head, arms and shoulders according to catheter insertion site. If the patient can't tolerate the supine position, assist him to semi-Fowler's position. During the test, all pressures are monitored with the patient in the same position.
- The catheter balloon is checked for defects using sterile technique, and all ports are flushed to ensure patency.
- The catheter is introduced into the vein percutaneously and directed to the right atrium. The catheter balloon is inflated so that venous flow carries the catheter tip through the right atrium and tricuspid valve into the right ventricle and into the pulmonary artery. While the catheter is being directed, the monitor screen is

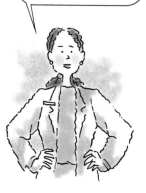

PA catheterization helps assess right- and left-sided heart failure. It also helps monitor fluid status in patients who have suffered serious burns or who have renal disease, noncardiogenic pulmonary edema, or acute respiratory distress syndrome.

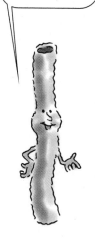

I don't know how much longer I can take all this pressure!

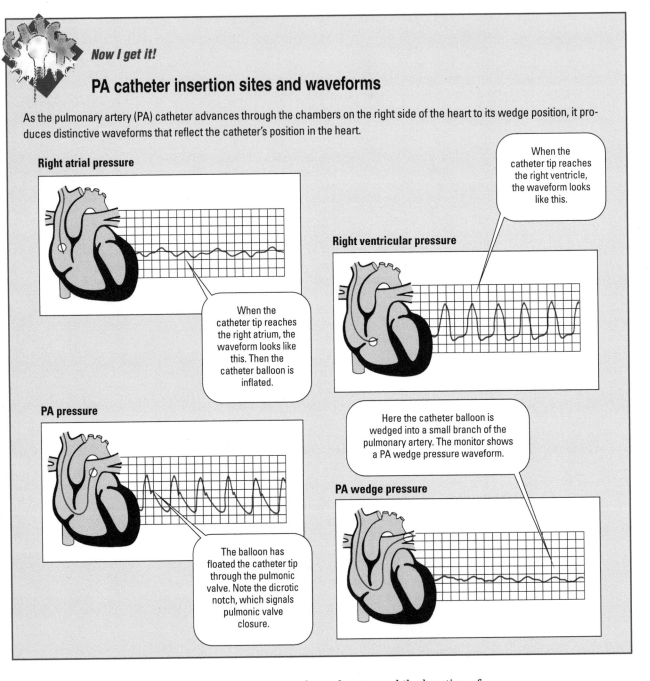

Now I get it!

PA catheter insertion sites and waveforms

As the pulmonary artery (PA) catheter advances through the chambers on the right side of the heart to its wedge position, it produces distinctive waveforms that reflect the catheter's position in the heart.

Right atrial pressure

When the catheter tip reaches the right atrium, the waveform looks like this. Then the catheter balloon is inflated.

When the catheter tip reaches the right ventricle, the waveform looks like this.

Right ventricular pressure

PA pressure

Here the catheter balloon is wedged into a small branch of the pulmonary artery. The monitor shows a PA wedge pressure waveform.

The balloon has floated the catheter tip through the pulmonic valve. Note the dicrotic notch, which signals pulmonic valve closure.

PA wedge pressure

observed for characteristic waveform changes and the location of the catheter tip is found. (See *PA catheter insertion sites and waveforms.*)

- Observe the monitor for any arrhythmias caused by catheter irritation. If this occurs, the catheter may be partially withdrawn or medication administered.
- To record PAWP, the catheter balloon is inflated with the specified amount of air (no more than 1.5 cc); the catheter tip should float into the wedge position, as indicated by an altered waveform on the monitor screen; then the pressure is recorded. If a PAWP waveform occurs with less than the recommended inflation volume, the balloon shouldn't be inflated further. Then the air from the balloon is allowed to return to the syringe, which is then deflated, allowing the catheter to float back into the pulmonary artery. The monitor screen is observed for a PA waveform. Then the system is flushed and recalibrated.

No overinflation

- The balloon catheter shouldn't be overinflated. Overinflation could distend the pulmonary artery, causing vessel rupture.
- When the catheter's correct positioning and function have been established, the catheter is sutured to the skin and antimicrobial ointment and an airtight dressing are applied to the insertion site according to facility policy.
- Obtain a chest X-ray to confirm catheter placement. (See *PA catheterization interference.*)

Stay on the ball

PA catheterization interference

Mechanical ventilators with positive pressure cause increased intrathoracic pressure, raising catheter pressure.

Miscellaneous tests

Electrophysiology studies

Electrophysiology (EPS) studies permit measurement of discrete conduction intervals by recording electrical conduction during slow withdrawal of a bipolar or tripolar electrode catheter from the right ventricle through the His bundle to the sinoatrial node. The catheter is introduced into the femoral vein, passing through the right atrium and across the septal leaflet of the tricuspid valve.

Possible complications of these studies include arrhythmias, phlebitis, pulmonary emboli, thromboemboli, and catheter-site hemorrhage.

What it all means

Normal conduction intervals in adults are HV interval, 35 to 55 msec; AH interval, 45 to 150 msec; and PA interval, 20 to 40 msec.

His or hers?

A prolonged HV interval (the conduction time from the His bundle to the Purkinje fibers) can result from acute or chronic disease. Atrioventricular nodal (AH interval) delays can stem from atrial pacing, chronic conduction system disease, carotid sinus pressure, recent MI, and use of certain drugs. Intra-atrial (PA interval) delays can result from acquired, surgically induced, or congenital atrial disease and atrial pacing.

What needs to be done

• Explain to the patient that EPS studies evaluate the heart's conduction system. Instruct him to restrict food and fluids for at least 6 hours before the test. Inform him that the studies take 1 to 3 hours.

A close shave

• Tell the patient that after the groin area is shaved, a catheter will be inserted into the femoral vein, and an I.V. line may be started.
• Have him void before the test.
• The patient is placed in the supine position. Limb electrodes and precordial leads are applied for ECG recording. The hair is clipped at the insertion site, and then the site is scrubbed and sterilized. The local anesthetic is injected, and a J-tip electrode is introduced I.V. into the femoral vein (occasionally, into a vein in the antecubital fossa). Guided by fluoroscopy, the catheter is advanced until it crosses the tricuspid valve and enters the right ventricle. Then the catheter is slowly withdrawn from the tricuspid area, and recordings of conduction intervals are made from each pole of the catheter, either simultaneously or sequentially. After recordings and measurements are completed, the catheter is removed and a pressure dressing is applied to the site.
• Monitor the patient's vital signs as ordered. If they're unstable, check every 15 minutes and alert the doctor. Observe for shortness of breath, chest pain, pallor, or changes in pulse rate or blood pressure. Enforce bed rest for 4 to 6 hours.
• Check the catheter insertion site for bleeding as ordered; apply a pressure bandage until the bleeding stops.
• Advise the patient that he may resume his usual diet.
• Make sure a 12-lead resting ECG is scheduled to assess for changes.

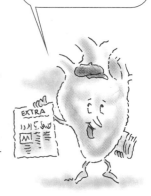

Read all about it! EPS studies help diagnose arrhythmias and conduction defects and determine the need for an implanted pacemaker, an internal cardioverter-defibrillator, and cardioactive drugs. Also, they evaluate the effects of these treatments.

Pulse oximetry

Pulse oximetry is a continuous noninvasive study of arterial blood oxygen saturation using a clip or probe attached to a sensor site (usually an earlobe or a fingertip). The percentage expressed is the ratio of oxygen to hemoglobin (Hb).

What it all means

Levels are normally greater than 95%. Hypoxemia with levels less than 95% indicates impaired cardiopulmonary function or abnormal gas exchange.

What needs to be done

- Explain to the patient that this test assesses oxygen content in the Hb.
- Make sure the patient has no false fingernails or nail polish.
- Place the probe or clip over the finger or other intended sensor site so that the light beams and sensors are opposite each other.
- Turn on the monitor and ensure that it accurately detects the patient's pulse and reads the percentage of oxygen.
- If the monitor is to remain on continuously, ensure that the skin remains intact under the probe or clip and that the circulation is adequate.
- After the test is performed, remove the probe and clean it with alcohol. (See *Pulse oximetry interference*.)

Stay on the ball

Pulse oximetry interference

Anemic conditions, vasoconstriction, certain drugs (such as vasopressors), hypotension, vessel obstruction, nail polish, or false nails may interfere with test results.

Pulse oximetry monitors oxygenation perioperatively, during an acute illness, and during testing for sleep apnea. It also helps determine bronchodilator effectiveness.

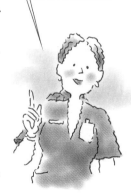

Pulmonary function tests

Pulmonary function tests (PFTs)—including volume, capacity, and flow rate tests—are a series of measurements that evaluate ventilatory function through spirometric measurements; they're performed on patients with suspected pulmonary dysfunction. Of the seven tests that are performed to determine volume, tidal volume (V_T) and expiratory reserve volume (ERV) are direct spirographic measurements; minute volume, carbon dioxide response, inspiratory reserve volume, and residual volume are calculated from the results of other PFTs; and thoracic gas volume (TGV) is calculated from body plethysmography.

Of the pulmonary capacity tests, vital capacity (VC), inspiratory capacity (IC), functional residual capacity (FRC), total lung capacity, and forced expiratory flow may be measured directly or calculated from the results of other tests. Forced vital capacity, flow-volume curve, forced expiratory volume (FEV), peak expiratory flow rate, and maximal voluntary ventilation are direct spirographic measurements. The diffusing capacity for carbon monoxide is calculated from the amount of carbon monoxide exhaled.

What it all means

Normal values are predicted for each patient based on age, height, weight, and sex and are expressed as a percentage:

- V_T: 5 to 7 mg/kg of body weight
- *ERV:* 25% of VC
- *IC:* 75% of VC
- FEV_1: 83% of VC (after 1 second)
- FEV_2: 94% of VC (after 2 seconds)
- FEV_3: 97% of VC (after 3 seconds).

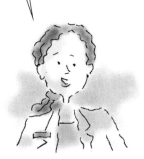

PFTs determine the cause of dyspnea, assess treatment effectiveness, and allow preoperative evaluation.

Reading results

Values such as these can be calculated at bedside with a portable spirometer. Results are usually considered abnormal if they're less than 80% of these values. (See *Interpreting pulmonary function test results.*)

What needs to be done

- Pulmonary function testing requires several areas of testing. Each requires its own procedure.
- Explain the procedure to the patient. Tell him not to eat a heavy meal before the test and not to smoke for 12 hours beforehand.
- Teach the patient how to operate the spirometer, and inform him that the accuracy of the tests depends on his cooperation. Just before the test, tell him to void and to loosen tight clothing.
- Inform the laboratory if the patient is taking an analgesic that depresses respiration. As ordered, withhold bronchodilators for 8 hours. After testing, instruct the patient to resume his usual activities, diet, and medications as ordered.

Tidal volume

- The patient is told to breathe normally into the mouthpiece 10 times.

Expiratory reserve volume

- The patient is told to breathe normally for several breaths and then to exhale as completely as possible.

Vital capacity

- The patient is told to inhale as deeply as possible and to exhale into the mouthpiece as completely as possible. This procedure is repeated three times, and the test result showing the largest volume is used.

(Text continues on page 424.)

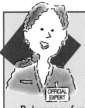

Advice from the experts

Interpreting pulmonary function test results

Pulmonary function test results are interpreted after data are collected and calculated. The implications are reviewed in this table.

Pulmonary function test	Method of calculation	Implications
Tidal volume (V_T): Amount of air inhaled or exhaled during normal breathing	Determining the spirographic measurement for 10 breaths and then dividing by 10	Decreased V_T may indicate restrictive disease and requires further testing, such as full pulmonary function studies or chest X-rays.
Minute volume (MV): Total amount of air expired per minute	Multiplying V_T by the respiratory rate	Normal MV can occur in emphysema; decreased MV may indicate other diseases such as pulmonary edema. Increased MV can occur with acidosis, increased carbon dioxide (CO_2), decreased partial pressure of arterial oxygen, exercise, and low compliance states.
Carbon dioxide (CO_2) response: Increase or decrease in MV after breathing various CO_2 concentrations	Plotting changes in MV against increasing inspired CO_2 concentrations	Reduced CO_2 response may occur in emphysema, myxedema, obesity, hypoventilation syndrome, and sleep apnea.
Inspiratory reserve volume (IRV): Amount of air inspired over above-normal inspiration	Subtracting V_T from inspiratory capacity (IC)	Abnormal IRV alone doesn't indicate respiratory dysfunction; IRV decreases during normal exercise.
Expiratory reserve volume (ERV): Amount of air exhaled after normal expiration	Direct spirographic measurement	ERV varies, even in healthy people, but usually decreases in obese people.
Residual volume (RV): Amount of air remaining in the lungs after forced expiration	Subtracting ERV from functional residual capacity (FRC)	RV > 35% of total lung capacity (TLC) after maximal expiratory effort may indicate obstructive disease.

(continued)

Interpreting pulmonary function test results (continued)

Pulmonary function test	Method of calculation	Implications
Vital capacity (VC): Total volume of air that can be exhaled after maximum inspiration	Direct spirographic measurement or adding V_T, IRV, and ERV	Normal or increased VC with decreased flow rates may indicate any condition that causes a reduction in functional pulmonary tissue such as pulmonary edema. Decreased VC with normal or increased flow rates may indicate decreased respiratory effort resulting from neuromuscular disease, drug overdose, or head injury; decreased thoracic expansion; or limited diaphragm movement.
Inspiratory capacity (IC): Amount of air that can be inhaled after normal expiration	Direct spirographic measurement or adding IRV and V_T	Decreased IC indicates restrictive disease.
Thoracic gas volume (TGV): Total volume of gas in the lungs from ventilated and nonventilated airways	Body plethysmography	Increased TGV indicates air trapping, which may result from obstructive disease.
Functional residual capacity (FRC): Amount of air remaining in the lungs after normal expiration	Nitrogen washout, helium dilution technique, or adding ERV and RV	Increased FRC indicates overdistention of the lungs, which may result from obstructive pulmonary disease.
Total lung capacity (TLC): Total volume of the lungs when maximally inflated	Adding V_T, IRV, ERV, and RV; FRC and IC; or VC and RV	Low TLC indicates restrictive disease; high TLC indicates overdistended lungs caused by obstructive disease.
Forced vital capacity (FVC): Amount of air exhaled forcefully and quickly after maximum inspiration	Direct spirographic measurement; expressed as a percentage of the total volume of gas exhaled	Decreased FVC indicates flow resistance in the respiratory system from obstructive disease such as chronic bronchitis, or from restrictive disease such as pulmonary fibrosis.

Interpreting pulmonary function test results (continued)

Pulmonary function test	Method of calculation	Implications
Flow-volume curve (also called flow-volume loop): Greatest rate of flow (V_{max}) during FVC maneuvers versus lung volume change	Direct spirographic measurement at 1-second intervals; calculated from flow rates (expressed in liters per second) and lung volume changes (expressed in liters) during maximal inspiratory and expiratory maneuvers	Decreased flow rates at all volumes during expiration indicate obstructive disease of the small airways such as emphysema. A plateau of expiratory flow near TLC, a plateau of inspiratory flow at mid-VC, and a square wave pattern through most of VC indicate obstructive disease of large airways. Normal or increased PEFR, decreased flow with decreasing lung volumes, and markedly decreased VC indicate restrictive disease.
Forced expiratory volume (FEV): Volume of air expired in the 1st, 2nd, or 3rd second of an FVC maneuver	Direct spirographic measurement; expressed as a percentage of FVC	Decreased FEV_1 and increased FEV_2 and FEV_3 may indicate obstructive disease; decreased or normal FEV_1 may indicate restrictive disease.
Forced expiratory flow (FEF): Average rate of flow during the middle half of FVC	Calculated from the flow rate and the time needed for expiration of the middle 50% of FVC	Low FEF (25% to 75%) indicates obstructive disease of the small and medium-size airways.
Peak expiratory flow rate (PEFR): V_{max} during forced expiration	Calculated from the flow-volume curve or by direct spirographic measurement using a pneumotachometer or electronic tachometer with a transducer to convert flow to electrical output display	Decreased PEFR may indicate a mechanical problem, such as upper airway obstruction, or obstructive disease. PEFR is usually normal in restrictive disease but decreases in severe cases. Because PEFR is effort dependent, it's also low in a person who has poor expiratory effort or doesn't understand the procedure.
Maximal voluntary ventilation (MVV) (also called maximum breathing capacity): The greatest volume of air breathed per unit of time	Direct spirographic measurement	Decreased MVV may indicate obstructive disease; normal or decreased MVV may indicate restrictive disease such as myasthenia gravis.

(continued)

Interpreting pulmonary function test results *(continued)*

Pulmonary function test	Method of calculation	Implications
Diffusing capacity for carbon monoxide (DL_{CO}): Milliliters of carbon monoxide diffused per minute across the alveolocapillary membrane	Calculated from analysis of the amount of carbon monoxide exhaled compared with the amount inhaled	Decreased DL_{CO} due to a thickened alveolocapillary membrane occurs in interstitial pulmonary diseases, such as pulmonary fibrosis, asbestosis, and sarcoidosis; DL_{CO} is reduced in emphysema because of alveolocapillary membrane loss.

Inspiratory capacity

- The patient is instructed to breathe normally for several breaths and then to inhale as deeply as possible.

Functional residual capacity

- The patient is told to breathe normally into a spirometer that contains a known concentration of an insoluble gas (usually helium or nitrogen) in a known volume of air. After a few breaths, the concentrations of gas in the spirometer and the lungs reach equilibrium. Then the point of equilibrium and the concentration of gas in the spirometer are recorded.

Thoracic gas volume

- The patient is put in an airtight box or body plethysmograph and told to breathe through a tube connected to a transducer. At end-expiration, the tube is occluded, the patient is told to pant, and changes in intrathoracic and plethysmographic pressure are measured. The results are used to calculate total TGV and FRC.

Forced vital capacity and forced expiratory volume

- The patient is instructed to inhale as slowly and deeply as possible and then is asked to exhale into the mouthpiece as quickly and completely as possible. This procedure is repeated three times, and the largest volume is recorded. The volume of air expired at 1 second (FEV_1), at 2 seconds (FEV_2), and at 3 seconds (FEV_3) during all three repetitions is also recorded.

Maximal voluntary ventilation

- The patient is instructed to breathe into the mouthpiece as quickly and deeply as possible for 15 seconds.

Stay on the ball

Pulmonary function test interference

- An opioid analgesic or sedative can decrease inspiratory and expiratory forces.
- Bronchodilators may temporarily improve pulmonary function.
- Lack of patient cooperation, hypoxia, and metabolic disturbances can make testing difficult or impossible.
- Pregnancy or gastric distention may displace lung volume.

Diffusing capacity for carbon monoxide

- The patient is told to inhale a gas mixture with a low concentration of carbon monoxide and then to hold his breath for 10 to 15 seconds before exhaling. (See *Pulmonary function test interference*.)

Sleep studies

Sleep studies, also know as *polysomnography*, help in the differential diagnosis of sleep-disordered breathing. They're helpful in diagnosing a breathing disorder in patients with a history of excessive snoring, narcolepsy, excessive daytime sleepiness, insomnia, cardiac rhythm disorders, or restless leg spasms. During testing the following are monitored: cardiac rate and rhythm, chest and abdominal wall movement, nasal and oral airflow, oxygen saturation, muscle activity, retinal function, and brain activity during the sleep phase.

For the patient with known sleep apnea, split-night studies may be required, such as monitoring the patient for the first half of the night, then using continuous positive airway pressure or nasal ventilation to open the obstructed airway during the second half of the night.

What it all means

Normal values include a respiratory disturbance index (or apnea-hypopnea index) of fewer than 5 to 10 episodes per study period. No ischemic change or arrhythmias appear on ECG. Impedance (chest and abdominal wall motion), airway (nasal and oral airflow), arterial oxygen saturation

> Sleep studies help to diagnose a breathing disorder in patients with a history of excessive snoring, narcolepsy, excessive daytime sleepiness, insomnia, cardiac rhythm disorders, or restless leg spasms.

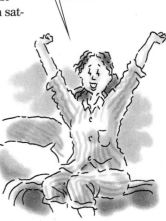

via oximetry, leg electromyogram (for muscle activity), electro-oculogram (for retinal function), and EEG (for brain activity) are normal.

Abnormal recordings suggest possible obstructive sleep apnea syndrome. Abnormal movement during sleep suggests a possible seizure or movement disorder.

What needs to be done

• Explain the purpose of the test to the patient and tell him that caffeinated products and naps should be avoided for 2 to 3 days before the test. Schedule the test for the evening and night hours, usually from 10 p.m. to 6 a.m.
• Advise the patient to maintain a normal sleep schedule so that he's neither deprived of sleep nor overrested.
• Tell the patient he may bathe or shower before the test.
• Secure electrodes to the patient's skin, depending on the type of monitoring being used.
• Make the patient comfortable and tell him that normal body movements won't interfere with the electrodes.
• Turn the lights off and monitor the EEG for a baseline reading before the patient falls asleep. The recording and video equipment record the sleep events as they occur.
• Monitor the patient during sleep until the test is completed. Monitor for respiratory distress during the study.

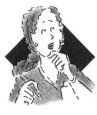

Quick quiz

1. A patient is undergoing external fetal monitoring. Which heart rate indicates fetal tachycardia?

    A.   140 beats/minute
    B.   165 beats/minute
    C.   115 beats/minute
    D.   60 beats/minute

Answer: B. Normal FHR is 120 to 160 beats/minute. FHR less than 120 beats/minute indicates bradycardia; above 160 beats/minute indicates tachycardia.

2. Which instruction should you give the patient before exercise ECG?
- A. Avoid caffeinated beverages for 3 hours before the test.
- B. Avoid smoking for 24 hours before the test.
- C. Avoid alcoholic beverages for 12 hours before the test.
- D. Avoid food and drink for 8 hours before the test.

Answer: A. Instruct the patient not to eat, smoke, or drink alcoholic or caffeinated beverages for 3 hours before exercise ECG.

3. After cardiac catheterization, how long should the patient remain on bed rest?
- A. 12 hours
- B. 8 hours
- C. 24 hours
- D. 36 hours

Answer: B. Bed rest should be enforced for 8 hours after cardiac catheterization.

4. Elevated right atrial pressure may indicate:
- A. pulmonary hypertension.
- B. constrictive pericarditis.
- C. ventricular septal defect.
- D. arterial hypotension.

Answer: A. Abnormally high right atrial pressure may indicate pulmonary disease, right-sided heart failure, fluid overload, cardiac tamponade, tricuspid stenosis and insufficiency, or pulmonary hypertension.

5. A PA catheter balloon should be inflated with no more than:
- A. 1 cc of air.
- B. 2 cc of air.
- C. 1.5 cc of air.
- D. 3 cc of air.

Answer: C. A PA catheter balloon should be inflated with no more than 1.5 cc of air.

Scoring

☆☆☆   If you answered all five questions correctly, outstanding! You're a testing titan!

☆☆   If you answered four questions correctly, not bad! You've passed the test!

☆   If you answered fewer than four questions correctly, don't get testy! Just keep at it!

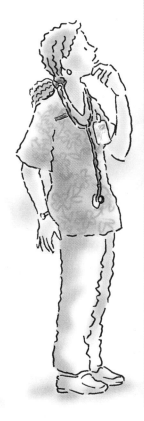

Appendices and index

Normal laboratory test values

This chart provides normal values for common laboratory tests, including chemistry, hematology, and coagulation tests. Where indicated, conventional and SI units are given.

Comprehensive metabolic panel

Laboratory test	Conventional	SI units
Albumin	3.5-5 g/dl	35-50 g/L
Alkaline phosphatase	45-115 U/L	45-115 U/L
ALT	Male: 10-40 U/L	0.17-0.68 µkat/L
	Female: 7-35 U/L	0.12-0.60 µkat/L
AST	12-31 U/L	0.21-0.53 µkat/L
Bilirubin, total	0.2-1 mg/dl	3.5-17 µmol/L
BUN	8-20 mg/dl	2.9-7.5 mmol/L
Calcium	8.2-10.2 mg/dl	2.05-2.54 mmol/L
Carbon dioxide	22-26 mEq/L	22-26 mmol/L
Chloride	100-108 mEq/L	100-108 mmol/L
Creatinine	Male: 0.8-1.2 mg/dl	62-115 µmol/L
	Female: 0.6-0.9 mg/dl	53-97 µmol/L
Glucose	70-100 mg/dl	3.9-6.1 mmol/L
Potassium	3.5-5 mEq/L	3.5-5 mmol/L
Protein, total	6.3-8.3 g/dl	64-83 g/L
Sodium	135-145 mEq/L	135-145 mmol/L

Lipid panel

Laboratory test	Conventional	SI units
Total cholesterol	< 200 mg/dl	< 5.18 mmol/L
HDL cholesterol	$\geq$ 60 mg/dl	$\geq$ 1.55 mmol/L
LDL cholesterol	< 130 mg/dl	< 3.36 mmol/L
VLDL cholesterol	< 130 mg/dl	< 3.4 mmol/L
Triglycerides	< 150 mg/dl	< 1.7 mmol/L

Thyroid panel

Laboratory test	Conventional	SI units
T_3	80-200 ng/dl	1.2-3 nmol/L
T_4, free	0.9-2.3 ng/dl	10-30 nmol/L
T_4, total	5-13.5 mcg/dl	60-165 mmol/L
TSH	0.4-4.2 mIU/L	0.4-4.2 mIU/L

Other chemistry tests

Laboratory test	Conventional	SI units
A/G ratio	3.4-4.8 g/dl	34-38 g/dl
Ammonia	< 50 ng/dl	< 36 µmol/L
Amylase	26-102 U/L	0.4-1.74 µkat/L
Anion gap	8-14 mEq/L	8-14 mmol/L
Bilirubin, direct	< 0.5 mg/dl	< 6.8 µmol/L
Calcitonin	Male: < 16 pg/ml	< 16 ng/L
	Female: < 8 pg/ml	< 8 ng/L
Calcium, ionized	4.65-5.28 mg/dl	1.1-1.25 mmol/L
Cortisol	a.m.: 7-25 mcg/dl	0.2-0.7 µmol/L
	p.m.: 2-14 mcg/dl	0.06-0.39 µmol/L
C-reactive protein	< 0.8 mg/dl	< 8 mg/L
Ferritin	Male: 20-300 ng/ml	20-300 mcg/L
	Female: 20-120 ng/ml	20-120 mcg/L
Folate	1.8-20 ng/ml	4.45-3 nmol/L
GGT	Male: 7-47 U/L	0.12-1.80 µkat/L
	Female: 5-25 U/L	0.08-0.42 µkat/L
Hb_{A1c}	4%-7%	0.04-0.07
Homocysteine	< 12 µmol/L	< 12 µmol/L
Iron	Male: 65-175 mcg/dl	11.6-31.3 µmol/L
	Female: 50-170 mcg/dl	9-30.4 µmol/L
Iron-binding capacity	250-400 mcg/dl	45-72 µmol/L
Lactic acid	0.5-2.2 mEq/L	0.5-2.2 mmol/L
Lipase	10-73 U/L	0.17-1.24 µkat/L
Magnesium	1.3-2.2 mg/dl	0.65-1.05 mmol/L
Osmolality	275-295 mOsm/kg	275-295 mOsm/kg
Phosphate	2.7-4.5 mg/dl	0.87-1.45 mmol/L
Prealbumin	19-38 mg/dl	190-380 mg/L
Uric acid	Male: 3.4-7 mg/dl	202-416 µmol/L
	Female: 2.3-6 mg/dl	143-357 µmol/L

Hematology tests

Laboratory test	Conventional	SI units
Hemoglobin	Male: 14-17.4 g/dl	140-174 g/L
	Female: 12-16 g/dl	120-160 g/L
Hematocrit	Male: 42%-52%	0.42-0.52
	Female: 36%-48%	0.36-0.48

Hematology tests
(continued)

Laboratory test	Conventional	SI units
Red blood cell	Male: 4.5-5.5 million/µl	$4.5\text{-}5.5 \times 10^{12}$/L
	Female: 4-5 million/µl	$4\text{-}5 \times 10^{12}$/L
Leukocytes	4,000-10,000/µl	$4\text{-}10 \times 10^{9}$/L
• Bands	0%-5%	0.03-0.08
• Basophils	0%-1%	0-0.01
• Eosinophils	1%-4%	0.01-0.04
• Lymphocytes	25%-40%	0.25-0.40
– B-Lymphocytes	270-640/µl	—
– T-Lymphocytes	1,400-2,700/µl	—
• Monocytes	2%-8%	0.02-0.08
• Neutrophils	54%-75%	0.54-0.75
Platelets	140,000-400,00/mm^3	$140\text{-}400 \times 10^{9}$/L

Coagulation tests

Laboratory test	Conventional	SI units
Activated clotting time	107 sec ± 13 sec	107 sec ± 13 sec
Bleeding time	3-6 min	3-6 min
D-dimer	< 250 mcg/L	< 1.37 nmol/L
Fibrinogen	200-400 mg/dl	2-4 g/L
INR (therapeutic target)	2.0-3.0	2.0-3.0
Partial thromboplastin time	21-35 sec	21-35 sec
Prothrombin time	10-14 sec	10-14 sec

Guide to less common diagnostic tests

Test and purpose	Description	Findings
Dexamethasone suppression test • Screens for Cushing's syndrome • Helps diagnose major depression and monitors its treatment	The patient receives an oral dexamethasone dose. Normally, dexamethasone suppresses blood levels of adrenal steroid hormones. In patients with Cushing's syndrome and some forms of depression, the drug fails to suppress these levels.	**Normal findings** Serum cortisol value is normally below 5 g/dl (SI, 140 nmol/L), indicating dexamethasone suppression. (However, a normal test result doesn't rule out major depression.) **Abnormal findings** Values above 5 g/dl indicate suppression failure, as in Cushing's syndrome, severe stress, and clinical depression.
Gallium scanning • Detects primary or metastatic neoplasms and inflammatory lesions • Evaluates malignant lymphoma and identifies recurrent tumors after chemotherapy or radiation therapy	The patient undergoes a total body scan 6 to 72 hours after I.V. injection of radioactive gallium citrate (Ga 67). Certain neoplasms and inflammatory lesions attract gallium; however, exact diagnosis requires additional tests.	**Normal findings** Normally, gallium activity appears in the liver, spleen, bones, and large bowel. Bowel activity results from mucosal uptake and fecal excretion of gallium. **Abnormal findings** Gallium scanning may reveal inflammatory lesions, discrete abscesses, or diffuse infiltration.
Liver-spleen scanning • Screens for hepatic metastasis and hepatocellular disease, such as cirrhosis and hepatitis • Detects focal disease in the liver and spleen, such as tumors, cysts, and abscesses • Demonstrates hepatomegaly, splenomegaly, and splenic infarcts • Assesses liver and spleen condition after abdominal trauma	A gamma camera records radioactivity distribution in the liver and spleen after I.V. injection of a radioactive colloid, most commonly technetium 99m. This substance concentrates in reticuloendothelial cells through phagocytosis. About 80% to 90% is taken up by Kupffer's cells in the liver, 5% to 10% by the spleen, and 3% to 5% by bone marrow. Without moving, the gamma camera images the liver or spleen instantaneously.	**Normal findings** Because the liver and spleen contain equal numbers of reticuloendothelial cells, they normally appear equally bright on the image. However, radioactive colloid generally has a more uniform distribution in the liver than the spleen. Although liver-spleen scanning may not detect early liver disease, it shows characteristic, distinct patterns as the disease progresses. **Abnormal findings** Metastasis to the liver or spleen may appear as a focal defect; confirmation requires biopsy. Because cysts, abscesses, and tumors fail to take up the radioactive colloid, they appear as solitary or multiple focal defects. Ultrasonography can confirm hepatic or splenic cysts. All abscesses require a computed tomography (CT) scan to confirm the diagnosis. Liver-spleen scanning can verify palpable abdominal masses and distinguish splenomegaly from hepatomegaly. Scanning can assess hepatic or splenic injury after abdominal trauma.

(continued)

Test and purpose	Description	Findings
Percutaneous liver biopsy • Diagnoses hepatic parenchymal disease, malignant tumors, and granulomatous infections	Under local anesthesia using a large-core needle, liver tissue is aspirated for histologic analysis. Such analysis can identify hepatic disorders after ultrasonography, CT scans, and radionuclide studies have failed to detect them. The biopsy may be done with or without the use of guided CT or magnetic resonance imaging.	***Normal findings*** Normally, the liver consists of sheets of hepatocytes supported by a framework. ***Abnormal findings*** Tissue examination may reveal diffuse hepatic disease, such as cirrhosis or hepatitis, or infections such as tuberculosis. Primary malignant tumors may be present but hepatic metastasis are more common. Nonmalignant findings with a known focal lesion require further studies, such as laparotomy or laparoscopy with biopsy.
Serum antidiuretic hormone (ADH) • Aids differential diagnosis of central diabetes insipidus, nephrogenic diabetes insipidus (congenital or familial), and syndrome of inappropriate ADH (SIADH)	A fasting blood sample is withdrawn and measured for ADH levels. The patient should limit physical activity for 10 to 12 hours before the test, and should be relaxed and recumbent for 30 minutes before the test. This test may be ordered as part of dehydration or hypertonic saline infusion testing, which determines the body's response to hyperosmolality states.	***Normal findings*** ADH values range from 1 to 5 pg/ml (SI, 1 to 5 ng/L). ADH may be evaluated along with serum osmolality; if serum osmolality is less than 285 mOsm/kg (SI, 285 mmol/kg), ADH is normally less than 2 pg/ml (SI, 2 ng/L). If serum osmolality exceeds 290 mOsm/kg (SI, 290 mmol/kg), ADH may range from 2 to 12 pg/ml (SI, 2 to 12 ng/L). ***Abnormal findings*** Absent or below-normal ADH levels indicate central diabetes insipidus caused by a neurohypophysial or hypothalamic tumor, viral infection, metastatic disease, sarcoidosis, tuberculosis, Hand-Schüller-Christian disease, syphilis, neurosurgical procedures, or head trauma. Normal ADH levels in a patient with signs of diabetes insipidus, such as polydipsia, polyuria, and hypotonic urine, may indicate the nephrogenic form of the disease (marked by renal tubular resistance to ADH); however, levels may rise if the pituitary gland tries to compensate. Elevated ADH levels may also indicate SIADH, possibly resulting from bronchogenic carcinoma, acute porphyria, hypothyroidism, Addison's disease, cirrhosis of the liver, infectious hepatitis, severe hemorrhage, or circulatory shock.

Test and purpose	Description	Findings
Serum prolactin • Aids diagnosis of pituitary dysfunction that may result from pituitary adenoma • Aids diagnosis of hypothalamic dysfunction regardless of cause • Evaluates secondary amenorrhea and galactorrhea	A blood sample is withdrawn and measured for serum prolactin level. The patient should restrict foods and fluids and limit physical activity for 12 hours before the test. He should be in a relaxed state during blood withdrawal.	**Normal findings** Normal values range from undetectable to 23 ng/ml (SI, 23 μg/L) in nonlactating females and 0 to 20 ng/ml (SI, 0 to 20 μg/L) in males. Serum prolactin levels normally rise tenfold to twentyfold during pregnancy and correspond to rises in human placental lactogen levels. After delivery, prolactin secretion falls to basal levels in mothers who don't breastfeed. However, prolactin secretion increases during breastfeeding. **Abnormal findings** Abnormally high prolactin levels, 100 to 300 ng/ml (SI, 100 to 300 IU/L), suggest autonomous prolactin production by a pituitary adenoma (Forbes-Albright syndrome). Rarely, hyperprolactinemia may result from severe endocrine disorders such as hypothyroidism. Idiopathic hyperprolactinemia may be associated with infertility. Decreased prolactin levels in a lactating mother cause lactation failure and may be linked to postpartum pituitary infarction (Sheehan's syndrome).
Serum vitamin B_{12} • Helps diagnose megaloblastic anemia • Helps identify central nervous system (CNS) disorders affecting peripheral and spinal myelinated nerves • Evaluates malabsorption syndromes	A fasting blood sample is withdrawn and measured for serum vitamin B_{12} level. This test is usually performed with serum folic acid testing because deficiencies of vitamin B_{12} and folic acid are the two most common causes of megaloblastic anemia.	**Normal findings** Serum vitamin B_{12} values ranges from 200 to 900 pg/ml (SI, 148 to 664 pmol/L). **Abnormal findings** Decreased values indicate inadequate dietary vitamin B_{12} intake, with malabsorption syndrome; hypermetabolic states such as hyperthyroidism; pregnancy; and CNS damage, such as posterolateral sclerosis or funicular degeneration. Elevated values may result from excessive dietary intake, hepatic disease, and myeloproliferative disorders such as myelocytic leukemia.

(continued)

Test and purpose	Description	Findings
Serum vitamin D • Aids diagnosis of skeletal diseases, such as rickets and osteomalacia • Helps identify hypercalcemia and vitamin D toxicity	A fasting blood sample is tested for serum 25-hydroxycholecalciferol level after this substance is separated from other vitamin D metabolites and contaminants. This test is commonly combined with serum calcium and alkaline phosphatase tests.	**Normal findings** Normally, serum vitamin D values range from 10 to 60 ng/ml (SI, 25 to 150 nmol/L). **Abnormal findings** A low or undetectable level may reflect vitamin D deficiency, which can cause rickets or osteomalacia (as from poor diet, decreased sun exposure, or impaired vitamin D absorption secondary to hepatobiliary disease, pancreatitis, celiac disease, cystic fibrosis, or gastric or small-bowel resection). Low levels may also be linked to hepatic diseases that directly affect vitamin D metabolism. 　Elevated levels may indicate toxicity. Elevated levels associated with hypercalcemia may stem from hypersensitivity to vitamin D, as in sarcoidosis.
Soluble amyloid beta protein precursor • Aids diagnosis of Alzheimer's disease and some forms of senile dementia	A cerebrospinal fluid (CSF) specimen is collected by lumbar puncture, and a small portion is tested using enzyme-linked immunosorbent assay (ELISA). Presence of the amyloid beta protein in senile plaques of the brain is a hallmark of Alzheimer's disease. CSF of some dementia patients contains smaller amyloid amounts than CSF of healthy people, making this test a useful diagnostic tool.	**Normal findings** Normal amyloid beta protein levels in CSF exceed 450 U/L, based on age-matched controls using the ELISA. **Abnormal findings** Below-normal CSF levels suggest a change in amyloid beta protein precursor processing and amyloid beta protein formation. Low levels of soluble amyloid beta protein precursor correlate with clinically diagnosed and autopsy-confirmed Alzheimer's disease.
Tensilon test • Aids diagnosis of myasthenia gravis • Helps differentiate between myasthenic and cholinergic crises • Helps monitor anticholinesterase therapy	The patient is observed after I.V. administration of Tensilon (edrophonium chloride), a rapid, short-acting anticholinesterase that improves muscle strength by increasing muscle response to nerve impulses.	**Normal findings** Fasciculations indicate absence of myasthenia gravis. **Abnormal findings** Improved muscle strength within 30 seconds of Tensilon administration indicates myasthenia gravis. (Results are inconsistent when myasthenia gravis affects only ocular muscles.)

Test and purpose	Description	Findings
Urine vanillylmandelic acid (VMA) • Helps detect pheochromocytoma, neuroblastoma, and ganglioneuroma • Evaluates adrenal medulla function	A 24-hour urine specimen is collected and measured for levels of VMA, a phenolic acid and the most prevalent urine catecholamine metabolite. VMA results from hepatic conversion of epinephrine and norepinephrine; urine VMA levels reflect endogenous production of these major catecholamines. The patient should restrict foods and beverages containing phenolic acid, such as coffee, tea, cola, bananas, citrus fruits, chocolate, and vanilla, for 3 days before the test. During the collection period, he must avoid stressful situations and strenuous physical activity.	***Normal findings*** Normal urine VMA values range from 2 to 7 mg/24 hours (SI, 11 to 37 µmol/day). ***Abnormal findings*** A catecholamine-secreting tumor can cause urine VMA levels to rise. A precise diagnosis requires further testing, such as urine homovanillic acid levels, to rule out pheochromocytoma.

Selected references

Bishop, M.L., et al. *Clinical Chemistry*, 5th ed. Philadelphia: Lippincott Williams & Wilkins, 2005.

DeGroot, L., and Jameson, J.L., eds. *Endocrinology*, 5th ed. Philadelphia: W.B. Saunders Co., 2006.

Fischbach, F.T. *A Manual of Laboratory and Diagnostic Tests*, 7th ed. Philadelphia: Lippincott Williams & Wilkins, 2004.

Ilkhanipour, K., et al. "Combining Clinical Risk with D-dimer Testing to Rule Out Deep Vein Thrombosis," *Journal of Emergency Medicine* 27(3):233-39, October 2004.

Kasper, D., et al., eds. *Harrison's Principles of Internal Medicine*, 16th ed. New York: McGraw-Hill Book Co., 2005.

Lim, D., et al. "Elevated Cardiac Troponin Levels in Critically Ill Patients: Prevalence, Incidence, and Outcomes," *American Journal of Critical Care* 15(3):280-88, May 2006.

Lippincott Manual of Nursing Practice: Diagnostic Tests. Philadelphia: Lippincott Williams & Wilkins, 2007.

Lynch, T., and Prahash, A. "B-type Natriuretic Peptide: A Diagnostic, Prognostic, and Therapeutic Tool in Heart Failure," *American Journal of Critical Care* 13(1):46-53, January 2004.

Nursing: Deciphering Diagnostic Tests. Philadelphia: Lippincott Williams & Wilkins, 2008.

Pagana, K.D., and Pagana, T.J. *Mosby's Diagnostic and Laboratory Test Reference*, 7th ed. St. Louis: Mosby–Year Book Inc., 2005.

Prue-Owens, K.K., LTC. "Use of Peripheral Venous Access Devices for Obtaining Blood Samples for Measurement of Activated Partial Thromboplastin Times," *Critical Care Nurse* 26(1):30-38, February 2006.

Smith, G.C., et al. "Pregnancy-Associated Plasma Protein A and Alpha-Fetoprotein and Prediction of Adverse Perinatal Outcome," *Obstetrics and Gynecology* 107(1):161-66, January 2006.

Stonesifer, E. "Common Laboratory and Diagnostic Testing in Patients with Gastrointestinal Disease," *AACN Clinical Issues* 15(4):582-94, October-December 2004.

Turgeon, M. *Clinical Hematology Theory and Procedures*, 4th ed. Philadelphia: Lippincott Williams & Wilkins, 2005.

Ye, W., et al. "*Helicobacter pylori* Infection and Gastric Atrophy: Risk of Adenocarcinoma and Squamous-cell Carcinoma of the Esophagus and Adenocarcinoma of the Gastric Cardia," *Journal of the National Cancer Institute* 96(5):388-96, March 2004.

Index

i refers to an illustration; t refers to a table; boldface refers to color pages.

i refers to an illustration; t refers to a table; boldface refers to color pages.